What Readers Are Saying
About *Time to Care*

"*Time to Care* has come at an opportune time given the present healthcare debate…It absolutely should be read by both the public and our political representatives."

— William S. Frankl, M.D., Author and Retired Clinical Professor of Medicine, Temple University School of Medicine

"We, as patients, can attest to the importance of a personal relationship with our doctor—one who listens to us, who talks to us, and gives us the feeling that he or she really cares. I urge everyone in the country to read this informative, provocative, and heartfelt book on today's medicine, and to join with Dr. Makous to create a new system to include a real, caring relationship between doctor and patient."

— Wilma Mills, Author, West Brandywine, PA

"Dr. Makous provides three hundred pages of fast-reading anecdotes about his sixty years of practice, before summing it up in fifty pages of reflection…The patients loved their doctor, in what was known as the patient-doctor relationship. But a strange thing was also true. The doctors loved their patients, the only group in society who seemed to care what the doctor was trying to do."

— George Fisher, MD, Author, *The Hospital That Ate Chicago*

"A well-written, thought provoking insight into the evolution of the healthcare system in our Country. A truly insightful vision for the future is found within the pages of this book."

— Dolores Hagerstrom, Marketing Professional and Community Activist, Exton, PA

"Many of us physicians of a bygone age understood Professor Peabody's admonition, '...the secret in the care of the patient is in caring for the patient.' In *Time to Care,* Dr. Makous draws on his rich store of experience to document what is possible when technical skill is combined with a caring heart."

— Harold A. Braun, MD, retired cardiologist, Missoula, Montana

"My wife and I immensely enjoyed reading Dr. Makous' anecdotes. It is hard to argue with the central importance of the doctor-patient relationship. Anyone who has been helped thorough illness by a caring doctor will find that his approach resonates deeply."

— William G. Kussmaul III, MD, Philadelphia cardiologist

"Dr. Makous has always been able to focus on the importance of the doctor-patient relationship in maintaining a successful medical outcome. The continuous doctor-patient relationship is the most rewarding experience both for the patient and the doctor. In *Time to Care,* he is to be complimented for presenting in detail the medical issues that face our society in this health care crisis."

— Richard B. Anderson, MD, retired pediatric psychiatrist and professor, University of Wisconsin Medical School, Madison, WI

"Those of us who don't do what physicians of Dr. Makous' generation did well—that is, take the time to get to know our patients and let them know we care—ought to at least take the time to read this great account of the evolution of American medicine as practiced at the front line over the last sixty years."

— Kenneth D. Goldblum, MD, general internist, Coatesville, PA

TIME TO CARE

PERSONAL MEDICINE
IN THE AGE OF TECHNOLOGY

Norman Makous, M.D. (signature)

NORMAN MAKOUS, M.D.

with Bruce Makous

TOWPATH
PUBLICATIONS

For further information, please contact:

TowPath Publications
PO Box 43522
Philadelphia, PA 19106

Book design by:

VMC Art & Design LLC
info@vmc-artdesign.com
www.vmc-artdesign.com

Printed in United States of America

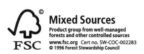

Mixed Sources
Product group from well-managed
forests and other controlled sources
FSC   www.fsc.org Cert no. SW-COC-002283
© 1996 Forest Stewardship Council

Makous, Norman.
    Time to care : personal medicine in the age of technology/
    by Norman Makous ; with Bruce Makous.
    p. cm.
    Includes bibliographical references and index.
    LCCN 2009930540
    ISBN-13: 978-0-9776686-1-8
    ISBN-10: 0-9776686-1-4

    1. Physician and patient. 2. Medical care.
    3. Medical technology. 4. Technology–Social aspects.
    I. Makous, Bruce. II. Title.

R727.3.M35 2009   610.69'6
                        QBI09-600099

I dedicate this book first to my patients and their families. I have learned and received more from them than I was able to give.

Secondly, I want to thank my family for your generous tolerance of my career-long practice of permitting patients in their need to intrude upon our private lives at home.

I thank all and I am most grateful.

TABLE OF CONTENTS

PREFACE

Who Cares?

Throughout my more than 62-year career in medicine, I have seen a steady decline in the level of personal care offered to patients by physicians. Over the years, I came to realize that this decline was related to the significant advances in medical technology.

People thrive on the personal attention of a physician. Today, they also expect the latest that technology offers. Valuable medical technology should be used to provide tools within the personal relationship between doctor and patient. The technology itself should not replace the personal aspects of medicine.

Late in my career, I received the following poem from a grateful patient:

Who Cares
By John Bongiovanni

Who gives you a good and thorough exam and doesn't rush you out?

Who is always pleasant and caring?

Who gives you his home phone number whenever you need him, and who is always courteous and never makes a patient feel uneasy about you calling him at home?
Who cares for the patient first and not the almighty dollar?

Who is not a stuffed shirt but a regular guy who makes you feel 100-percent better after you leave his office?

And here's the payoff. Who allows you to call the farm where he goes once in awhile for a little R & R?

> There are not many doctors you can get in an emergency,
> but not this guy.
> Who is this guy? I'll tell you who. Norman Makous, that's
> who.

John's poem reinforces my observations. It expresses what many people today miss in their medical treatment: personal care. This is the key inspiration for writing this book.

This is the story of how I came to understand the importance of the physician's relationship with the patient, and how I worked to hold onto my commitment to patient care, despite the powerful changes in medicine going on around me.

This work is directed to anyone who is interested in how medical care evolved in the late 20th century, affecting patients and practicing physicians. It may also be of interest to healthcare professionals who want to know more about the art of providing personal medical care. For the convenience of anyone reading the book, I have included a glossary as Appendix 2. Terms appearing in bold at first mention are included in the glossary.

My observations are based on a career that started with four years of medical school during World War II, and went on to nine years of post-graduate training, a two-year stint on active duty with the US Army, US Navy, and US Marines during the Korean War, and 48 years of solo private practice in four different locations, ending in 2006.

My views were also shaped by my activities as a student or faculty member at four medical schools, my participation in a number of professional medical organizations, and my involvement with several government agencies. A detailed chronology of my professional experience is shown in Appendix 4, following the conclusion of this book.

Many of my patient anecdotes, shown in italics, are included to help capture the essence of personal care. Others provide a basis for some understanding of the changes in care, especially based upon the concentration on science and technology, and the resultant cost. To protect patient privacy, I have changed patient names; and, where necessary, I have modified specific identifying details.

My observations are based on accumulated recollections frequently revisited over the years. Some of the information is based on my records, or from medical or other literature, and I have provided additional reading in Appendix 5. While memory can be faulty, the details are of less importance than the overall impression that the experience has conveyed.

Commentary is based on my own running meta-analysis of the medical literature and events throughout my career. I'm sure some may disagree, not only with my opinions, but also with my interpretations of this information. However, these are my views, as derived from my vantage point as a professional involved in the delivery of personal medical care for more than six decades in the latter half of the 1900s.

INTRODUCTION

I Can't Jitterbug Anymore

John Bongiovanni was one of those appreciative patients who make a physician's devotion to medicine worthwhile. He was a grocer who had owned his own food market. Shortly after he retired in his early 60s, he came to see me for the first time.

"I get chest pain, Doc," he said off-handedly.

"Where, exactly, in your chest?" I asked him.

"Right in the middle," he said, spreading his fingers and holding his hand over his breastbone.

"When do you feel it?"

"Occasionally when I bowl. And I can't jitterbug anymore."
He said he bowled regularly, and he used to take his wife out dancing several times a week.

*After I examined him and did an **electrocardiogram**, I was sure that the pain was caused by poor circulation in the heart muscle from **hardening of the arteries**.*

*"You have **angina pectoris**," I told him. "Heart pain that occurs during exertion."*

I prescribed medication along with changes to his diet, and the chest discomfort improved. He continued to bowl and to take his wife dancing, finding he could once again jitterbug without chest pain.

John required regular care. Soon, he brought his wife in to see me, and she became one of my patients, too. Over time, I became very familiar with both of them and many aspects of their lives.

I treated John for several years, but he eventually needed heart surgery. After the procedure, I was both surprised and disappointed. His heart sounds were the most distressed of any patient I'd ever followed after heart surgery. Despite this apparent failure, he returned to his activities with greater vigor than before the surgery, and without chest pain.

*Over time, John's chest pain returned and gradually became worse. Eleven years after his surgery, his wife died of **Alzheimer's disease**. They had been married for 56 years. Despite his loss, he continued his bowling, and in time, returned to his weekly dancing.*

I took care of John for more than 20 years before I retired from patient care.

Upon my retirement, he wrote to me. "You did wonders for me, Doc," he explained, and said I would be sorely missed.

After that, like a few of my other patients, he still called me several times each year to see how I was doing or to see what I thought of his treatment under his new cardiologist.

*Four years after I retired, John required a **pacemaker**. He died a year later at the age of 91, which was 23 years after his heart surgery. He'd been out dancing the prior week.*

The John Bongiovanni story is a good example of personal medical care. The emphasis is on the "personal" part. It really involves doctors taking the time to develop meaningful and caring relationships with their patients. Once a patient experiences this type of medical care, it is, as John wrote, "sorely missed" if no longer available. Even those who have never experienced this degree of personal attention, still need the reassurance that this type of care provides.

—∿—

In the absence of personal attention, patients demand more testing, but testing does not satisfy the need for personal interaction.

Individualized care, which involves the use of science-inspired technology, is not personal care. Alone, it is incomplete. It does not provide the necessary reassurance that can only be provided through a trusted physician who focuses upon the totality of the person and not just upon a narrow technological application to a disease. Time and personal commitment are needed to build the mutual understanding and trust that are fundamental to personal care.

Medical practice is an "Art based on science." This succinct characterization by Sir William Osler, a highly regarded physician from the early part of the 20th century, still holds today. Were it not for individual variation, Osler also noted, medicine would be a science rather than an art. While personal care today is still more art than science, it does require the judicious use of science-based technology.

The 20th century is regarded by many as the "Golden Age" of medical practice. During this time, medical science advanced more than in all of past history. The 1940s was perhaps the most significant period in this advancement. It was a watershed decade in medicine. The traditional anatomical paradigms in medical science were being replaced by new physiological and biochemical ones. As a result, the technological advances in medical care began to accelerate.

Since then, the continued acceleration of science, technology, and cost has intruded on personal care in our country. This has also occurred during a time in which American individualism and its accompanying sense of entitlement have become more of a cult than ever before. In the absence of personal attention, patients demand more testing, but testing does not satisfy the need for personal interaction.

—⁂—

Most people today have some type of medical insurance coverage, enabling many to pay for care. As a result, more people today have higher expectations and higher levels of anxiety than in the past. They therefore seek medical attention earlier than they did in the days in which patients were personally responsible for their own medical costs. For doctors, the personal contact upon taking a history and performing a physical examination is less rewarding in early disease. This reinforces the belief among many less experienced physicians that these contact procedures have little to offer and that testing is far superior to examination.

The indirect financial commitment through third parties creates another serious obstacle to overcome in establishing and maintaining the personal relationship between doctor and patient.

Consequently, taking the history and even conducting the initial physical examination are frequently delegated to medical assistants. This approach neglects the fact that obtaining a complete history and performing a hands-on examination initiates the all-important personal relationship of trust and reassurance. Thoroughness helps to demonstrate competence. Unsatisfactory outcomes without personal relationships breed the dissatisfaction that adds fuel to the cultural appetite for lawsuits.

Today, individuals in our no-fault society are not only too willing to go to court, they also feel that they should not have to bear the cost of medical care. They may not mind paying for it if the cost is hidden, when others such as the government, employers, and insurers pay the providers of medical care. The indirect financial commitment through third parties creates another serious obstacle to overcome in establishing and maintaining the personal relationship between doctor and patient.

—֍—

This book investigates the issues related to the breakdown of personal care, the role of this trend in the declining quality of personal care, and the growth in the cost of technology. It also explores possible outcomes in the future of healthcare in the US. One key issue is the growing need to ration care through healthcare regulation as well as the underwriting process.

The following six sections of this book largely parallel phases of my career:

- **Part I, Do No Harm: Traditional Medical Practice and Training**, looks at medical education and care prior to the technological revolution.

- **Part II, The Art of Personal Care**, discusses how care was provided primarily by solo general practitioners or small groups of physicians in the same specialty, and how this impacted the personal relationship between doctor and patient.

- **Part III, Life-Saving Technology**, looks at the dramatic shifts in medicine resulting from several key technological innovations.

- **Part IV, Advances in Art and Science**, deals with the impact of technical changes and other innovations on medical practice, using the field of cardiology as the primary example.

- **Part V, Paying the Price**, addresses the involvement in medical care by the government, hospitals, organizations, and insurers, and the ongoing attempts to manage the cost of care. The current and future practices in the rationing of care are discussed.

- **Part VI, Conclusion: Personal Care Is Key**, provides insights into the future of healthcare delivery.

PART I

Do No Harm: Traditional Medical
Practice and Training

CHAPTER I

The Brickyard

Medical facts are the basis of medicine and medical care. When I entered the University of Wisconsin Medical School in Madison in 1944, medical training consisted of first learning the fundamental facts of human anatomy, physiology, and chemistry. Bacteriology, the pathology of diseases, their causes, and their treatments followed.

Standards for applying this information came from the experience of experts and **preceptors,** teachers who are practicing doctors. This formed the basis for observation and innovation in treatment of the individual patient.

"Do no harm," from the Hippocratic Oath, was the traditional underlying standard.

The practical standards of care were derived from similarities of responses in groups of similar patients, and were frequently controversial. It was not until much later that sophisticated scientific studies of large numbers of patients made up the widely accepted standards of today.

"By the end of your third year," Dr. William Middleton, dean of the Medical School, once told us, "you will know more medical facts than at any other time in your career."

Medical facts are like bricks in a brickyard. They do not in themselves create an effective structure to form a basis for the delivery of good medical care.

At the time, dictums were used a great deal. "Common things most commonly occur," was repeated by just about every instructor, as was, "when you hear hoof beats on a dark street at midnight, don't assume it's a zebra."

3

"Except when you are at a referral or teaching hospital," I wanted to add. Only difficult or unusual cases were referred for treatment at our academic facility.

Dr. Harris, head of obstetrics, made his points with preposterous animal similes. "That's about as likely to happen as the survival of a celluloid mouse chased by an asbestos cat in Hell," was one of his favorites.

Dean Middleton had served as chief medical consultant in the World War II European Theater of Operations. As a military man, he was a notoriously exacting teacher. He covered subjects in the Socratic style, by asking questions.

"What's the first step in the treatment of any condition?" was his most common question.

"Prevention!" was the required answer, whether this was possible or not.

The dean had instituted "The Brown Derby Award." Any student who didn't answer, "Prevention," or who came up with an outlandish answer or a guess, won the award. Each winner signed the derby and wore it in class until relieved by the next awardee.

Dr. Erwin Schmidt, head of surgery, was a tall, silver-haired gentleman referred to as "The Great White Father" by the students. His dictum was that a student's first response to a question concerning the treatment of any disease should be, "Diagnosis."

A doctor cannot cure an illness until the cause is known. Therefore, treatment should not be attempted until the diagnosis is known.

Dr. Schmidt's fourth-year students got to "scrub in" and stand at his operating table with arms aching from holding a retractor to keep an abdominal incision open. Often, this was as the third or fourth assistant, a position from which we often were unable to see anything of the surgery.

In pharmacology, Dr. Tatum impressed upon us that the amount of a drug used in treatment had to be tailored to the specific individual. "The dose of a drug is enough but not too much."

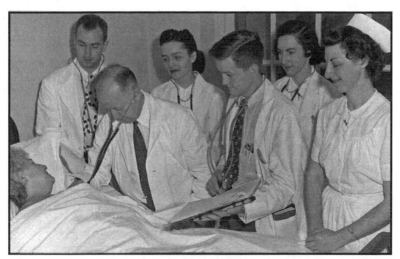

*Dr. William Middleton, Dean of the University of Wisconsin Medical
School, conducts bedside rounds in 1945 as students observe*

This dictum still holds true but has evolved over the years.
Today, it goes, "start low and go slow."

Our first exposure to patient care was actually in the second
year of medical school, when we had physical diagnosis for an
hour each week. There was no white-coat ceremony as is common
today. The coats were short. Only the staff physicians were
allowed to wear long coats. However, when the new sophomores
first received their white coats and diagnostic equipment, several
would parade off campus, down State Street, and around the
Wisconsin State Capital Square.

Junior year was the most difficult to endure. We had lectures
from 8:00 a.m. until 5:00 p.m., except for several hours devoted
to "working up" patients on the hospital wards. We would have to
take a history, examine the patient, and write this up for review by
a faculty member.

Since the University's facility, Wisconsin General Hospital,
accepted only cases referred to it by other hospitals and doctors,
it provided little in the way of acute care. Therefore, the medical

conditions in the cases we observed in the Hospital were usually complicated. Many were chronic, and the diseases were often rare.

Some patients in that era waited until their condition had become extreme before seeking medical attention. They would then be referred to Wisconsin General Hospital.

Cancers were often far advanced. One such man had been in the Hospital for nine months. Over half of his face, including the jaw and facial bones, had been invaded by a neglected skin cancer. He was still undergoing extensive reconstructive surgery when I was assigned to follow his care.

A great deal of plastic reconstruction had been completed, but with only half his face remaining, he was a horror to see without bandages. Next to him, the Phantom of the Opera was good looking and less tragic. He did eventually leave the hospital but had to return a number of times for further surgery. Successful surgery of that extent was unusual at the time.

As with many academic hospitals, the unusual case is the norm. These cases are good for teaching disease mechanisms, but the experience is poor for teaching the detection and treatment of conditions that are more apt to be seen in a community.

Thus, through my three years of classroom education, I stocked up my brickyard of medical facts, but I hadn't even started to build a structure to guide me in medical care. I was looking to build a framework for each disease condition, which I could then adjust based on my accumulating experience.

This was just the beginning. A great deal of hands-on, practical experience was needed before I had built a structure upon which I could rely with confidence.

CHAPTER 2

Learning What Not to Do

While my patient-care experiences at the Wisconsin General Hospital itself did not help me gain any idea of the prevalence of a particular disease in the general community, my experiences outside of the Hospital were more instructive and important in this regard.

Senior students spent three months around the state outside of both Madison and Milwaukee counties under the supervision of preceptors.

My three-month preceptorship in the summer of 1946 was in Eau Claire, Wisconsin. I was assigned to a four-doctor group, one each in pediatrics, ear-nose-throat (ENT), urology, and surgery. All did some general practice in addition to their specialties. I spent the afternoons in their offices when they were seeing patients.

I and the other students stayed at nearby Sacred Heart Hospital as "externs." There were no interns at the Hospital, so we were given interns' work.

Dean Middleton required that we keep a log of our daily experiences. Part of my first day's entry was, "Interesting operating room procedure. Some surgeons wear street clothing with shirt off and gown over. Masks of all but the nursing staff customarily cover only the mouth. Nose is left exposed to facilitate breathing or to keep glasses from getting steamed."

The nurses were the only ones following the proper procedure. The patient-care experience was supposed to be instructive and it was, but largely in a negative way. I was learning a lot of what not to do.

The general surgeon for my preceptorship, Dr. Mason, took me with him when he consulted with physicians and did surgery in small-town hospitals near Eau Claire. He no longer performed kitchen-table surgery in patients' homes, as he had done for years.

He explained that in those situations, the **anesthesia**, which was **ether**, would be given by a family member. It was dripped from a can onto a cloth covering the mouth and nose. When necessary, the patient would have to self-administer the anesthetic. The patient could not overdose, since the can of ether would fall out of the patient's hand when the patient became unconscious.

Dr. Mason was always ready with a story. He had attended North-Western Medical School in the early part of the century. The lecture on urine was one of the more memorable ones he had attended.

His professor placed a large container of urine on a table next to the lectern. He described various causes and characteristics of the urine in great detail. He noted what had been known for centuries—that the urine of patients with untreated **diabetes** tastes sweet because it contains sugar.

The professor finished the lecture by demonstrating the final test of urine with a flourish. This was "the taste test." He proceeded to dip his finger into the urine and lick.

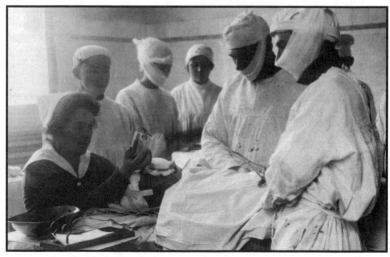

A nurse administers ether as the surgical team stands by during a post-World War II procedure
Image provided by the U.S National Library of Medicine

He then invited the students to file past and do the same. Most did so, despite reservations.

After they took their seats again, he then explained that this was really a test of observation, not fortitude. He had dipped his middle finger into the urine but had licked his forefinger.

"And," he might have added, "be cautious with your trust."

—∿∿—

At Sacred Heart Hospital, a number of patients had unusual presentations that I found remarkable in my inexperience. For instance, there was a 66-year-old **cachectic** woman, whose body was wasting away due to cancer. She was riddled with cancerous lumps, which were palpable and visible under the skin on her abdomen, chest, arms, and legs. She had hard masses in her abdomen. Her ancient but vigorous mother visited daily and sat by her bedside.

Another patient, a man with a tremendous excess of body fluid from congestive heart failure, seemed dehydrated. He had congestion in his lungs and abdomen, but his skin was wrinkled from dehydration. This was a paradox, as far as Dr. Middleton was concerned when he read my notebook, after my stint in Eau Claire. But several years later, a study presented in the medical literature pointed out that this was caused by depletion and imbalance of body salts.

—∿∿—

*The first time I prescribed **digitalis** for the treatment of congestive heart failure was tragic. Charles was an elderly man who had been in the hospital for several days. He had received his first dose of the medicine that morning.*

That evening I made rounds. Charles was sitting in bed in no distress as I approached.

As I felt for his pulse in his wrist, I asked, "How do you feel?"

"I feel fine," was his chipper response.

But I couldn't find any pulse in his wrist, where I knew it had been present previously. As I lifted his gown to listen to his heart,

Charles' neck vessels began to pulsate irregularly. He had a seizure and died.

All I could do was run helplessly around the room then out into the hall, seeking assistance. Nothing could be done for him.

Charles had developed **ventricular fibrillation**, a chaotic heart rhythm that cannot sustain life. It's an emergency condition requiring immediate heart resuscitation. The **defibrillator** technology that accomplishes this today would not be available for nearly 20 years.

I was concerned that an excess dose of digitalis may have been the cause, but there was no test to determine this. His dosage was appropriate based on the recommended standards for dosing at the time.

For a long while after that, I took few pulses, and when I did, it was with some apprehension. I wasn't sure what I had learned, other than the death of a patient in my presence is more distressing than in my absence.

—w—

*A 17-year-old fellow had legs so severely ulcerated that only a strip of skin, several inches wide extending from behind his knees to the heels, remained. I suspected **amyloidosis**, a condition in which an insoluble substance infiltrates and compromises the function of vital organs.*

For diagnosis, I decided to make a "Congo Red" solution from a powder I found in the chemistry laboratory. Amyloid in the tissues would absorb the Congo Red dye. After injection, the blood level would fall abnormally fast. We could measure this. I explained my proposed procedure to the attending physician.

"Go ahead with the test," he told me.

The lab supervisor stopped me. "Why take the risk?" She said. The boy might develop a serious reaction, and nothing could be done for the condition anyway.

I had lucked out. I had been stopped from undertaking something for which I might have been sorry.

—ɷ—

That summer, there was a national **poliomyelitis** epidemic. Minneapolis, 90 miles west of Eau Claire and across the Mississippi River, was particularly hard-hit, but Eau Claire had its share of cases as well.

At the time, the infectious viral cause of polio had not yet been established. At Sacred Heart, the nuns and nurses were frightened, correctly regarding it as a contagious disease. They were reluctant to spend more time with these patients than absolutely necessary. However, they seemed to be unconcerned about asking me to attend to such a patient, which I had no qualms about doing, in my ignorance.

These were among my first experiences in patient care. They helped most in learning what not to do, which still forms a basis for a key precept of the Hippocratic Oath, "Do no harm." I realized that many years of experience were needed to build the practice framework of proactive efforts—those which I should undertake to care for my patients with confidence.

CHAPTER 3

Hospitals Are Where You Go to Die

By the time our class graduated in 1947, Dean Middleton had arranged most of the internships for us. We didn't have to find our own. This was as uncommon in that era as it is today.

For my internship, I ended up at Research Hospital in Kansas City, Missouri. The name had been changed in 1916 from German Hospital. Anything "German" was, of course, unpopular during World War I. "Research" was a strange choice for a new name, since the hospital wasn't affiliated with a medical school, and no research was actually conducted there. It was a well-reputed teaching hospital, however.

Research Hospital was located on Kansas City's "Hospital Hill," across the street from the segregated all-white Kansas City General Hospital and down the street from Kansas City General Number Two, for African-Americans.

Research had 250 beds, but the census was usually more than 300 during the three years I was there. This was common during and immediately after World War II when no new hospitals or additions were being built. The overflow patients were placed in beds in hallways with screens around them.

I arrived in Kansas City on a Saturday. This was a week early by request of Hospital management. Most of the eight interns in the previous group had departed to take state board examinations, and the Hospital had no medical or surgical residents at the time. So, on Sunday, the day after I arrived, I covered the entire 300 beds alone until late afternoon.

The building was "H" shaped. The emergency room and surgery were on the sixth floor. Two floors of a wing had units for the severely ill run by teams of skilled nurses. These were the

Intensive Care Units of the time. The only high-tech equipment we had were two **iron lung respirators** and a number of oxygen tents. Even air-conditioning was limited to only a few private rooms.

One of the obstetricians told us that the hospital's front entrance and one of the delivery rooms were models for the clinic Ernest Hemingway describes in his book, *A Farewell to Arms*. The author had been a reporter at the time for *The Kansas City Times*. The obstetrician had allowed Hemingway to watch a delivery. I doubt that the patient was asked to give permission for this.

The internship was categorized as "mixed, not rotating," because we had no pediatric service. The newborn nursery was part of obstetrics. The few children admitted for medical procedures were placed on those respective services, not pediatrics. A parent usually stayed with his or her child in a private room.

During my first year, the house staff at Research consisted of eight interns, a pathology resident, and several radiology residents. All of the residencies were approved for training and board certification. We served eight weeks each on medicine, surgery, and obstetrics. We were not on-call every other night, as required in many internships, but had duty every third night.

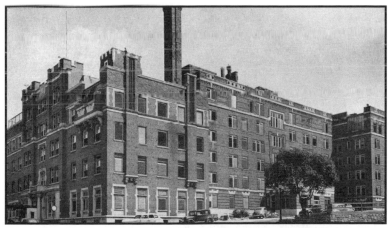

Research Hospital, Kansas City, Missouri, 1945

Today, a great deal of concern exists about physician errors, including those attributed to house-staff fatigue from long hours. Many states now regulate the hours. Continuous duty for more than 18 hours is generally considered excessive. One downside is that the reduction of errors from fatigue on the one hand, is offset in part by an increase in errors due to decreased continuity of care previously provided by a single, house physician.

Prior to the mid-1940s, medical care had precious little in the way of effective medical treatment to offer the patient. Despite this, hospital care could provide life-saving procedures, both technical and non-technical.

I realized that personal care, even without
medicine, can be a critical component
in curing patients.

---

*Upon my arrival at Research, for example, there was a patient who had been diagnosed with the highly fatal **Rocky Mountain spotted fever**. An antibiotic specific for this infection had just been developed, but was not widely available as yet.*

The patient did not receive the antibiotic, but survived largely due to the 24-hour care by a few dedicated nurses.

Often, in fact, all we really had to offer patients in hospitals in that era was bed rest and good nursing care. I realized that personal care, even without medicine, can be a critical component in curing patients.

All intravenous injections and fluids had to be started by doctors. Some older physicians still questioned the wisdom of giving fluids intravenously. Nurses were not allowed to start fluids intravenously, but were allowed to start them by **hypodermoclysis**, that is, **subcutaneously**, under the skin. Many fluids, such as 5-percent glucose and normal saline, were given this way. Infrequently, fluids were given via retention enema.

These approaches were useful when a doctor was not available or when vein access was difficult. Subcutaneous fluid administration was discontinued in the early 1950s, after it was shown that this approach could throw an occasional patient with marginal kidney function into kidney failure.

A service, now quaint, offered to nearly all patients in most hospitals every evening, was a back rub by a nurse. After spending so much time on their backs, it was much appreciated. This welcome attention and nicety disappeared during the 1950s. It demanded too much nursing time and was not thought to be cost-effective.

Bedpans were usually used by the bed-fast. Those who were allowed out of bed used a bedside commode, even if they could have been helped to a toilet. Many of the older hospitals had no such facility in the room.

It was usual hospital practice then, less common now, to place bed rails on each side of the beds of many older patients and those tending to be confused, especially at night. The heights of some of the beds were not adjustable and falls could be very dangerous. The rails could be lowered so nurses could attend to the patient more readily.

Some confused or angry patients would climb over the rails and were in danger of falling and breaking a hip. This was true especially if nursing and aide supervision was inadequate. Such patients were strapped by one or even both wrists to the bed.

I went to see one older man and found him dead on the floor at his bedside. He had been trying to climb back into bed after he'd had a rather large bowel movement on the floor in the corner of the room. Assuming the call button was accessible to them, some patients were still too proud to ring for such help, even if they were inclined to use a bedpan.

Surprisingly, as recent as the 1990s, an occasional elderly person who had never been hospitalized would be reluctant to go to the hospital for an elective admission. They remembered from their youth that hospitals were places where their family and friends went to die. Even today, some consider hospitals to be places where one may be exposed to potentially fatal infections.

The fear of hospitals in that period was valid. Prolonged bed rest could have and still has potentially deleterious and even fatal effects. A blood clot that originates in a leg vein is one such complication. One of these can break off and float to a lung as a **pulmonary embolus** that can be fatal.

The patient at greatest risk was the one who had been in the hospital for more than a week.

Vein inflammations can also cause blockage and swelling of the lower limbs. Pregnant women after delivery were especially prone to this complication, which can be chronic and debilitating.

These silent blood clots in the veins were difficult to detect until a patient became active again. Especially devastating were those that formed after successful surgery and caused a patient's death during discharge from the hospital.

Hospital-acquired infections may not have been as well appreciated back then, but may still have been less common in those days as compared to recent years. Resistant infections from antibiotic overuse were not yet a problem, of course, since **penicillin** had only recently been made available. And in the absence of antibiotics, aseptic precautions may have been more carefully followed at that time, than they have been in recent years.

Certain underlying complications in patients who were generally improving were more apt to go undetected during long hospital stays that exceeded a week. As the acute episode subsided, the detailed daily examination was often neglected. Abdominal tumors, abscesses, and other masses could develop undetected by the attending doctors and nurses.

Such an instance occurred in a middle-aged man who was admitted with abdominal pain, the cause of which could not be determined. Because of his lessening discomfort and apparent improvement, the routine daily physical examinations by the physicians became cursory. If the detailed daily examination had been continued, the gradually enlarging abdominal mass from an aortic bulge, which in this case was an **aneurysm**, would have been found before it ruptured and killed him.

Routine treatment without ongoing testing was another risk of longer hospital stays back then. Admitting doctors would often give more attention to the newer or more serious patients, while longer-term patients would be attended to by nurses, interns, and hospital laboratory staff.

Ongoing re-examination was important in preventing premature discharge and early readmission, but it was often overlooked. For this and other reasons, I realized that the patient at greatest risk was the one who had been in the hospital for more than a week.

The postmortem examination of a patient who died was extremely important in understanding the reason the treatment had failed and whether this type of failure could be prevented in the future. The autopsy rate at Research Hospital was more than 60 percent, which is considered very good and up to the level necessary for teaching.

Autopsies are rarer today. Now, the advanced technology for testing provides physicians with most of the answers pre-mortem. Despite this, some recent studies have found that two-thirds of patients' **pathology** is not related to the final illness, and goes undiagnosed.

Near the end of my year of internship, I found that I had learned some effective standards for practicing internal medicine, which I decided to adopt as a specialty. I elected to continue as a medical resident at Research Hospital for one year, which turned into two years.

One very important factor in the decision, of course, was that I had become engaged to a student nurse at the hospital. Dorothy Bowlin and I were married when she finished her training, two months after I had started my residency. At the time, we could only have imagined the long and happy marriage—and the many new family members—that this union would bring about.

CHAPTER 4

Roundsmanship

The Research Hospital medical staff presented a range of expertise, but by and large, as in my preceptorship, I learned more of what not to do in given situations...versus learning the right things to do.

The heads of the departments at Research Hospital were mostly honorary positions and were rotated every few years. The head of radiology administered the house-staff programs, except for pathology. Surprisingly, the chief of medicine played no role in our program.

I was one of three medical residents, and we were basically unsupervised. I designed my own course of study, spending time in the laboratory, pathology, radiology, and with **subspecialists**.

Dr. Ira Lockwood, the head of radiology, had been president of the American Roentgen Ray Society, the professional association of x-ray specialists. His group had an office in a downtown professional building. They serviced a number of clinics and small hospitals in a wide area. I regarded them as "radiologists on horseback."

These radiologists were not only specialists but also general consultants. They provided outstanding help to the clinicians by interpreting the x-rays in conjunction with the entire medical problem. Often they were more up-to-date in a specialty area than some of the certified specialists in that field.

Some radiologists with whom I'd come in contact elsewhere were narrow, that is, they only provided very limited information. They would interpret the x-ray shadows only in terms of diagnostic possibilities with little or no regard for clinical input. When the clinical concerns are considered, however, the number of diagnostic possibilities decreases and the probability of a specific diagnosis increases.

—w—

Dr. Carl Ferris was the best general internist, and his young associate, Dr. Martin Mueller, the sharpest. Dr. Ferris would spend several hours discharging a patient from the hospital. He personally took care of the instructions, appointments, and all of the other arrangements. I was appropriately impressed by such attentive and personal care.

Most of the other physicians discharged patients themselves, but they usually did not take the time that Dr. Ferris devoted to each patient. Several of the surgeons would have their nurses discharge their patients. Today, physicians usually delegate this to special nurses. At times, the patient isn't even sure whether or not the physician is even in the loop on the details.

—w—

During my residency, I had many more opportunities to learn what to avoid. One handsome, perfumed general practitioner had a large practice, mostly women. Often, he and his nurse would make house calls separately until 11:00 p.m., following a full day and evening in the office. They kept in contact by phone—and this was decades before cell phones were available.

The house staff considered him a "shot doctor," and he had separate rooms in his offices with different motifs for each of the various types of shots. There was a room for Solu-B, a multivitamin replaced in the 1950s by vitamin B-12 as the dominant "feel good" shot; a **calcium gluconate** room; a hormone room; and a penicillin room.

During the three years I was at Research, this particular doctor admitted more than a dozen women with acute **hepatitis**, inflammation of the liver, which undoubtedly came from contaminated needles used in his office. He mentioned to me one time that those with arthritis had less joint pain when they became **jaundiced**, or yellowed, from the hepatitis.

At the time, drug company reps would comment on the similarity between the bile salts in the blood from the inflamed liver, and the adrenal gland's anti-inflammatory hormone, **cortisone**. I suspected they had pointed out the association to this doctor, since he had become aware of this ironic benefit of the jaundice. Shortly thereafter, in 1949, cortisone became available for use in the treatment of arthritis.

—⟋ⲙ—

The chief of medicine officially interpreted all of the electrocardiograms. Before he read them, I would write my interpretation on the back. He didn't like it.

"That isn't necessary," he told me one day.

On several occasions, he had missed the abnormalities of atrial flutter and fibrillation.

I didn't stop this practice of writing my interpretation on the back. He never said anything again.

My considerable respect for one particular cardiologist was lessened by an incident in which he interpreted one set of 10 **electrocardiogram tracings** I had shown to him. "Tracings" are the printouts from the electrocardiogram, showing the electrical activity of the heart. These were from a man with a **myocardial infarction,** a heart attack. The man was having chest pain over a two-week period.

The cardiologist was not familiar with the case. As he examined the 10 tracings, he started to explain how a blockage had formed in a certain small branch of a major heart artery, which showed on the tracing, followed by a blockage in another branch, which he said also had a specific effect on a later electrocardiogram. When I pointed out that he was reading the tracings in reverse chronological order, without batting an eye, he started explaining them all over again with equal detail. The explanations were quite precise and imaginative.

—⟋ⲙ—

Dr. Williams, a **gastroenterologist**, had trained at Rush Medical College under the well-known Bertram W. Sippy. The Sippy Diet of hourly milk and cream, along with calcium carbonate at less frequent intervals, was a standard treatment for **peptic ulcers** of the stomach and **duodenum**. The regimen eased symptoms. It seemed to promote healing despite the fact that peptic ulcers are caused by an infection, as we know today. The regimen was later found to cause premature heart disease and kidney stones.

One of the older nurses related that she had seen Dr. Williams in the distant past, walking through the halls after doing a rectal exam. He had a specimen of feces on the end of his ungloved index finger, and was on his way to the lab to test it for blood. This was definitely not a standard practice, even then. Today, this test can be done at the bedside and even by people at home, so there's no need to transport specimens at all.

—␣␣—

Dr. Long, a fellow intern from Arkansas, told stories that were peppered with local color. He frequently used expressions like, "happy as a pig in mud," and, "that went down like a turd in a cistern."

As a medical student, he had done a diagnostic **sigmoidoscopy**, *which is a partial colon exam by way of the rectum, on a woman with nondescript abdominal pain. The exam was negative, but he found that he had inadvertently perforated the colon with the rigid scope used at the time.*

Though conscious, the patient was oblivious to the complication, as it caused no discomfort. An abdominal X-ray showed air under her diaphragm indicating that the air from within the bowel had gotten into her abdominal cavity through the perforation.

Despite this potential source of infection, "she never turned a hair," in his words. She had no fever or other signs of infection. In fact, her abdominal pain was gone and she was greatly improved.

"Dr. Long, thank you for that wonderful treatment! You've cured me!" She said enthusiastically each time he walked in the room to see her.

We regarded this as fulfilling the "law of unintended conse-quences."

—∞—

Patients certainly can become worse upon admission to the hospital, but not necessarily from complications of a disease. Infrequently, one would become unresponsive, appearing and remaining semi-comatose. Examination and testing could not determine what, if anything, was wrong.

Personal care at home can triumph over the more technical care which hospitals can offer.

With such patients, at times, displaying a little roundsmanship for the benefit of the house staff, I would perform a "diagnostic procedure." I'd have the patient lifted out of bed and into a chair.

Frequently, patients would suddenly open their eyes, become alert, "bright-eyed, and bushy-tailed," to use one of Dr. Long's expressions.

I suspected that many such patients had intentionally feigned a comatose state out of fear. And some did so because they found that they could learn more about their condition from careless, garrulous caregivers if they were regarded as unconscious.

Occasionally, sending a seriously and incurably ill patient home prematurely would result in a rapid, amazing improvement, and even remission of an incurable disease at times. They had more hope, more family love, and often better care at home.

I was impressed that, at times, personal care at home can tri-umph over the more technical care which hospitals can offer.

CHAPTER 5

Infections and Epidemics

Infections and their complications are intrinsic to all medical specialties. Most infections are recognizable, but some are subtle and produce atypical symptoms and signs. Among the best examples are **tuberculosis** and **syphilis**, which can be acute or chronic in onset and have been called the "Great Imitators."

The type of infection and the organs involved in a specific patient can lead to many different conditions. The traditional use of symptoms and signs helps in limiting the number of conditions that must be considered, but the diagnosis ultimately relies on testing.

Prior to the 1940s, tests were available to diagnose the type of infection, but they were not of much help. Usually, no specific cure was available. After the introduction of penicillin, and later, other antibiotics, determining the specific type of infection became very important. Each antibiotic had its own spectrum of infections for which it was more effective than the other antibiotics.

The bacteriology textbook by Dr. Zinnser that we had used in medical school included maps showing the distribution in the US of the **bubonic plague** bacillus in ground squirrels. This bacteria caused the infection that led to the Black Death of Medieval Europe. Around 1900, the infestation in the US was limited to ground squirrels along the West Coast. By the 1930s, the bacillus had moved eastward to squirrels in the Great Plains.

Therefore, one of my expectations upon going to Kansas City was that I would see a case of bubonic plague. As it turned out, I didn't even hear of any cases, much less see one at Research Hospital. A few rare cases were found in humans before 1950, but not many more since. The ground squirrel infestation has not moved much further east in the past 50 years.

Tuberculosis was a scourge of mankind throughout history and had reached epidemic proportions worldwide in the 19th century. In medical school, we spent several weeks at a state tuberculosis sanatorium in a rural area in Waukesha County, Wisconsin.

These types of facilities were traditional for the non-specific treatment of tuberculosis through environmental control. The isolation also reduced the risk of infecting others. These sanatoriums disappeared over the next 10 to 15 years as the benefit of newly introduced anti-tuberculosis drug therapies became established.

Another international scourge which started at least as early as the Renaissance was **syphilis**, also known as "lues." Columbus was accused of bringing it to Europe from the New World. Traditional **mercury** and **arsenic** preparations controlled the chronic disease, but didn't cure it. The medical dictum for infected men was that, "for one night with Venus, you spend two years with Mercury."

In the early 20th century, in search of a "Magic Bullet" for a more effective treatment of syphilis, Dr. Paul Ehrlich had tested and discarded a number of arsenical preparations. He found that one effective compound, **arsphenamine**, was too toxic for use.

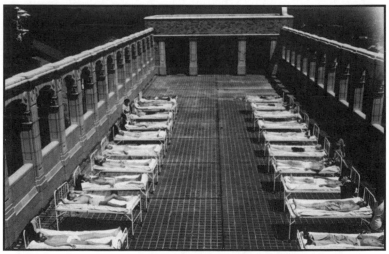

Poliomyelitis and arthritic patients at a sanatorium on a deck for sunshine and fresh air therapy circa. 1940
Image provided by the U.S National Library of Medicine

The claim to fame for Dr. Tatum, our pharmacology professor at the University of Wisconsin Medical School, was that he had methodically re-evaluated many of the compounds Dr. Ehrlich had tested and discarded. Dr. Tatum found that **mapharsen**, which was one-half of the arsphenamine double molecule, was less toxic and more effective than arsphenamine. Mapharsen became the US Armed Forces' standard treatment for syphilis, until penicillin replaced it.

Penicillin, an antibiotic produced by a bread mold, first became clinically available during World War II. It significantly reduced deaths and amputations among Allied Forces. Also, it was the first drug that could actually cure syphilis. The US Armed Forces controlled all penicillin in the country until the end of the War. After the War, penicillin was released in very small amounts for use by the civilian population.

The penicillin supply at Wisconsin General Hospital was rationed in the Department of Medicine by one of the faculty members. It was injected in doses of 100 to 200 units every three to four hours. These tiny doses might have been lifesaving for many **pneumonia** cases, but only served to increase bacterial resistance for other infectious conditions.

As a student, I followed the first case of **endocarditis**, a heart-valve infection, which was being treated with penicillin at Wisconsin General. These infections were uniformly fatal prior to the introduction of penicillin. The standard, minute doses of penicillin were eventually increased to more than 1,000 units every three hours, but this was still inadequate. The patient died from the infection eight to nine months later.

Soon, we learned that these infections were curable, but much larger doses of penicillin were needed. Inadequate amounts of antibiotics tend to produce bacteria that become resistant to the drug's effect. Today, doses as high as 200 million units a day may be given for some conditions.

Penicillin is eliminated from the body within three to four

hours, which greatly limits its effectiveness. At first, in order to prolong its availability in the body, it was mixed with bees wax. This was injected deep into the buttock muscles once daily. This use was discontinued when doctors determined that patients requiring treatment over a long time period began to develop large pliable masses of wax under the skin at the junction of their buttocks and thighs. These had to be removed surgically in some instances. It wasn't long before the need for injections was eliminated by the development of an oral form of penicillin, which was effective when swallowed.

—⚱—

While I didn't see any cases of bubonic plague at Research Hospital, I did encounter a number of other infectious diseases, many of a type I never saw again. They all provided diagnostic challenges to determine exactly what kind of infection, if any, was present. Growing the bacteria from the patient or watching for a change in the level of a specific blood test over time helped zero-in on the type of infection present.

In addition to the case of Rocky Mountain spotted fever, a type of tick-transmitted disease, I encountered a case of **histoplasmosis**. This is a fungus infection that usually presents as a mild unrecognized chest cold, but which I saw as a chronic tonsillitis. **Tularemia**, or "rabbit fever," presented as an abdominal skin ulcer with high fever in a rabbit hunter from downstate Missouri. I also saw several cases of **brucellosis**, which is caused by brucella, an infectious bacterium that causes abortion in cattle.

Each of the five cases I saw of tuberculosis, called "consumption" before the bacterial cause was discovered, presented with a different pattern of symptoms and signs. Usually, tuberculosis causes a lung infection and is found by a chest x-ray in non-hospitalized patients. Our cases, however, presented atypically, most involving organs other than the lungs. They were therefore diagnostic challenges and the patients had to be admitted to the hospital. All five cases had fever. One had primary involvement of the kidneys; another, the brain; and in a third, the lymph glands. In the fourth, the infection could not be localized to a single organ.

*The fifth case, a patient named Florence, had a galloping consumption, also called **Florida Phthisis**. This is a form of lung involvement that isn't localized to a relatively small area of the lung, which is the more common form of tuberculosis. Instead, it was a more extensive pneumonia that involved most of both lungs.*

While her chest x-ray was startling, Florence did not seem as ill as the ordinary patient with pneumonia. In fact, she was feeling rather good and appeared euphoric. She had a facial flush and high fever between 103 and 104 degrees. Her heart rate was around 100 beats per minute and was disproportionately slow. Given the level of fever, it should have been about 130 per minute. These symptoms are characteristic of this type of tuberculosis.

—ᵡᵡ—

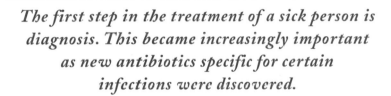

The first step in the treatment of a sick person is diagnosis. This became increasingly important as new antibiotics specific for certain infections were discovered.

At Wisconsin General Hospital, during medical school, I had seen a similar dissociation between the severity of the fever and heart rate.

Tess was a 16-year-old girl whose temperatures consistently ran from 103 to 105 degrees and higher at times, any time of the day or night—whether taken orally or rectally, under mild sedation, or even when taken under the continuous observation of a nurse. Her pulse, however, was a normal 70 to 80 per minute, and she did not appear ill.

*Tess had only one laboratory test abnormality, and that was a prolonged **prothrombin time**, the time it takes the blood to clot. This test is usually abnormal because of severe liver disease,* *blood conditions, or from the drug **dicumarol**. This is similar to **Coumadin**, also known as **warfarin**, which is prescribed to reduce blood clotting. Its effectiveness is determined by measuring the blood-prothrombin time. She had none of these conditions. As it turned out, Tess had been taking dicumarol surreptitiously.*

Tess's other problem was violent "seizures." Curiously, these only occurred when her temperature was taken.

She was finally placed under very heavy sedation and her temperature was taken. Now her "seizures" were in slow motion. The observers were able to detect Tess's adept attempts to switch the glass thermometer during her thrashing movements. They came to find that she had hidden six mercury thermometers, each with an elevated temperature, in and around her bed.

*I never did learn her actual psychiatric diagnosis, but I came to regard her condition as a form of **Munchausen Syndrome**, the feigning of a disease in order to receive medical attention or hospitalization.*

—⟋⟍—

These are but a few examples of diagnostic problems that fever and infection present to the doctors. They vividly demonstrated why in medical school Dr. Schmidt had emphasized that the first step in the treatment of a sick person is diagnosis. This became increasingly important as new antibiotics specific for certain infections were discovered.

New tests and technology seemed to negate the need for the traditional reliance upon symptoms and signs to provide direction in treatment. Some doctors simply wanted to use every available test. Despite an ongoing reduction in cost per test, it became apparent that the increasing number of possible tests could become cost prohibitive. Nonetheless, the practice of "shotgun testing," which is the overuse of available tests as is so prevalent today, would begin to take hold.

Chapter 6

Pregnant 'til Proven Otherwise

Doctors Harris and Harper gave the lectures on obstetrics in medical school. Rotund Dr. Harris was the head of the department. The standing joke among his students was, when he was talking to a pregnant patient at the end of the hall in silhouette, we couldn't be sure which one was the patient and which one was the doctor.

White-maned Dr. Harper practiced in Madison, but not at Wisconsin General Hospital. We obtained all of our practical obstetrical experience in Chicago and at preceptorships around the region.

Dr. Harper emphasized that, "Any woman between the ages of nine and ninety who walks through your office door should be considered pregnant 'til proven otherwise."

As a consultant, he had seen too many instances of pregnancies misdiagnosed as uterine or pelvic tumors, leading to unnecessary **hysterectomies** and unintentional termination of the pregnancies. Today, such tumors can be readily diagnosed by **ultra-sound**, but this method would not be introduced into medicine for another 25 years.

Since Wisconsin General Hospital was a tertiary-care facility primarily accepting only complicated cases, I might have concluded from my training there that the most common form of delivery of a baby was by **Caesarean section**. The obstetrical staff had only a small practice of faculty wives and a few others. When a woman came in for a normal delivery, it frequently took place in an amphitheater before a large audience of students.

In order to gain firsthand experience in delivering babies, we were sent to Chicago. We spent one week at the University of Chicago Lying-in Hospital and three weeks at the Maxwell Street Maternity Center.

Just after I arrived at the Lying-in Hospital, a woman was admitted with fluid swelling in her legs and high blood pressure from a toxic state of pregnancy called **pre-eclampsia**. A senior resident had a theory that this might be due to sensitivity to a pituitary gland hormone, so he gave her a steady intravenous drip of the pituitary hormone **pitressin** to "desensitize" her. This worthless procedure caused her to convulse. She and the baby were all right, but he appropriately caught hell from the attending obstetrician.

The Maxwell Street Maternity Center was located in the middle of the Southside Chicago slums. Cut-rate stores and flea markets abounded in the neighborhood. If you knew merchandise, one could find real "steals," which was also how some of the goods got there.

The Center provided free obstetrical care. The prenatal care, if any, was done at the Center, but the deliveries took place at home by medical students. If needed, an obstetrician with a car was on call to rush to the assistance of the students and to determine if the patient needed to go to a hospital.

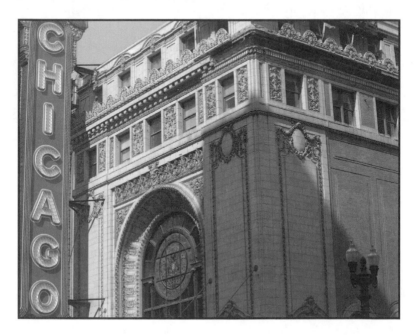

The Center's infant mortality rate of eight to nine per 1,000 was considered astoundingly low, less than half that of hospital deliveries anywhere in the country at that time. The maternal mortality rate was correspondingly low. Both rates would still be very acceptable today.

The students performing these deliveries were from Northwestern and Marquette Universities as well as Wisconsin. Two students went out on each delivery. The first week at the Center, the junior student would have to carry the larger and heavier of the two bags on a streetcar, which was our mode of transportation. Getting to some houses took more than an hour, particularly those located south of 110th Street.

Many of the deliveries were in the slums. The housing was poor, and as it was during World War II, largely overcrowded... even though many people had jobs and money. Affluence was often evident from the numerous suits and evening gowns hanging on lines across a room where closet space was inadequate. Frequently, they had an expensive electric refrigerator or a console radio-phonograph.

Nobody was mugged while I was there, but several weeks before my arrival, an attending student had been threatened with his life if the baby or mother died. The husband, a Black Muslim, sat in the room with a knife across his lap. The baby and mother did exceedingly well. I don't know about the attending student's psyche, however.

On one delivery in the middle of the night, we had to thread our way over a dozen people sleeping on the floor of one room and the hall of a tiny, two-room apartment. The woman in labor occupied the single bedroom. The only bathroom and the running water were located in a closet down the hall.

Drapes for the patients' beds frequently consisted of newspapers that they had been instructed to collect in preparation for their labor and delivery. Nobody actually boiled water, as frequently depicted in many old movies.

Of the 11 calls I attended during my two weeks there, eight of them were false labors. Two of these had **pseudocyesis**, or false pregnancy. The patients weren't actually pregnant but thought they were. They had not sought any prenatal care.

Some of the difficult and prolonged labors, usually with first-time mothers-to-be, were brought to successful completion by an older woman acting as a midwife. She would finally persuade the young "doctor" to allow the mother out of bed to assume a squatting position on the floor. This facilitated the natural delivery mechanics that usually resulted in rapid appearance of the baby. Women had been having babies in this position since time immemorial.

Most of the deliveries were of women who'd had a number of prior pregnancies. For those, there were no mechanics of delivery at all. The babies didn't "travel" down the birth canal as we had been carefully trained. They just appeared. We would joke with each other that our job was to catch the babies before they hit the floor.

—m—

The next experience I had in obstetrics was during my internship at Research Hospital. I wasn't allowed to deliver a baby myself, so I would get up at night to help two doctors in particular, the only ones who made an effort to teach me anything.

A third doctor, Dr. Guffie, an ancient obstetrician, only allowed his own nurses to help him. Some older nurses claimed that while in practice some years before, Dr. Guffie had to be prevailed upon to use rubber gloves for pelvic exams and surgery. He reputedly could do a Caesarean section skin-to-skin in eight minutes. It was 11 minutes the two times I was allowed to assist him.

As of the early 1940s, hospital confinement following a normal delivery ranged from 14 to 18 days. By the end of World War II, the hospital stay was down to eight days and even six days, depending on the facility. Some doctors regarded this as a dangerously short period of hospitalization.

More dangerous was that most of the hospital time was spent

in bed, frequently causing the "milk leg" of **thrombophlebitis**, the dangerous inflammation of veins from circulatory stagnation. While this could lead to the sometimes fatal pulmonary embolus mentioned earlier, more commonly, the leg swelling became permanent and incapacitating.

—ɯ—

I saw a few women who were similar to the locally well-known lady in Kentucky, who reportedly appeared annually with a stack of reading material at her nearby hospital for delivery of her baby. While in for her 16th child, a representative of the Margaret Sanger Institute, an early promoter of family planning, tried to convince her of the need to space her pregnancies and have fewer of them.

"Lordy me, no!" She protested. "Ah look forward to this time here every year. It's the only time ah have to myself!"

The hospital stay served as her annual vacation.

—ɯ—

A few years later, my first delivery as a **locum tenens**, or substitute doctor, had a tragic outcome. I relieved two general practitioners in northern Wisconsin while they took a two-month vacation, their first time off in five years.

At 5:30 a.m., the morning after they left, I was called by a woman near term when she started to bleed. She was in the hospital by 6:30 a.m. The hospital had no obstetrician, and none were in the area.

The consulting surgeon I was told to call when I needed help saw her by 7:00 a.m. The woman had a **placenta previa**, which means the placenta is located in the lower part of the uterus covering the cervical outlet. These are prone to bleed at the onset of labor, endangering the baby more than the mother. The baby showed no signs of distress at that time, so, unwisely, the surgeon did not choose to do a Caesarean section right away, as is required for a placenta previa. I didn't know enough to argue the point.

The surgeon waited until the baby showed signs of distress at 9:00 a.m. By the time he did the Caesarean section, the nine-pound baby boy had died. I was very distressed by the outcome.

—⚬—

The only other delivery I had at that practice started with another infrequent complication, but the outcome was quite satisfying. This woman arrived at the hospital, ready to deliver her fifth baby. She had what I came to call the "220 Syndrome." Her weight was 220 pounds, her blood pressure was 220 over 90, and her blood sugar was 220 milligrams per deciliter, all of these abnormally high. On top of that, the baby was **breech**, with its bottom, not the head, presenting first.

I anticipated any of a number of possible bad results, so I called the same general surgeon I had contacted for the earlier case. I interrupted his supper with a plea for help.

After the phone call, I barely got back into the delivery room in time to literally catch the baby, which was coming out feet first. Mother and baby were fine.

I was back on the phone in 20 minutes to report an uncomplicated delivery and a healthy baby, canceling the surgeon's trip. He hadn't even gotten up from the supper table as yet.

—⚬—

Infant and mother mortality had improved tremendously in the previous hundred years. The advances were due to the general acceptance of the germ theory and the use of aseptic techniques. In time, antibiotics would also have a major impact.

Heart disease was a significant cause of death in pregnant women. Before heart surgery, one of the main causes of death was valvular disease, especially **mitral stenosis**. This is a narrowing of the valve separating the left atrium and left ventricle, caused by **rheumatic fever**. This is easily missed when occurring as an isolated condition.

One woman named Zelda was pregnant and had mitral stenosis. I saw her weekly as a cardiac consultant during her last trimester. Each time she came to see me during her latter months of pregnancy, Zelda told me about a recurring dream in which she was climbing a very long flight of stairs. Each night, she was closer to the door at the top, but had to stop because she was breathless.

"What do you think will happen when you reach the top of the stairs and open the door?" I asked.

Zelda didn't respond.

"Do you think you're going to collapse and die?"

She nodded.

Before she got to the top of the stairs, I put her into the hospital. Zelda had her baby uneventfully. Mother and baby did well.

Others with undiagnosed mitral stenosis usually went into acute heart failure. Some of these died.

Many women with severe valvular or congenital heart disease get pregnant despite advice to the contrary. Most obstetricians at the time advised termination of the pregnancy.

In my experience, those who didn't follow this advice and led a very sedentary life did very well. Those who couldn't rest much because of obligations to care for young children didn't do well, despite medical therapy. Today, corrective heart surgery during pregnancy can help many, but this option wasn't available or utilized until after the 1950s.

Infant and mother mortality had improved tremendously in the previous hundred years. The advances were due to the general acceptance of the germ theory and the use of aseptic techniques. In time, antibiotics would also have a major impact.

CHAPTER 7

Vocal Anesthesia and Unusual Surgical Methods

Surgery started to change significantly in the early part of the 20th century. One sea change, for example, had occurred around the turn of the century, when surgeons were simply urged to wear rubber gloves routinely.

Dr. Mason, my medical school surgery preceptor, told me about a style of surgery practiced in the early 1900s by a renowned abdominal surgeon at Northwestern University. He operated Monday, Wednesday, and Friday from 6:00 a.m. to 6:00 p.m., using three operating rooms. While he was starting an operation in one room, assistants were still closing the abdomen of the preceding patient in another room. The next patient was being prepared and the abdomen opened by assistants in the third room.

He accepted only those patients in whom he had a special interest. At times, he had not examined the patient beforehand. In those cases, if an assistant attempted to explain the problem, he would reportedly protest, "Don't tell me! Let me find it!"

He made abdominal incisions from the breast bone to the pubic bone at the lower end of the abdomen. Then he explored the abdominal cavity systematically, beginning under the diaphragm. As he found pathology he would remove or correct it. He left postoperative care to the assistants.

—⁂—

Progress in anesthesia aided neurosurgery in the 1920s and thoracic surgery in the 1930s. This marked the beginning of an era of rapid surgical progress.

By the 1940s, Frederick Mohs at the University of Wisconsin started his microscopically controlled excision of skin cancers. A long time passed before this first effective cancer treatment could outlive the stigma of the numerous quack, cancer-cure clinics that used salves and ointments, turning the curable into the incurable. The **Mohs Method** is still an acceptable, alternative form of skin cancer treatment today.

Progress in anesthesia aided neurosurgery in the 1920s and thoracic surgery in the 1930s. This marked the beginning of an era of rapid surgical progress.

The first cardiothoracic surgery at the University of Wisconsin was in 1945 with the correction of a **coarctation**, a ring-like constriction of the aorta. A **patent ductus arteriosus**, which is a congenital connection between the aorta and pulmonary artery, was also corrected at that time. This procedure had first been performed successfully in the late 1930s.

—◠◠—

Prior to the 1940s, surgeons supplied their own instruments. After that time, hospitals started providing the instruments, but some surgeons still preferred to use their own.

During my internship, I helped a surgeon perform a **thyroidectomy** *on a 16-year-old girl. Sarah had a very overactive thyroid gland that, as of the day of surgery, was still inadequately controlled by medication, which was an important prerequisite for the surgery.*

The surgeon gave Sarah a local anesthetic. He used his own instruments, one of which was a notorious **hemostat**. *This is a surgical clamp used to stop bleeding, but this particular one had a defective ratchet. The hemostat would automatically disengage from the ratchet every few minutes, pop up, and fall into two pieces, allowing the bleeding to resume. The surgeon would then reclamp it without comment.*

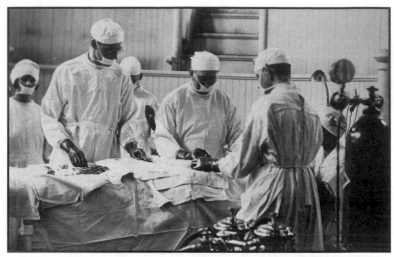

*Operation taking place in 1914 in
the University of Virginia Hospital amphitheater*
Image provided by the U.S National Library of Medicine

*The surgery took about two hours, but the local anesthesia
wore off after an hour.*

*All he would give Sarah after that was vocal anesthesia. "Now
don't give me no trouble, girl! I'm almost done!"*

*He refused to give her any more anesthetic, so I had the circu-
lating nurse give Sarah a quarter grain of* **morphine** *without the
surgeon's knowledge. This, along with her exhaustion, allowed
Sarah to sleep during the skin closure, which is, of course, very
painful when local anesthetic is not used.*

*For a week after the ordeal, Sarah had a tremendous "thyroid
storm." Her temperature went as high as 107 degrees and her
heart rate hit 200. We packed her in ice and opened the windows
to the winter cold. Because of her youth and generally good health,
Sarah survived this frequently fatal complication.*

—⟐—

One of the surgeons at Research was a minimalist. He had admitted a middle-aged woman for a surgical procedure. I was assigned to take her history and examine her preoperatively.

*Among many other questions, I asked about her obstetrical history. She explained that she had a **hysterectomy** by the admitting surgeon. She then recounted her two pregnancies with dates.*

Astounded, I asked, "Are you sure of the dates?"

"Yes. I'm sure."

"You had two children after your hysterectomy?"

"Well, yes."

I was intrigued until later, when I had the opportunity to assist this surgeon with one of his hysterectomies. The mystery was solved. He would remove only the top portion of the uterus above the fallopian tubes. Thus, most of the uterus remained intact and apparently still functional in some women.

Around that time, the removal of the gall bladder carried a national mortality rate of 10 to 15 percent. At Research Hospital, however, it was only 2 to 3 percent. Surgeons generally at the time preached "adequate exposure," based on the belief that, without high visibility during the procedure, mistakes were prone to be made. They would have cringed at the keyhole abdominal **laparoscopic surgeries** of today.

Some surgeons would keep enlarging an incision, if necessary. On one occasion, I saw an incision extended not only from the **xiphoid** at the lower end of the breast bone to the pubic bone at the lower end of the abdomen, but also completely across the middle of the abdomen, flank to flank. The patient did eventually recover.

One of the surgeons only performed colorectal surgery. Once, he reported at a national surgical meeting that he had done 100 resections of part of the colon and had lost only two patients.

The very low mortality rate compared to the national average was received with some skepticism. He attributed his success not primarily to adequate exposure or his meticulous technique and attention to detail, but to the fact that he gave at least two blood transfusions to every patient preoperatively, whether they were **anemic** or not.

Around this time, improvements in the understanding of physiology, increases in the number of effective new medicines, along with the development of new surgical techniques, created many opportunities for innovative methods in all aspects of medicine.

In medical school, we also had a several-week stint in anesthesiology under Dr. Ralph Waters, considered the dean of American anesthesiology. At that time, **cyclopropane** was beginning to supplement and replace ether and **chloroform**.

Dr. Waters casually mentioned during one of my operating room sessions with him, that he had tried giving oxygen intravenously to patients. He was investigating whether this might provide the promise of supplementing, if not replacing, the lungs in patients who needed it. He found that up to 60 milliliters, or two ounces, of oxygen could be dissolved in the blood this way. This was not nearly enough to replace the amount supplied by the lungs.

For a time in the 1950s, an intravenous injection of carbon dioxide was used for outlining the right side of the heart for the x-ray diagnosis of **pericardial effusion**, the collection of fluid around the heart. Carbon dioxide is absorbed rapidly, much faster even than oxygen, and causes no problems.

Researchers knew that when air under high pressure is absorbed by the blood, it creates serious problems. This is because it is 80-percent nitrogen. Unlike oxygen and carbon dioxide, nitrogen is poorly absorbed and forms bubbles in the tissues, which can be painful and potentially fatal. This is what happens in **"the bends,"** an affliction of people working under conditions of high environmental pressure such as deep-sea diving.

Air bubbles in the blood are a complication during surgery that also can prove fatal. When large amounts of air get into the blood stream, the blood froths and blocks blood flow through the right side of the heart to the lungs. Death will result. Most people can be saved if they are turned onto their left side. The gas bubbles rise in the heart and the blood flows under the froth into the lungs. Incidentally, the amount of air injected from a syringe is too small an amount to cause death, as occasionally depicted in murder mysteries.

Around this time, improvements in the understanding of physiology, increases in the number of effective new medicines, along with the development of new surgical techniques, created many opportunities for innovative methods in all aspects of medicine.

As part of the development process, most new surgical techniques and operations in that era were tested on animals before they were tried on people.

Many medical advances at the time were made by thoroughly studying single patients, or by studying small groups of patients with similar problems. These innovations did not have the **controls** that are standard today. A "control" is a participant in a research study who is given a placebo, and his or her response to the inactive medication is compared to the response of the individuals in the study who are given the active drug or treatment. In the earlier times before large studies were required, individual patients often served as their own controls, with the doctor comparing the patients' responses to the active drug, to their condition prior to taking the medication.

This small-sample approach of studying single patients or small groups of patients was risky, but not necessarily as risky as the shotgun application of treatment standards today based on data derived from large groups. The traditional method of individualized innovation in diagnosis and treatment was tailored specifically for the single subject at hand. Though not applicable to broad groups of patients, such innovation was more personal with respect to that particular patient.

CHAPTER 8

Heroic Innovations

In the late 1940s and early 1950s, many new lifesaving therapies became widely available. Since the potential medical benefits of these new methods were unproven by today's standards, however, physicians frequently put patients at risk. Doctors applied their best medical judgment in weighing the value and risk of an untested but potentially lifesaving procedure. Generally, the risk from using a treatment should be lower than the risk from not using it, and also lower than the risk from using any other treatment.

On one occasion, a 19-year-old named Earl was transferred to Research Hospital from an osteopathic hospital where he had been for a week. A reaction to a sulfur drug he was taking for a cold caused his kidneys to shutdown. Earl was given the sulfur drug because he was allergic to penicillin. Neither drug had ever been indicated for treating a cold.

The big challenge came during the evening of the day Earl arrived, when he had a fever of more than 105 degrees. He had developed pneumonia and couldn't tolerate anything taken by mouth because of his kidney condition.

*Two new antibiotics aside from penicillin had recently become available. One was **Chloromycetin**, which was found to be effective in **typhoid fever** and **typhus** infections, but was only available in an oral capsule at the time. The other was **Aureomycin**. It was out in an oral capsule and had just become available for injection, too. Some experimental animal work had suggested that **tetracyclines**, of which aureomycin was one, also had a fever-reducing effect, similar to aspirin.*

To give Earl the amount of injectable Aureomycin that he needed would have cost more than $300 a day, about $2,600 in *today's dollars. But that amount of injectable drug wasn't available, so the cost question was moot.*

*On the expectation that Earl was going to die that night if something wasn't done immediately, I emptied the contents of four, oral Aureomycin capsules, amounting to a total of one gram, into a saline-filled syringe. I injected this into his **IV** tubing, and watched as some insoluble, white particulate matter rolled down the tubing into his vein. Earl's temperature began falling within four hours and was completely normal in 12 hours. It cured him.*

*The next morning, I was able to reach a drug company rep. He was appalled at my innovative, off-label use of the drug. He explained, however, that the insoluble particles in the capsules were a relatively innocuous soap-like **triglyceride, sodium fluoride**, and a **diphosphate**.*

After several days, Earl's kidneys started to function spontaneously, and he began voiding several gallons of urine every 24 hours. We were barely able to keep up with the fluid loss and the salt imbalances, but we did.

In any event, due to an innovative application, Earl survived an otherwise certain death.

I tried this approach on two other occasions with less spectacular results. One was for a patient with acute **diverticulitis** and an **abscess of the sigmoid colon**, sometimes referred to as the "left-sided, acute appendicitis." He responded in days, not hours, but did get well faster than he would have when penicillin was the only antibiotic available.

The third occasion was for a woman who had a **Pel-Ebstein fever**. This is a high relapsing fever that appears for three to 10 days, then subsides for three to 10 days recurrently over many months. Possible causes such as a **lymph node** tumor or a **collagen disease of the connective tissues** could not be diagnosed in her at the time.

She didn't respond to the Aureomycin. Finally, five months later, the source of the fever became evident. Her chest x-ray showed the development of a lymph node tumor in her chest adjacent to her heart.

None of these patients had any adverse reaction, save some mild vein inflammation at the injection site.

Generally, the risk from using a treatment should be lower than the risk from not using it, and also lower than the risk from using any other treatment.

—ɯ—

At the other extreme, however, were situations in which doctors used unnecessarily risky innovations on patients whose life was not in immediate danger. One instance involved a teenage girl with mild infectious **mononucleosis**, also known as the "kissing disease." A staff internist, on a hunch, gave her an early anti-cancer drug, one which was not indicated for that disease. Giving her the drug caused no harm, but it did expose her to the risk of damage to her bone marrow.

On another occasion, the same doctor stuck a six-inch needle into a young woman's chest cavity in an attempt to aspirate a small cystic mass in her lung. He started near the spine after freezing the skin. When several efforts failed, he became impatient and stuck the needle deep into the chest at a half dozen unanaesthetized places, beginning in the back and working around to the front between the same two ribs.

He finally **aspirated** a small amount of infectious material containing the single cell protozoan parasite, **trichomonas**, which probably came from a bronchial tube. This organism is common in the intestinal and genital tracts as well as the bronchial tubes, and does not necessarily cause any problem.

Except for the discomfort of the patient, there were no complications such as air around the lung or bleeding. I'm not sure about the young woman's psyche, however.

Outcomes were not as fortunate in all of the non-standard treatments tried. One man named Jethro was hospitalized with a diffuse, raw, and oozing rash on his back. His doctor ordered **boric acid** *packs. By the end of the week, his body was red all over, like a broiled lobster, his kidneys shutdown completely, and he developed shock. Within a week, Jethro died. This was the clinical picture of boric acid poisoning, the danger of which had recently been emphasized in the medical literature.*

Boric acid had been used as eyewash and a home remedy for rashes. It was used in the newborn nurseries as a mild antiseptic for diaper rashes. About this time, hospitals banned its presence in the newborn nursery. It often was mistaken for powdered milk and inadvertently used as baby formula, resulting in the same kind of "broiled lobster" death in babies as occurred in Jethro.

While boric acid has no special merit, it is not harmful for small, localized rashes, as only inconsequential amounts are absorbed by the body. In diffuse rashes, however, it can be absorbed through the skin in large, toxic amounts.

Another patient, Fred, was 26 years old. He came in from the country with **hypertension** *and severe kidney failure. He was making urine, but his kidneys weren't doing much of anything else, which included his not being able to keep the blood cleared of* **creatinine**, *a product of metabolism resulting from the breakdown of protein. This type of kidney failure causes or can be caused by high blood pressure, and it increases the risk of stroke.*

Normal creatinine levels are below 1.4 milligrams per deciliter in the blood. Fred's creatinine levels started at 5.0 milligrams and gradually rose to a high of 27.0. By restricting protein intake and pushing intravenous fluids, we increased his urine output and gradually brought his creatinine back down to 5.0 over several weeks.

Fred went home to convalesce further, which to him meant hunting and not working. He did this for six months, at which time he returned to the Hospital with a massive stroke that unfortunately proved fatal within the week.

—ᴠᴠ—

In the late 1940s, **peritoneal dialysis** for kidney failure was reported to be feasible. Fluid flushed through the abdominal cavity was supposed to remove the wastes that the kidneys would ordinarily remove. This was being tried at some hospitals.

Through each patient encounter, I often learned more from the patient than from my colleagues or any other source. These encounters were especially important in learning the art of personal care, and they helped me develop my own standards of care that would serve me and my patients throughout my career.

Jerry Murphy, a surgical resident, tried this innovative method when a woman's kidneys shut down after an otherwise uncomplicated abdominal operation. He had only read about the technique and had never tried it even in an animal, but the situation was desperate.

He sterilized two huge 50-liter jars and filled them with a special sterilized fluid he had prepared. He ran this fluid into her lower abdominal cavity through a tube inserted into one side. It was drained by another tube emerging from the other side.

Unfortunately, all that it did in this instance was slow the rise of the creatinine and overload her with fluids. She died within several weeks.

The autopsy showed that the kidneys were not the normal fist-size. Due to damage from earlier disease, each kidney was about the size of a walnut—too small to sustain life.

Extra-corporeal renal dialysis, the kidney machine, which would have been indicated here, became an effective reality over the next 10 years. A kidney transplant, another possible solution for her, was not done successfully until 1961.

New techniques in medicine, combined with a better understanding of physiology and biochemistry, would help relieve doctors of some of the need to try untested new procedures. This improvement, however, would come at a price.

With the influx at that time of effective new methods of treatment, and fewer generally accepted standards of care, doctors were able to apply innovations much more freely than today. Physicians generally developed their own standards of care by trial and error based on results with an individual patient.

After my internship and residency, I began to apply what little I had learned to a broader base of patients. Through each patient encounter, I often learned more from the patient than from my colleagues or any other source. These encounters were especially important in learning the art of personal care, and they helped me develop my own standards of care that would serve me and my patients throughout my career.

PART II

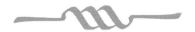

The Art of Personal Care

CHAPTER 9

Cat Fever, Retired Generals,

and Irreproducible Findings

My residency at Research Hospital ended in 1950, and the following two-and-a-half years were uncertain and hectic at times. Dorothy and I moved several times and covered much of the Western World, it seemed. The medical experience I gained, however, made the inconvenience all worthwhile.

Initially, I went to the University of Vermont's Division of Experimental Medicine in Burlington as a research fellow in cardiovascular diseases under Drs. Wilhelm Raab and Eugene Lepeshkin. I spent about eight hours daily in the lab, five days a week, and attended or held conferences at the Bishop DeGoesbriand Hospital. I had no patient-care responsibilities.

Dr. Raab's area of interest was with the effects of **adrenaline** and other **catecholamines** on the cardiovascular system. I did a study of the effects of adrenaline on the hearts of rats when deprived of oxygen.

We also went to a state mental hospital to evaluate the effects of intravenous adrenaline on patients' cardiovascular systems. The only informed consent we had to obtain was from the director of the hospital. I spent my spare time during the next several years examining the changes produced on the electrocardiograms of these subjects.

Dr. Lepeshkin's forte was electrocardiography. He had left Russia with his family shortly after the Revolution. His father had been a botanist and a curator at a natural science museum in Leningrad. The family escaped from Russia in a boxcar by bribing railway officials with the alcohol used to preserve museum specimens.

After this, Dr. Lepeshkin studied medicine. While still a medical student, he began writing the first definitive European textbook on electrocardiography. He had been to libraries in five capitals in Europe collecting his references.

On coming to this country, he rewrote the book in English. In 1946, while visiting his publisher in New York City, his car was broken into and his leather briefcase containing the only copy of the manuscript was stolen. It was never recovered. Dr. Lepeshkin was still rewriting it when I joined him four years later. He kept his notes on three-by-five-inch file cards, usually only a few lines of almost illegible scratching on each, which was enough to give him total recall of the article.

—∿∿—

Several months into my fellowship, I received a phone call from an irate US Navy Commander. After World War II, I had stayed in the Naval Reserve on inactive duty. I was still in the reserve while in Kansas City.

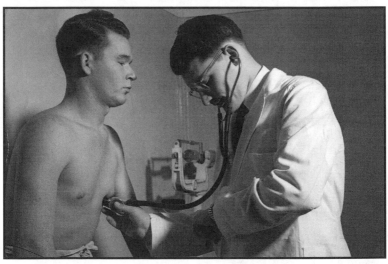

US Navy Lieutenant Norman Makous, MD, examines patient at US Army Field Hospital, Wurzburg Military Post, Germany, 1950 (US Army photograph)

"We've been looking all over the country for you!" The Commander said. "You were supposed to notify us when you changed your address!"

My service with the Navy actually had begun years earlier. One month before starting medical school, I was called into active duty at the Great Lakes Naval Training Station in Illinois. I was excused from boot training and assigned to ship's company at Camp Smollet. Of the 14 boot camps at Great Lakes, two of them were segregated African American camps, where inductees received basic training for six weeks. Camp Smollet was one of these two camps.

I served in the entirely Caucasian ship's company of the dispensary. Sick recruits could be kept in the dispensary for up to three days, after which they were sent back to training or transferred to the Naval Hospital. Most of them had "cat fever." That was the Navy jargon for **catarrhal fever**, which consisted of a sore throat or bronchitis. Venereal disease, primarily **gonorrhea**, was also a common reason for admission.

Every 10 days, a new group of trainees arrived in camp. They required a half-dozen inoculations, including typhoid, **tetanus, yellow fever**, and others. We gave these in a Quonset hut drill hall the size of a football field.

Corpsmen stood on each side of the line of recruits, giving them the shots in each arm. Some, with prominent Southern drawls, would at times throw the syringe with needle into the arm like a dart. The African American recruits were not reticent about demonstrating their anxiety, but none of them fainted. A corpsman who had spent time in one of the Caucasian boot camps claimed that one out of every six of the supposedly macho white boots fainted during the standard administration of shots.

Even more atrocious was the behavior I observed on one occasion in which three corpsmen told an African American recruit that the treatment of his venereal disease required an injection into a testicle. The injection was to be made with a huge ear-lavaging syringe to which a large oilcan spout was taped.

Every time the corpsmen made out that they were about to make the injection, the subject flinched. They would give him a tongue lashing and then repeat the torturing farce. This went on for some 20 minutes before they ended it, blaming the recruit for the "failure" of the treatment.

—◊◊◊—

In 1950, after the Navy interrupted my fellowship in Vermont and put me back into active duty, I spent the next eight months with the US Army. They assigned me to the Army Hospital in Wurzburg, Germany. Aside from hospital duty as a ward physician, I helped man outpatient clinics for the servicemen and their families.

We'd see patients in the general medical clinic and refer them to a subspecialty clinic if necessary. Some were dismayed that the same doctor who had referred them was now the specialist who was seeing them. We had less time to spend with patients in the general clinic than in the clinics for specialized care, so often by referring a patient, more time was available to provide better treatment.

—◊◊◊—

The medical problems were not exotic. The most common problems were **psychosomatic**.

A 35-year-old sergeant complained of vomiting after every meal.

The mess sergeant standing at the door of the hall would ask him, "how was your meal?"

He'd vomit and say, "see for yourself!"

This had been going on for months, but he remained overnourished. He lost no weight. The problem was not life-threatening and did not interfere with his duty.

Obviously, he was not really sick. I could only conclude that he either had a psychosomatic illness or was lying in order to get special treatment.

On another occasion, we had some difficulty in getting a staff sergeant's severely enlarged heart taken seriously. We had to transfer him to the Army General Hospital in Frankfurt. He would have been discharged from the service if he were sent back to the States.

—⁂—

One of the German doctors was amused by the fact that the American doctors did extensive testing for collagen disease of the connective tissues on patients with chronic fever. Any European doctor or even medical student, he said, would have known at a glance that the temperature chart was that of a patient who was suffering from typhus.

While typhus was very common in post-War Germany, it was much less common than collagen disease in the US. As I had learned in medical school, where one is located makes a big difference in the diseases that one should expect to see.

While in Germany, I attended an Army medical conference in Nuremberg. An Army surgeon at the Munich General Hospital reported on the treatment of a man who had undergone surgery for the construction of a bowel-to-stomach connection. It didn't start functioning for 36 days.

Ordinarily the patient would have lost weight and died from starvation. The surgeon got adequate calories into him by administering daily ethyl alcohol intravenously. High calorie lipid infusions were not yet available. Surprisingly, neither the patient nor the doctor became an alcoholic.

—⁂—

After eight months with the army in Wurzburg, my orders returned me to the Navy and the States. This time I was assigned to the US Naval Hospital on the Camp Lejeune Marine Base in North Carolina.

The Hospital had a 1,100-bed capacity but only about 600 beds were filled at the time. Approximately 200 of those patients would have been kept in a civilian hospital, even in those days. Marines needed to be ready for full duty upon returning to their unit, however, so they were kept in the hospital longer to convalesce.

At first, I was in charge of the infectious disease ward with some 30 beds. The dominant disease was hepatitis picked up in Korea. **Malaria** relapses were nearly as common.

Next, I was transferred to a general medical ward. Every Saturday morning, the Captain inspected the wards.

On one occasion, the inspection party came to my ward just after a marine was brought in. He had been bitten by a snake and it was presumed to be a rattler.

After a rapid preliminary assessment, I directed the marine to come to attention for the Captain with the rest of us.

He had no ill effects from the minor delay in treatment. In fact, he required no treatment at all, since the snake bite was found to be non-poisonous. He suffered no adverse effects but had a good story about a Navy doctor giving a Captain's inspection higher priority than his potentially fatal snake bite.

—∿—

After my four-month stint at the general medical ward, I took over the sick officers' quarters, which was known as the "SOQ." This provided many interesting medical experiences.

*A routine blood sample from a retired Marine Air Force General—who came in for an annual checkup—revealed a strange creature in the blood smear. It was a **trypanosome**, which is a mosquito-transmitted parasite. Two types of trypanosomes exist, one originating in Central America and the other in Eastern Asia.*

When chronic, the trypanosome appears in the blood mostly at night and only for about five years after the initial infection. This was 1952, and the General's history revealed that his only exposure had been in Guatemala for six months in 1931 and he had spent 15 minutes refueling in the Philippines in 1944.

After making him nearly anemic with numerous blood tests, we couldn't repeat the finding. By the time the slide specimen arrived at the Naval Research Lab on the Base, its characteristic markings denoting the geographical type of the parasite had been marred, so that identification of its origin was no longer possible.

The General wasn't ill and had no symptoms, so we decided that the best course of action was to ignore the finding.

—∿—

Another retired Marine General came in with gastro-intestinal discomfort that he'd had for years. It proved to be functional, not due to anything serious. I gave him the standard antispasmodic, **tincture of belladonna.**

He was elated. "It cured me!"

"In all of your years in the Marines, it's never been prescribed for you?"

"No."

I found that surprising, since this was the standard symptomatic treatment of the era.

The General was so grateful that he said he was going to write me a letter of commendation for my Navy file.

These years at military clinics and hospitals provided experience with a different spectrum of diseases than I'd seen in the civilian hospitals. Also, patient care in the military was much more standardized and less personal. As a doctor who has worked in both types of hospital settings, the disadvantages to a less-personal style of care were easy to see.

CHAPTER 10

I Just Stopped in for a Blood Pressure Check

My two-year stint in active duty with the Navy was over in October of 1952. Before I resumed my interrupted cardiology training, I worked as a locum tenens, or temporary substitute practitioner, for two months in Baron, Wisconsin. Baron is located 100 miles northeast of Minneapolis, and 60 miles north of Eau Claire, Wisconsin, where I had done my medical school preceptorship.

I was substituting for a general practitioner team, Dr. Gerald Fostvedt and his wife, Dr. Lucille Radke. Three years earlier they had taken over the practice from a bachelor who had been seeing about 60 patients a day. He moved to Alaska because it was less crowded and the hunting and fishing were better. This was the Fostvedts' first vacation while there. They provided me with their house, one of their cars, and a stipend of $1,000 per month.

Dorothy and I, along with our one-year-old son, were greeted in Baron by a 26-inch snowfall. This was beautiful but inconvenient. The car they had left us had no chains or snow tires. In fact, none of the eight doctors in town used either of those items. They simply kept a shovel and sand bags in the trunk. Snow clearance was so superb that snow tires were unnecessary.

Plows were always out on duty with the first dark cloud on the horizon and a forecast of snow. By morning, they had the roads plowed wide—even though trees, limbs, and poles with wires might be atilt, broken, or toppled by the weight of the snow.

After our arrival, the owners stayed at home for about one week, several days longer than they had planned. I'm sure it was because I looked like a high school kid to them, and they weren't sure I could handle the practice. The town had a population of 2,000, but it drew from a valley of 100,000 people. The hospital was at Rice Lake, 20 miles away.

The two pharmacies in town were hurting. Dr. Fostvedt had been with a pharmaceutical company in North Jersey. He had a pharmacy of his own in the office and would dispense generic medicines to his patients for free.

Although of brief duration, this office-based experience with general medical practice in a small rural community of 2,000 people would prove very worthwhile. It was entirely different from the hospital-based training in urban centers I'd had previously. It would prove to be of value no matter what type of medicine I eventually practiced.

According to one of the pharmacists, the previous doctor had written about 180 prescriptions a day, which were filled by the two pharmacies. He had used syrup of white pine as a vehicular base for most of his prescriptions.

One pharmacist said, "There's a hogshead of that stuff in my basement! That's enough to supply the whole state of Wisconsin for the next fifty years!"

—∿∿—

One 96-year-old patient named George came to see me. He was as yellow as a gourd from serum hepatitis he'd acquired from a blood plasma transfusion following prostate surgery several months earlier. He should have died from it, but he didn't turn a hair.

I asked George the inevitable question put to any nonagenarian. "To what do you attribute your long life and good health?"

"I always sit down and eat three meals a day, no matter how I feel," he replied.

And that's what saw him through the hepatitis, I'm sure. The earliest and most common symptom from hepatitis, other than the loss of a desire for cigarettes in smokers, is loss of appetite. But George ate every meal, three times a day—even though, as he admitted, he had no appetite. Maintaining good nutrition can be more important in acute liver disease than in many other conditions.

—⁓—

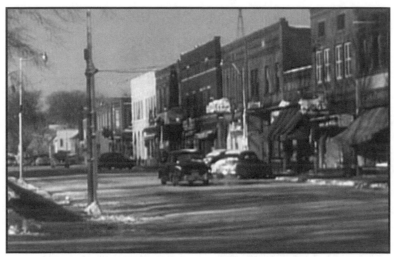

Main Street in Baron, Wisconsin, 1952

Resistance by patients to good medical practice was common. Records had been kept on three-by-five cards and little was written on them. Most needed a physical examination.

When I pointed out to patients that they'd not had an examination in eight or nine years, I'd hear, "Old Doc So-and-So knew what was wrong without examining me."

Others would say, "I don't have time for an exam right now. I just stopped in for a blood pressure check."

Or, "I was shopping and I have to pick up the kids from school in a half an hour and then pick up my husband from work."

Sometimes good care wasn't readily accessible. One severely depressed woman was brought in by her husband. There were no effective medications for treatment. The nearest psychiatrists and facility were two hours away. He never took her there as advised, and sadly, she committed suicide a week later.

The one aspect of the area and the practice I thought most notable was the fact that I had never seen so many people in their 80s and 90s in excellent as well as in ill health. Many of them were farmers of Scandinavian descent.

Although of brief duration, this office-based experience with general medical practice in a small rural community of 2,000 people would prove very worthwhile. It was entirely different from the hospital-based training in urban centers I'd had previously. It would prove to be of value no matter what type of medicine I eventually practiced.

CHAPTER 11

Shotgun Coronary

In January of 1953, after the temporary medical practice in Baron, I resumed my cardiovascular training. This time, it was at Pennsylvania Hospital in Philadelphia under the sponsorship of Dr. Joseph Vander Veer, who was head of cardiology there.

In 1952, Pennsylvania Hospital had provided one of 11 approved cardiology residencies in the country. In 1953, it was one of 36. This increase was a response to the introduction of successful cardiac **catheterization** laboratories and of successful cardiac surgery. Cardiological technology was about to take off.

I was paid nothing during the first 12 months of the residency and supported my wife and child on savings from the two years on active military duty. The second year, I obtained a National Institutes of Health clinical fellowship, which provided a stipend of $300 per month.

The Pennsylvania Hospital Heart Station was on the ground floor and consisted of six large, high-ceilinged rooms, three on each side of a wide hall. A large steam duct that was part of the City's central heating system ran under the floor of the hallway. This supplied volumes of steam heat year-round to the hospital and other buildings.

Summers in Philadelphia were generally hot and humid. The addition of the steam heat made the Heart Station almost unbearable. There was no air conditioning and opening windows was of little help, as the heating duct vented just below one of them. A new heart station with a catheterization laboratory opened just after the end of my fellowship.

One other fellow was in cardiology at the same time, my senior fellow Frank Boyer. Fellows did consultations on the wards, which contained most of the beds in the hospital. We also attended a long-standing Thursday night cardiology clinic, and several cardiology subspecialty clinics. These included a prenatal clinic, a peripheral vascular clinic, and a children's heart clinic.

In addition, I attended the general medical clinic once a week. We ran all of the Hospital's in- and out-patient **anticoagulation** treatment programs for both private as well as ward patients. This practice had started in the late 1940s, when the Hospital had participated in the Irving Wright multi-hospital study of anticoagulation treatment of **acute myocardial infarction**.

The Pennsylvania Hospital cardiology clinic was started in the early 1920s. It was held every Thursday evening at 5:00 p.m. after a cardiology conference. Doctors from as far away as Central Pennsylvania to South Jersey attended the conference. After the conference, we had supper and saw patients in the clinic.

At its peak, more than 325 patients were seen at the clinic weekly, but this included those who came in to receive **mercurial diuretic injections** for congestive heart failure as often as three times a week, or for monthly penicillin injections for **rheumatic fever** prevention. The number of clinic patients gradually declined to about 275 a week in 1959.

This was due, at least in part, to the introduction of the first potent oral **diuretic, chlorothiazide**, in 1958. This reduced the need for frequent mercurial diuretic injections. It was also due to the fact that Ms. McDougal, a very dedicated nurse nearly 60-years old who had kept the clinic running for years, left when she married for the first time.

Ms. McDougal had the important personal touch. She would phone patients who missed appointments, and would even go to their homes to find out what could be done to help them. The Hospital was actually run at that time by about a half-dozen such dedicated women, known to the house staff as "The Vestal Virgins."

The L-shaped open medical wards were located in the oldest parts of the Hospital building. Ward I on the first floor was for men. Women were on the second floor in Ward III. Located in the middle of the "L" in each ward were the nurses' station, a single-patient room for the acutely ill, a treatment room, and a laboratory where house staff did most of the routine lab work on their assigned patients. These were adjacent to the elevator and a wide flight of stairs.

The hallway in the short leg of the "L" had about half the number of beds compared to those of the longer hallway, and was for the sicker patients. This was the medical intensive care unit of the time. The longer hallway had a row of large, hollow, heated Doric columns down the center of the hall. Under the windows on each side, were about ten curtained beds. The attending staff physician made bedside rounds almost daily, while grand rounds were made weekly by the chief of medicine or his designate.

—◊◊—

On one occasion, the chief of medicine's designate Perry McNeil, a glib and entertaining "roundsman," was holding court on Ward I at his weekly grand rounds. It was attended by many interns, residents, fellows, students, and nurses. All were congregated around one of the beds in the long hallway, flowing over the feet of not only the adjacent beds but also those across the aisle.

The elderly man in question had a heart murmur, low-grade fever, anemia, and weight loss—the classic findings of **bacterial endocarditis***, which is an infected heart valve. He had been under scrutiny of the cardiac fellows for more than a week. We were unable to establish the diagnosis, which would be made definitively if cultures of the patient's blood had shown a growth of bacteria. But, the numerous cultures had remained unexpectedly negative, and our diagnosis indefinite.*

While an intern ran through the pertinent medical facts, Dr. McNeil finished his cursory examination and stood by, listening tolerantly. After the intern had finished presenting the background information, Dr. McNeil pronounced authoritatively

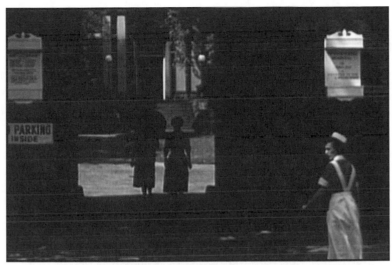

*A student nurse enters the 8th Street Gatehouse entrance of
Pennsylvania Hospital in 1954*

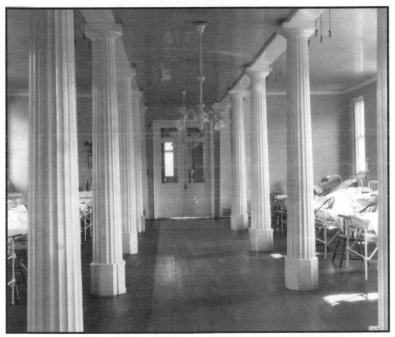

The mens' ward at Pennsylvania Hospital in 1950

and unreservedly in his own inimitable manner that, "This man has bacterial endocarditis."

The two cardiac fellows regarded this with considerable skepticism.

With little or no urging, Dr. McNeil went on to explain that, "One of the **pathognomonic features** of endocarditis is the presence of these long, splinter-like **hemorrhages** under the fingernails." He held up the man's hand.

As Dr. McNeil continued with his expostulation, the South Philadelphia patient became increasingly animated, finally getting Dr. McNeil's attention.

"Hay ya, Doc!" The patient said in a thick accent. "Doze are schplintas! Ahm a cabinet maker!"

His survival over the following year established that the patient indeed had not had endocarditis, a 100-percent fatal disease if untreated. We had to be satisfied with a diagnosis of **prostatitis**, an inflammation of the prostate gland.

—ɯ—

I found that I no longer was learning only what not to do. Through the various specialty training programs, conferences, and clinics, I was beginning to learn what should be done.

Besides being a glib, entertaining, and extemporaneous speaker, as well as raconteur and martini lover, Dr. McNeil was also a duck hunter. Early one morning, he fell behind the others in his hunting party on the way to a duck blind on the Delaware Bay. The others had looped around a marshy area. Dr. McNeil took a shortcut across the marsh in order to catch up with his hunting party.

Halfway across, he realized he'd gotten into quicksand. With a mighty effort, Dr. Mcneil made his way to firm ground, still hanging onto the two heavy and expensive Belgian shotguns *he was carrying. Being the Scotsman he was, the idea of tossing aside the guns to save his life had never entered his mind.*

On reaching the duck-blind, he dropped to the ground, exhausted, weak as a kitten, drenched in sweat, and short of breath. Sometime later, his breathing, weakness, and sweats were no better.

Finally, when he was unable to raise his gun to fire at some approaching ducks, he allowed the others to take him to the Hospital. He was having an acute myocardial infarction, a heart attack. His recovery and convalescence were uneventful—and he still had his precious shotguns.

—⚏—

In my Pennsylvania Hospital fellowship, despite the influence of some of the negative role models, I found that I no longer was learning only what not to do. Through the various specialty training programs, conferences, and clinics, I was beginning to learn what should be done.

I began to develop a basic system of medical management that I could alter as new information and research changed medical care and more scientifically based standards were available. These changes began happening quickly over the coming years.

CHAPTER 12

Doc, How Often Should a Man My Age Have Sex?

After my two years of fellowship, I was in a dilemma. I knew I didn't want to be a "hospital bum" forever, yet I didn't know where I wanted to practice. I had no strong urge to return to any of the communities in which I had trained. They all had their positive and negative aspects.

I recalled a Northwestern student I'd met when I was at the Great Lakes boot camp in the Navy, before starting medical school. I had pitied him at the time. He already knew he'd go back and practice in his home town in Ohio. He was not interested in exploring the country to see where he would most like to practice. Now I envied him.

Fortunately, I was able to postpone making this decision when I was offered the chance to become the director of a new cardiac catheterization laboratory at Kansas City General Hospital in Missouri. I remained in that position for a year and a half.

Finally, in 1956, after my stint at the catheterization laboratory, I was nine years out of medical school, married with three kids and a mortgage. I knew I could put it off no longer. I had to go to work and start a real practice.

General practitioners usually had no difficulty in starting up a practice. Small communities trying to attract a family doctor often helped with setting up an office. Also, doctors were generally considered a good credit risk. Borrowing from a bank was not difficult, and equipment companies were eager to lend them money to purchase the company's products.

Specialists, however, had to stay in larger communities. Many would set up an office in a professional building in the hub of a metropolitan area. Others started out as an employee of an established physician in the same specialty, often with partnership as the aim. They would attract patients from all 360 degrees of the surrounding area. They would only need a few patients from each geographical sector to survive.

—〽—

Early in 1956, Dr. Stanley Morest asked me to join him in his practice in Kansas City. He was a board-certified internist who was generally regarded as a **peripheral vascular disease** specialist more than a cardiologist.

Stan had a new office in a building with a number of other physicians. He gave me an office rent-free and the help of his secretary, Dolores. Our agreement was that I was to see each of his hospital patients daily and was to work with him in the office in the afternoons. He paid me $10 to take a history from one of his patients and $5 for an examination.

The best way for a specialist to build a practice was to spend as much time as possible in the area hospitals. If you were seen there, the emergency room physicians and other doctors would refer patients to you and call for your help because of your availability.

Initially, I got three or four referrals from other doctors. The patients were either deadbeats or **hypochondriacs**…"No-Pays" in any case. Then there were no further referrals. Everybody just leaned back to see whether I was going to make it on my own. I soon realized that I would need three years to build the same size practice that a generalist could build in six months in his hometown.

After six weeks, while sitting at my desk, Stan sidled in, laid an envelope on my desk, and walked away without saying a word. It was a "Dear John" letter, notifying me that our engagement was unilaterally terminated. Stan didn't think it was going to work. The arrangement was costing him about $200 a week.

This was a real shock. I scrambled. To make ends meet, I spent several months doing examinations at the homes of applicants for the Metropolitan Insurance Company. For picking up a urine specimen and mailing it to the company, I was paid 50 cents. The occasional complete history and physical examination brought me $15, and lesser amounts for limited examinations. I was making about $250 a month—not enough to support my family.

—ɯ—

Within several weeks of my dismissal, I found an office to share with a general practitioner who had an extra room in his stand-alone medical building. Dr. Morest's secretary, Dolores, volunteered to come and work for me. She thought that I needed her help more than he did, and she wasn't happy about continuing to work for him, especially after the way he had treated me. I was uncertain about being able to pay her, but she had no doubt that I'd be able to do so. She was right.

My first patient in the new office was Jerry, an 84-year-old gentleman with a blue, painless, great toe. He had called me late one afternoon, and I had him come right in. I found that Jerry was in stable condition with no other complaints. The problem was one of inadequate blood circulation to his legs, which is usually due to atherosclerosis or hardening of the arteries. I gave him a prescription for a blood vessel dilator and told him to come back in a week when I would be able to give him a comprehensive examination.

When I examined Jerry a week later, he was in mild congestive heart failure. On taking a more complete history, I found that he'd had indigestion involving the upper abdomen and chest that had awakened him one night a week before his first visit. His electrocardiogram revealed a recent myocardial infarction. I also found moderately severe atherosclerotic disease of the lower abdominal aorta, the primary reason that his toe turned blue. His aortic obstruction was not so severe that it required surgery.

*One of the label warnings on the **vasodilator** I had prescribed was that it might cause heart failure. The combination of the drug, a lower blood pressure from his damaged heart, and the hardening of his arteries now made all of his toes turn blue from inadequate circulation. I changed his treatment, and he did well at home.*

About a month later, Jerry came in for another visit. He wanted to know, "Doc, how often should a man of my age have sex?" I was so dumbfounded that I neglected to ask him how often he was having it now. I mumbled some textbook generalizations. The real reason for the question was that he'd become impotent from the reduced circulation to the pelvis caused by the blockage of his aorta.

—〰—

Several months after being dismissed by Dr. Morest, I became the attending physician for the non-pulmonary medical care of tuberculosis patients in the city sanitarium located between Kansas City and Independence, Missouri. I made rounds there two to three times weekly.

This experience was rewarding in several respects. I learned to sharpen my clinical skills and work without immediate laboratory support. Testing was available, but the specimens were sent to a city lab, and it would take nearly a week for the results to come back. Therefore, I frequently was forced to make assessments and prescribe a treatment plan based entirely on clinical findings and judgment, without the benefit of any test results.

Another rewarding aspect of this opportunity was that I was able to see some cardiac patients. The most prevalent cardiac problem at the sanitarium was that of tuberculosis involving the **pericardium**, which is the sac around the heart. In these patients, collected fluid compresses the heart, called **cardiac tamponade**. The compression caused a **pulsus paradoxus**, an adverse effect on the blood pressure that could be assessed by measuring the pressure during inspiration and expiration.

As much as one, two, or even three pints of fluid might distend the pericardial sac. This large amount usually was apparent in x-rays. Typically, the fluid accumulated gradually over days and weeks. It could be removed through a needle inserted through the chest wall.

Most fascinating was that some patients would go into and out of this heart compression within hours. In fact, when heart enlargement was not evident by x-ray, which suggested a smaller quantity of accumulated fluid, withdrawal of as little as two ounces would cause the tamponade to disappear within minutes. Such a rapid response was unexpected in my experience.

—⚏—

Soon, I was on the staffs of nine hospitals, including the Independence Sanitarium and Hospital. Some days I'd cover well over 100 miles in my travels. At times, I'd drive 30 miles south to Richards-Gebaur Air Force Base, where I was a consultant. Then from there, I'd drive 60 miles to north Kansas City to do an insurance exam. On the way, I'd see patients at as many as six hospitals.

When I acquired the electrocardiogram interpretation concession, as I called it, at the Independence Sanitarium and Hospital, I closed my office in Kansas City and opened one in Independence. I persuaded Dolores, my secretary, to buy a car and come with me to my new practice. I covered much less territory after I moved my family to a home in Independence, on the opposite side of Kansas City.

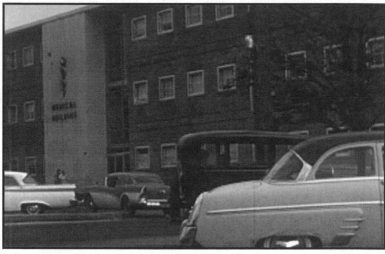

In 1958, Norman Makous moved his offices to Independence, Missouri

Some of the older physicians at the Independence Sanitarium and Hospital still retained some quaint practices from the distant past. You could always tell when one particular general practitioner had a patient in the hospital. The smell of vinegar permeated the floors where he had his patients. He prescribed vinegar gargles for sore throats. Those with aches and pains had vinegar hot packs and compresses.

He also used vinegar in surgery. I'm not sure whether he washed his hands in it, probably did, but he always poured a little vinegar into the abdomen and incision on closing the wound. His patients never had any wound infections.

His son was a surgeon who returned from training just before I arrived in Independence. He monitored his father's patients and practice. Finally, he put a stop to his father performing any more surgery, before any hospital sanctions were made against the use of vinegar in patients.

—ɯ—

I would advise those who hadn't been seeing a doctor very frequently that, "I'll be seeing you more often than you are currently being seen. In several months, you'll be better. I don't know how much better, but you will be better. Then you won't have to come in to see me as often."

I became too busy after confining my practice to Independence. While I was practicing primarily as a cardiologist, I was called upon to do a great deal of internal medicine. At the time, I was the only board-certified internist east of Kansas City in an area of 125,000 people. People who wanted an internist usually went into Kansas City some 10 miles away.

Within a year, I was seeing 30 to 40 patients a day—15 to 20 in the hospitals, and the same number in the office in the afternoons. On some days, I also visited nursing homes and made house calls.

Unlike the physicians in Philadelphia, almost all doctors in the Kansas City area, including those in general practices, felt that they had to have a hospital practice. Doing so was not only a matter of prestige and pride, but it maintained the continuity and therefore the quality of care of the patient. Most physicians made hospital rounds of their patients in the morning and held office hours in the afternoon.

Only one family practitioner I knew in Independence rejected hospital practice. He saw patients in the office all day and referred those in need of hospitalization to other doctors. He said hospital practice was time consuming and inefficient, and he could make more money in the office, which he did.

I found that many patients had been seeing a general practitioner weekly and receiving only a few minutes of a cursory interaction with no examination. The doctors made no attempt at a diagnosis and gave only symptomatic therapy. I regarded these as "turnstile practices."

As a result of providing full examinations, I would find many previously undiagnosed conditions. In one two-week period, in fact, I picked up eight cases of previously undiagnosed **lupus erythematosus**, a serious collagen disease that can involve the arteries of most organs, especially the kidneys.

I would advise those who hadn't been seeing a doctor very frequently that, "I'll be seeing you more often than you are currently being seen. In several months, you'll be better. I don't know how much better, but you will be better. Then you won't have to come in to see me as often."

CHAPTER 13

Personal Care versus Heart Care

In the summer of 1959, my wife Dorothy and I vacationed in the East. I visited my sponsor for my cardiology fellowship, Dr. Joseph Vander Veer, in Philadelphia. Shortly after that visit, he asked me to join him in his cardiology practice and serve on the staff of Pennsylvania Hospital.

As I mentioned earlier, I realized I was too busy in Independence. I was spending less and less time with the family, which now included five kids with another on the way. I frequently missed dinner and family activities. I thought this new situation would give me more time with them. I wanted to accept the offer. Dorothy agreed, so we returned to Philadelphia in 1959.

In my new position, I had time for some academic pursuits, which I had missed in Independence. That December, I attended a conference in New York City on "Salt, Water, and Electrolytes." The first presentation was on the structure of water. I knew I'd been away too long. The structure of water? Wasn't water one of the four basic elements, along with earth, air, and fire? Obviously I'd never taken physical chemistry.

I was on the full-time cardiology staff at Pennsylvania Hospital. Besides helping in the catheterization lab, I supervised the residents at the Heart Station, managed the cardiology clinics, made anticoagulant rounds, performed consults, did my stint as one of the attending physicians on medical ward rounds, and served on staff committees. Soon, I joined the staff at Bryn Mawr Hospital, and was required to attend the cardiac clinic there, too.

I started building my office practice. Patient care outside the hospital setting is a creative challenge. There was a difference in practice style between the East and the Midwest. The communities of the East were older. Therefore, offices were apt to be in old houses or buildings in or near residential neighborhoods, or in business locations more accessible to patients by public transportation. Specialists often were on hospital campuses.

In the newer communities of the Midwest, doctors' practices were usually housed in office buildings that required an automobile for access. Physicians generally felt that having their offices closer than a mile or two from the hospital placed them at risk of being "taken over." And there was a sense that those actually housed on a hospital's campus had "sold out," giving in to the temptations of the bigger system, and not wanting the added work involved with an outside practice.

I also noticed other regional differences between Kansas City and Philadelphia, possibly due to my limited experience. For example, in the Midwest, I saw a number of patients whose chest pain mimicking a heart attack arose from sensitive "trigger" points in the musculo-skeletal tissues of the chest wall, spine, and especially the neck. This experience was infrequent in Philadelphia.

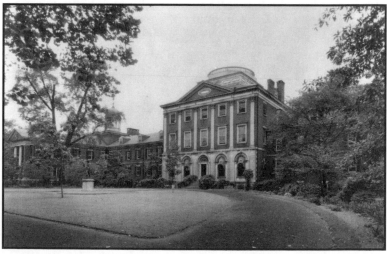

Pennsylvania Hospital, 1954

The use of medications, both new and old, often was different between the regions. Part of that was due to the common practices and recommendations of regional experts, and part was due to the regional differences in promotion by drug company representatives.

As time went on, I realized that my practice was best characterized as "primary care cardiology." I found that taking care of people with heart conditions was more rewarding for both of us, than just taking care of peoples' hearts.

Dr. Vander Veer allowed me to see patients in his office rent free. His office was located directly across the street from Pennsylvania Hospital. This made me "geographic full-time." I could walk to the hospital and did not have to drive to other locations like some other staff doctors.

Contrary to the Midwest practice, I preferred to see patients in the office in the morning and make hospital rounds in the afternoon. First, the laboratory results from tests on the hospital patients from that morning were back in the afternoon, and the results were only six to 10-hours old, rather than 24-hours old—as it was when one made rounds in the morning. Also, in Philadelphia, I found that most patients preferred to come to the office in the morning instead of the afternoon. Older patients generally wanted to get out in the morning. Travel was easier and they were not returning home from Center City during the late afternoon rush hour or in the dark.

Setting up a referral practice, the lifeblood for a specialist, is much easier in a hospital-based setting. And it's important that referred patients go back to their referring doctors, or those doctors will stop sending them. Referral patterns were frequently generational. The younger doctors were often more up-to-date on technology and were immediately available in the hospital.

Soon, they began to dominate some specialties, especially the acute illnesses and those requiring special diagnostic or invasive techniques. They were becoming "hospitalists," which is now regarded as a specialty unto itself.

In general, I found I could attend to patients' cardiovascular problems and prevent complications more effectively if I saw the patients frequently, and was aware of every change in their health status. "Chest colds" or "flu" misdiagnosed by their family physician, on occasion were actually from heart failure or even heart attacks. "Indigestion" might originate from a heart condition. The same is true of pain in the lower jaw that is sometimes misdiagnosed as dental pain. In the throat, it may be misdiagnosed as a "sore throat."

Also, medication can be adjusted and tailored to the individual patient much more efficiently with frequent examination. I don't understand the cardiology practice in which patients are seen only once every three to six months.

As time went on, I realized that my practice was best characterized as "primary care cardiology." I found that taking care of people with heart conditions was more rewarding for both of us, than just taking care of peoples' hearts.

CHAPTER 14

Give Him All the Eggs He Can Hold

The critical first step in conducting a complete medical examination is taking the patient's history. This consists of discovering the information that people tell the doctor about how they feel. This can require "a good ear."

After all of the specialists' attention to this patient, the procedure that cured him was taking his history.

Claude Farley was a generalist I worked with at Research Hospital. Like many generalists of that period, Claude felt that specialists had little more to offer patients than he did.

One story that illustrated this point was about a patient with a chronic, pussy nasal discharge. He'd had this condition for years, and been to innumerable ear, nose and throat specialists without any help.

When Claude received this patient, the first thing he did was take a history. He learned that, several years earlier, the man had been chopping and hauling wood when he slipped and fell face down into the woodpile. The nasal discharge started a short time later.

Claude probed around the floor of the man's nose and found the end of a wood sliver. He pulled out the splinter, which was several inches long.

After all of the specialists' attention to this patient, the procedure that cured him was taking his history.

— ∞ —

The problem in securing a good history from a patient was illustrated most vividly to me while I was director of the Cardiac

Work Evaluation Unit. The American Heart Association started sponsoring the Unit in 1951 to determine whether cardiac patients could work safely without aggravating their heart condition.

At the time, physicians usually told employees not to return to work after being diagnosed with heart disease. Many employers were reluctant to allow their employees to continue to work, and would never hire a cardiac patient. I was placed in charge of the Unit in 1961 when it moved to Pennsylvania Hospital from the Philadelphia General Hospital.

The subjects were employed people from the area referred by cardiologists for study in the Unit as outpatients. A team of professionals consisting of a cardiologist, a registered nurse, and a vocational counselor, did the evaluations, and each took his or her own history. They then discussed their findings as a group.

I was intrigued by the marked differences in the individual history obtained on occasion by the team members from the same patient. For example, the nurse or counselor would, at times, obtain a more relevant medical history than the physician. A portion of this was the result of a difference in semantics and the style of questioning. Words mean different things to people of different backgrounds and training. The nurse or counselor may have been communicating better with the patient.

Another key factor was that some patients have poor recall. The process of questioning jolts the memory, so a subsequent examiner, while taking the history, obtains better information.

Culture, background, and education make a big difference in obtaining an adequate history. Questionnaires are thought to save time. They tend to be oversimplified, often skewing the patient's interpretation of what they believe the doctor wants to hear.

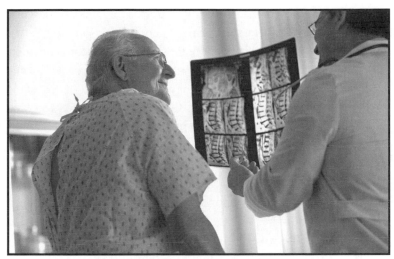

A doctor explains x-ray results to his patient

Some patients deliberately withhold information about their symptoms. They want to see if the physician can objectively detect the heart condition or other problem. At times, the physician may have spent more than a half-hour obtaining a detailed history. Then, upon reviewing the findings from the examination and several tests with the patient, the patient or spouse would frequently come forth with an entirely different version of the essential part of the history. This could easily change the significance of the other findings, and thus modify the conclusions and recommendations.

Culture, background, and education make a big difference in obtaining an adequate history. Questionnaires are thought to save time. They tend to be oversimplified, often skewing the patient's interpretation of what they believe the doctor wants to hear. This leads to omissions and misunderstandings.

Questionnaires and physicians use terms that are derivatives of those the patient uses. Patients may call a sensation in the chest, "Indigestion," "gas," "an ache," "pressure," or "shortness of breath." A poorly designed questionnaire may refer to the chest symptoms only as "pain."

Some patients think primarily in terms of anecdotes. They will deny any of a list of symptoms. Then, when asked to recount a specific event or what happened, they will describe, in considerable detail, the symptoms that occurred while eating or with some other activity. Their description may include some of the same words and symptoms about which they had just been asked, and the presence of which they had denied.

Many physicians leave much of the information gathering to an assistant, who in time may become more adept in obtaining a history than the doctor. Other physicians tend to review the history in a cursory manner. An important opportunity to build a rapport, as well as to build the patient's confidence in the doctor, is lost.

The difficulty experienced by physicians in obtaining a meaningful history has been increasingly evident in hospital emergency room records, which I have reviewed over the past 40 years. In one example, an admitting clerk recorded the complaint as, "chest pain." The triage nurse wrote, "chest pressure." The physician's notes registered "gas," without adequate expansion, exploration, or explanation of the symptom in view of the prior notes. As a result, a heart attack from an acute myocardial infarction was missed. There were many similar situations.

This reflects the contemporary emphasis on technology and testing rather than patient history and physical examination. At times, unfortunately, not even the required tests are done.

—⁂—

Good communication and avoidance of misunderstanding is a constant challenge, and isn't confined to obtaining an adequate history. Getting patients to comprehend instructions can also be a problem.

Semantics play a role along with differences from cultural and occupational expectations. Often what is effective instruction for one person is entirely ineffective for another. Recitation helps some patients to understand and remember, but even then many forget what the doctor said. Writing instructions and making a chart of medications helps some, but others, even those who can read, prefer oral instructions and ignore written ones. Many doctors do not take the time to ensure understanding, turning this over to an aide.

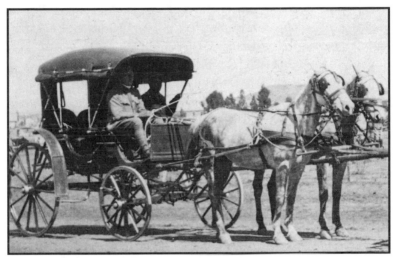

Horse and buggy medicine circa. 1900

The 90-year-old Dr. Harper, father of our obstetrics professor in medical school, made this clear during senior year when I spent a week at the Wisconsin State Health Department. One of his anecdotes addressed the importance of making instructions to patients crystal clear.

Dr. Harper had started practice in Madison near the end of the 19th century. Just after telephones had come into use, he answered a frantic call from the wife of a prosperous farmer named Ole who lived not far from Madison. Ole's wife said he had mistakenly swallowed Calomel, a bi-chloride of mercury solution used as a disinfectant, which he kept in the barn. The Doc knew he needed to rush out and pump Ole's stomach.

Swallowing raw eggs was a common antidote, and, of course, most farmers had chickens. The rationale was that the egg whites bind with the mercury and slow the absorption until the stomach can be emptied. So Dr. Harper told the wife, "put him to bed and give him all the eggs he can hold."

The Doc harnessed his horse to the buggy and trotted as fast as he could to Ole's farm. As he went up the lane, Ole's wife was plainly visible in her white apron, anxiously waiting on the porch.

Dr. Harper hopped out with his not-so-little black bag, containing, among many other things, the equipment to pump out Ole's stomach. He followed the wife up the stairs to the bedroom. There, in his high, four-poster bed, sat Ole, bolt upright, in his night gown and nightcap. His big, gnarled hands were stretched out in front of him, palms up, and fingers widely spread. Just as instructed, his hands were piled high with "all the eggs he could hold." Fortunately, Ole suffered no ill effects from the deficient instructions.

Good communication and avoidance of misunderstanding is a constant challenge, and isn't confined to obtaining an adequate history. Getting patients to comprehend instructions can also be a problem.

—⟶⟵—

When oral medications didn't work or were not available, I prescribed rectal suppositories, and would recall Dr. Harper's lesson very clearly. People who had never used a suppository, often didn't follow the instructions on the container. If they neglected to remove the silver foil wrapper, the suppositories were completely ineffective.

One patient, in fact, told his doctor: "For all the good these damn things did me, Doc, I might as well have shoved them up my ass!"

Instead of using them correctly, he had swallowed them.

CHAPTER 15

Psychiatric Cardiology

For patients, choosing a doctor is like choosing a future spouse. It should be someone with whom they are compatible and comfortable. Of course, they also want someone who is knowledgeable.

The combination of personal care and individualized technical care builds patient confidence. Some don't mind doctors with cold personalities, if they are on the cutting edge of medical-care science. Most, however, prefer doctors who understand them and with whom they can communicate. Competence is important, but to many, this is secondary.

The definition of a "good doctor" varies. Many patients regard the good doctor as one who is up-to-date on new technology and uses extensive testing. Some physicians regard the good doctor as one who knows his own limitations.

Some general practitioners delivering personal care pride themselves on their ability to determine when a patient has a transient illness, or when he or she is really sick. They make sure that their patients receive the proper treatment, usually by referral to a specialist. Many nurse practitioners are better at providing initial assessments than physicians.

The comprehensive initial examination is critical in building patient confidence in the doctor. An occasional patient, who was in for the first time, would claim that the physical examination I had just done was the most extensive one he or she had ever received. I found that hard to believe. Afterwards, when I started to talk about some of the tests I wanted done, these patients would want to know why they needed tests when I hadn't found anything wrong on the physical examination. They felt completely reassured by the hands-on examination.

When I started in my career, authoritarian medical care was the norm. "I'm the doctor. You're the patient. Do as I say." Patients were minimally included in their own care. Some physicians still practice this way, and some patients complain that this type of one-sided care is all they're getting.

In recent years, I have experienced the indignity that many patients feel. On one occasion, a super subspecialist eye doctor talked to a trainee about me. Not once did he answer my questions or direct a comment to me until the end of the examination. Then all he said was, "You're all right."

Over the course of my career, I learned to treat patients as I would like to be treated under similar circumstances. Rather than authoritatively telling them what to do, demanding that they say nothing, and handing them a prescription as they leave, I made sure that I included them in the decision-making process.

On another occasion, I was scheduled for some minor surgery. The surgeon had spoken with the referring doctor but not with me. Two technicians told me what he was going to do. When I began questioning them, in order to clarify some points that differed from my understanding of the procedure, the surgeon came into the room. He'd been listening from the hall.

On directing the same questions to him, he suddenly became very annoyed. He felt I was questioning his judgment, which I wasn't. He then went into a subdued rage and suggested that perhaps I didn't want him to operate on me. I agreed that I didn't. He followed me out with a tirade over my arrogance. I was simply dissatisfied that I wasn't included in decisions about my own care.

—⁂—

One of my surgeon colleagues was known to be very efficient. He used five operating rooms at once. He was a "hale fellow, well-met" socially, but professionally he was terse and to the point—even cold.

The surgeon made rounds in the hospital before patients were awake. This way, he avoided questions. One patient, for example, kept trying to catch him, but he was always gone before she could wake up enough, even when she had prepared a written list of questions.

One of my doctor friends had a surgical diagnostic procedure done by this surgeon colleague and was waiting to hear the results. Several days later, he was walking down the street when a sleek, black sports car slowed at the curb, and the heavily tinted window went down.

The surgeon, sitting behind the wheel, waved to him and said, "You're all right!" Up went the window and off sped the car.

Another doctor friend had gone to the same surgeon's office twice and found that his two visits totaled 140 seconds. Physicians understand this approach, but patients do not.

Over the course of my career, I learned to treat patients as I would like to be treated under similar circumstances. Rather than authoritatively telling them what to do, demanding that they say nothing, and handing them a prescription as they leave, I made sure that I included them in the decision-making process.

At the time I started practicing, involving patients in their own care was a style that was used by a minority of physicians, and not appreciated by all patients. One patient who was sent to me by a retiring general practitioner said, "Gee, I never had a doctor who talked to me before." She never came back.

At first, I was frustrated in communicating the results of an evaluation with my patients. At the end of the detailed explanation using language I regarded as very simple, some patients would say, "I know, doc, but what's wrong with me?"

I turned to a senior colleague, who had a very large practice of satisfied patients, for advice. He said he still got this reaction from some patients, and suggested a particular approach, which I tried on a patient named John.

After my initial examination, I explained the origin of John's heart pain in simple, non-technical language.

John said, "I know, Doc. But what's wrong with me?"

I put my hand on his arm and said, "John, it's your heart. You got a bad heart."

The lights went on, and John turned to his wife. "Doc says I got a bad heart...a bad heart."

—ɯ—

I learned that sometimes, that which seems the most medically irrelevant to the doctor, is most important to the patient.

One day, a woman brought her 16-year-old daughter Robin to see me. Robin had raised pink blotches on both shins.

*I conducted a complete evaluation. In addition to the history and physical examination, this included a blood count, a red-blood cell sedimentation rate test, a skin test for tuberculosis, and a chest x-ray. All were normal. I decided she had **erythema nodosum,** a condition which is self-limiting and requires no treatment.*

Robin and her mother returned to the office after I received the test results.

I told Robin, "I've found nothing wrong with you and I don't know why you have the condition. But I'm sure it will go away without treatment."

Robin was still very troubled.

I was at a loss as to what else to tell her, then I recalled one other thing I could say for certain. I had read a recent article in the Journal of the Archives of Internal Medicine *which indicated that erythema nodosum was never associated with cancer.*

I added, "Although I don't know why you have the condition, I am certain of one thing. You do not have cancer."

Robin suddenly broke out with a beaming smile, let out a sigh,

and became animated for the first time. "That's such a relief!"
She said. "That's what was worrying me most!"

Cancer does occur in 16-year-old girls, but it is unusual, and addressing that issue did not occur to me at first. Only after the fact did I appreciate the anxiety that is generally so much higher in teens than in adults. When one is ill, many people fear the worst.

In medical school, this was referred to as the "sophomore syndrome." When the medical student or trainee in other medical disciplines, such as nursing, begins to learn about different diseases, many are sure they have each new disease they study. One research study concluded that medical professions attracted people with more than the ordinary level of anxiety over their health.

—ɷ—

Anxiety and depression affect a large proportion of patients seen by cardiologists. This includes those with imagined as well as real heart disease. At one point, it seemed, I was "curing" more patients with anti-depressant medications than with cardiac medicines. I kidded my colleagues that, "I'm in the practice of psychiatric cardiology."

A large number of patients whom I saw over the years had chest symptoms that caused them to believe that they had heart disease. Some with anxiety attacks would feel their heart pounding, or would sense a jolt from a "skipped beat." They would wonder, "Is it my heart?"

Many people are overly sensitive to any left chest discomfort. These sensations often are of muscular-skeletal or gastro-intestinal origin.

Muscular-skeletal aches or tenderness in the chest wall, so called "trigger points," are often mistaken for heart pain. Frequently, these are due to tenderness of the cartilage connecting the ribs to the sternum. As anxiety increases one's awareness of a particular part of the body, normal sensations ordinarily ignored are now felt. These sensations may actually feel painful.

Because most people realize that the heart is in the left chest, they become concerned about sensations located there. They ignore pain in the right chest, although true heart pain on occasion may be felt on the right side as well. Interestingly, the only patient without **angina** who ever complained to me of pain in the right side, was left-handed.

—⸙—

At Camp LeJeune, a young Marine named Charley was hospitalized for study because of an ache over his heart and upper left abdomen. It occurred upon exertion, especially when carrying a heavy knapsack. He was quite anxious as he was sure he had heart trouble.

He had a six-inch band of overly sensitive skin, extending from his heart, under his left armpit, and to the spine. This resulted from strain in this area of his spine, causing pressure on a nerve. It was due to a curvature from a lower-spine deformity.

Charley's heart was normal. This relieved his mind, but I don't know whether he was ever able to return to full duty. At least he didn't return for further treatment.

—⸙—

Many people go from doctor to doctor with the same chest-pain complaint. The doctors all assure them that they have no heart trouble. They are not reassured by the comment that "Your heart is normal." The best reassurance is relief of the pain. This requires a diagnosis of the problem, the determination of the cause of the problem, and relief by treatment. Then they are convinced.

Some patients look to technology for reassurance. They don't want to participate in their own care, especially as it might involve a change in habits and lifestyle. Occasionally, I would hear from the technology-oriented, those who feel that medicine is all science. They would say, "Doc, don't bother me with my disease. Just cure me."

Many patients with this attitude go directly to the surgeon, the procedural specialist. Many of these interventions are awesome and can be life-saving. Other times, they are merely temporizing and do not address the underlying disease.

CHAPTER 16

The Laying on of Hands

I found that the duration of the follow-up visit was an important aspect of addressing anxiety. Of course, this varied with the individual patient. I scheduled 20 minutes for these appointments, but I gave each person the time he or she needed—even a half-hour or more. One study found that the average patient of a family practitioner was satisfied with an eight-minute visit.

In the examining room, I always made a point of sitting down and appearing at ease, even if, or especially if, I felt rushed. I found that if I didn't take the time, even if only a brief visit was required for medical reasons, patients would be dissatisfied and would let me know. If I did sit down as if unrushed, I would avoid any potential complaint about a "hurried visit." Then a relatively brief encounter would often prove sufficient for both of us.

Doctors must convey a sense of complete attention to the patient. They must not give all of their attention to the chart or whatever electronic recording device they currently are using. People need the reassurance of the doctor's undivided attention.

A good laugh is important for many patients. Julia was middle-aged and saw me every month. We always had a pleasant visit. Once she complained that, "I got so mad after I left your office the last time! I had a list of questions I was going to ask you but you made me feel so good, I forgot to ask them."

Most people will choose a doctor who enjoys their company.

For many years, I did a complete physical examination on almost all patients, old as well as new, including retina, head, neck, extremities, chest, and abdomen. Sometimes I would see one of my regular patients, and within a week or so, this patient would return early with some anxiety—maybe about the medication I prescribed or some other detail from the previous appointment. After addressing the problem, I would start to leave the room, when the patient would ask, "Aren't you going to examine me?"

Under the circumstances, this was unnecessary, I thought.

The brief contact from "laying on of hands" during the examination made patients feel much better and reassured. Several studies have demonstrated that patients with muscular complaints respond significantly better to treatments requiring direct contact of the therapist. Massage or manipulation, for example, may be more effective than standard physiotherapy or medication with a program of exercise.

The comprehensive annual health examination reassures the well and is particularly reassuring to the "worried-well," those who are anxious about their health. Its value in finding unknown disease, however, has been controversial. One study of a large number of annual examinations over a period of 10 years revealed that most of the abnormalities that were discovered were already known to the subject. Nonetheless, screening for specific conditions such as breast cancer has been found to be both worthwhile and cost-effective.

In addition to consultative cardiology, my mentor, Dr. Vander Veer, conducted executive health examinations in his office for a number of companies. These included three banks, two national accounting firms, and several small companies of various types. When I joined his practice, he had me help with these company examinations, and when he gave up his office in Center City, he turned some of them over to me.

During a 30-year period, I performed several hundred of these examinations each year. They included a brief health history since their previous examination, a physical examination, electrocardiogram, and blood tests. Up until the early 1980s, I conducted **fluoroscopic** examinations of the chest in my office. After that time, chest x-rays were done at longer intervals. A more extensive panel of blood tests was included in the exams. One thing that was not done routinely until the 1970s was a **proctoscopic examination**, one of the most valuable screening procedures for well people.

Most of the time, unknown disease of significance was detected only in subjects who had been symptomatic for a week or two, and had put off seeing their personal physician because they knew they were scheduled for their annual company examination. On one occasion, a vice president of a bank had just returned from a two-week vacation on a Caribbean isle where he'd had the "flu" and had not completely recovered.

Upon fluoroscoping his chest, I was astounded to find that his heart was extremely enlarged. This proved to be due to an **effusion**, a collection of fluid in the pericardial sac around his heart. He'd had some vague chest discomfort with the acute illness which was from inflammation of the pericardial sac and the collection of fluid. This type of inflammation ordinarily caused severe chest pain.

The generational difference in the health status of executives of banks and partners in several national accounting firms demonstrated a change that seemed to be based on level of education. The younger ones overall had higher educational levels, and their health was a lot better—lower weight, lower blood pressure, normal blood sugars, and lower cholesterol levels. I attributed this to better health habits—more exercise, less smoking, less drinking, and a better diet.

In addition to any effects one's level of education may have had, the health status of the CEO also had an effect on the employees' health, as determined by one's lifestyle and habits. Their health risk factors reflected the CEO's standards and often the CEO's appearance. If the CEO over-ate, drank, and smoked, so did the employees. If the CEO didn't change his lifestyle, no one else did either, even if recommended by the chief medical officer of the company.

Patients usually don't attempt to do what has been suggested at the prior examination—lose weight, exercise, reduce fat and salt in their diet, and stop smoking—until a short time before their annual examination. Then they stop any efforts immediately following the annual exam. I came to regard the chief value of annual examinations as a reminder to the individual to change habits and lifestyle as had been recommended in previous years.

CHAPTER 17

Bugs in the ICU

Emotional issues for patients and their families can affect outcomes and require special attention from their doctor.

When a long-time patient of mine stopped following my directions and started causing herself harm, I transferred her to an internist friend for care. As it would turn out, she fell in love with him, and then began harassing him at the office and calling his home frequently.

Sexual harassment of patients by doctors is considered very newsworthy today. Sexual harassment of doctors by patients, however, is considered an occupational hazard to which all physicians are probably subjected at some point.

Another woman came in to see me for the first time. I had taken care of her husband for a number of years and had met her when she accompanied him.

Patients were instructed to strip to the waist and to put on an examination shawl. She did that, but didn't stop at the waist. She had totally disrobed and sat on the edge of the examination table with legs crossed, wearing only the short examination shawl.

I ignored her lack of attire, and she didn't say anything. She came back twice with the same behavior, and then never came to see me again.

On another occasion, when a baby in heart failure took a turn for the worse, I offered to see the baby at home. The mother began making suggestive overtures over the phone, so I convinced her that it was best if she brought the baby into the office to see me.

At times a patient might admit that she didn't want her husband intruding on her day at lunchtime. As the saying goes, "I married him for richer or for poorer, but not for lunch."

Some extended this to retirement or illness. One patient who had just retired resignedly noted that his wife made him leave the house before 9:00 a.m. every day and wouldn't let him return until after 4:00 p.m.

Another of my patients, who was age 66, had been a widow for 15 years. She then married a 71-year-old man. I asked her why. "He's still good in bed," she said.

After a few years, he started to become enfeebled, and she learned he was actually 81 when they got married. The burden of care proved more than she had expected. She divorced him and moved away.

For several years, she would come back to visit the area every summer and take him on a cruise with her. Apparently he found the sea air invigorating.

—∿∿—

Physician safety was of some concern at times. Occasionally, you'd see a story in the newspapers about a patient walking into a doctor's inner office and shooting him without warning. The victims were usually psychiatrists.

While at Independence Hospital, I was asked to see a postoperative middle-aged man who was not cooperating with the nurses. He was lying in bed with a silly grin on his face. When I started talking to him and asking him questions, he suddenly gave me a roundhouse blow to the side of my head, knocking off my glasses. Thankfully, I was uninjured. We both recovered.

The only time I was truly concerned for my safety was when the daughter of a patient threatened me. Her father had progressive disability from many small strokes. She and her family had taken excellent care of him at home. Then he had another stroke episode, and I admitted him to the hospital.

At one point, he became furious with the nurses when they refused to let him sit up due to his condition. They insisted that he be fed lying on his back. He aspirated food, developed pneumonia, and died a few days later.

After his death, his daughter was very distressed and appropriately furious with the nursing staff, blaming them for her father's death. At the time, nursing was experiencing a difficult period, so I decided to support them.

The daughter glared at me and said, "I'll take care of you later!"

She would not leave his body and accompanied him to the hospital morgue. The pathologist finally separated her from her father's remains.

At midnight, several months later, a few days after the assassination of President Kennedy, the daughter called me at home. "Well, Dr. Makous, how does it feel knowing you are a murderer?"

I was quite troubled by her comment, but I didn't know what to say.

"I'm going to call you from time to time to remind you," she added, and then hung up.

I started giving parked cars and shrubs a wide berth, especially when walking from the car into the house at night.

I received one more call the following month, and then the calls stopped.

—⟨⟨⟩⟩—

At one point, a member of a Gypsy sect from West Virginia was referred to me. Soon I was seeing a number of members from his sect. After a while, I admitted one of their leaders to Pennsylvania Hospital with unstable angina. We had little to offer but bed rest.

He held court with his numerous followers all day and most of the evenings, despite our pleadings that he not do so. Finally, we put our foot down and made the visitors leave.

The leader's angina quieted some, and he signed himself out. Almost immediately, he was admitted to another hospital. To my knowledge, I never saw another member of his sect.

—⟨⟨⟩⟩—

A patient named Tony was admitted to the intensive care unit at Pennsylvania Hospital for treatment of complications from a myocardial infarction. He kept complaining about "the bugs in the ICU."

Because of this seemingly paranoid fear of insects, and on the recommendation of a psychiatrist, I transferred him to a locked psychiatric ward.

Immediately, Tony's family and friends were swarming all over the place almost around-the-clock. I thought they were concerned about his care situation.

Then I learned that this was allegedly a Mafia family who was reportedly under investigation by the FBI at the time. As it turned out, Tony's concern about the "bugs" was completely rational, not delusional. He was referring to FBI listening devices.

The family was convinced that this move to the psychiatric ward was an FBI ruse to question him or to secretly tape his conversations.

I moved Tony back to the regular ward for an FBI-surveillance-free recovery, as far as I knew, and an eventual discharge from the hospital.

CHAPTER 18

Take Two Aspirin and Call Me in the Morning

Good personal care requires that patients be able to contact their physician by phone or even by email when they have the need. I always provided them with my home phone number, which was printed on my prescriptions. I found that the calls at home were not burdensome. A few new, anxious patients would call me frequently, but this soon stopped when they became assured that I was as available as I claimed.

Today, coverage of doctors during off-hours, by another physician, nurse triage, or even a phone-answering service, too frequently results in the referral of people to an emergency room for their medical attention. This increases the unnecessary use of these facilities.

A colleague of mine, when handling my calls, never tried to determine the nature of a problem over the phone. He routinely referred my patients to our emergency room where he would see them. Another colleague, who spent a great deal of time out of town, gave up on coverage by other physicians. He took his own calls, which he had automatically forwarded to his cell phone—no matter where in the country he happened to be located.

—◆◆◆—

After World War II, many clinics were started by general practitioners. In some, even the specialists with the clinic were expected to take all calls from patients.

I knew a doctor who took separate years of specialty training in pediatrics, internal medicine, obstetrics, and general surgery. He decided to specialize in thoracic and cardiac surgery. Then, when he joined a general medical clinic in suburban Kansas City, he was required to take general night and weekend phone calls on his rotation, like everyone else. When patients called at night or on weekends because of a cold or any other problem, no matter how minor, they were getting advice from a board-certified cardiac surgeon.

Another of my colleagues, one of my co-interns at Research Hospital, had gone directly into general practice with an established physician.

One of the calls he'd gotten the first few months of practice was from an anxious couple with their first baby, who was just a few weeks old. "We got up to give the baby her 2:00 a.m. feeding and her diaper was still dry. What should we do?"

My colleague told them, "Give the baby an ounce of water every 15 minutes until the diaper is wet." He knew his instructions would keep them up for a while.

Not caring about the anxiety of the new parents, he told me that he was thinking, "You woke me, now you can stay awake too."

Some doctors would make sure their answering service could track them down no matter where they were. If a doctor got paged for an emergency phone call in a public place like a theatre or ballpark, it was considered good, free, and ethical advertising. The Kansas City baseball park stopped paging doctors by name when one doctor, who incidentally was thought by some colleagues to have underworld connections, was paged over the public address system at every ball game, whether he was attending it or not. After other doctors complained, paging was done by an assigned number.

During the 1960s while in Philadelphia, I was becoming embarrassed by the frequency with which I was being called by name from meetings at which no other doctors were paged. I had several imaginative and persistent patients who were able to track me down, even when my answering service couldn't find me.

One phone call I received from a patient in the middle of the night was not only a little annoying but also very amusing.

A neighbor woman I knew only slightly phoned me at 3:00 a.m.
She had never been a patient of mine and I knew nothing of her
complicated medical history.

"Doctor, I don't know what to do," she explained.

After she went over the details of her concern, I asked about
her medications. She was taking many for a number of medical
conditions.

I asked her, "Have you tried to get hold of your regular physi-
cian? Is he away, or something?"

"Well, no."

"Why didn't you call him?"

"I didn't want to wake him. He works so hard!"

Ultimately, people make their own medical
treatment decisions. These are not always the
correct ones. That's why they consult with a
physician. The same can be said of physicians'
decisions at times, too, however. These are
often just educated guesses.

The better the physician knows the patient and
incorporates the personal element of care, the more
educated the guess. That is one reason medicine is
still referred to as "the practice of medicine."

Karl, another patient of mine, also called me at home late one night.
He was an ex-chairman of the board of a barge-hauling company.
He was 82 at the time, and still drove every day for nearly an hour
from his home in Delaware to his office on the Delaware River near
Philadelphia.

When Karl first came to see me a few years earlier, I found that he had a valvular heart condition that required no special treatment. Later, he developed an abnormal heart rhythm that required a permanent pacemaker. After one was put in, he had no more problems until the evening of the call.

At 11:00 p.m. on this particular evening, he called me and complained that, "I've got a funny feeling in my chest."

He had never had evidence of coronary artery blockage, but at his age it was possible that this was the early stage of a heart attack. I told him, "Get to the emergency room at your nearest hospital."

"I really don't want to do that," Karl said.

I knew that he distrusted the local medical care. This was one reason he had been coming all the way to Philadelphia to see me. As expected, he refused to go to his local hospital, and he had no one who could drive him to Pennsylvania Hospital, which was more than an hour away.

He had no heart medicine or **nitroglycerin** *on hand. Aspirin, however, reduces the progression of a clot if one is forming in one of the arteries of the heart, and can actually prevent complete blockage and a heart attack in many people. It's one of the first things that should be given at any hospital emergency department for a possible heart attack.*

Everyone at that time had aspirin at home, so I said, "If you're going to take your chances and stay home, the only thing you can do is to take two aspirin " then I added, consciously, "—and call me in the morning." I explained the reason to do so.

In the morning, I still was concerned, so I didn't wait for Karl to call me. I called him. He'd had an uneventful night and a good sleep. He hadn't had a heart attack, although it was possible that one was prevented.

Every time Karl came into the office after that, we would chuckle over my instructions when he may have been having a heart attack. "Take two aspirin and call me in the morning," of course, is the infamous punch line of many comedians' jokes about doctors.

*Over time, Karl became interested in **chelation therapy**, a popular unproven alternative medical treatment for **coronary artery disease** and **arteriosclerosis** that is still recommended by a few doctors today. The treatments consist of intravenous injections of a combination of medications that are supposed to dissolve fat and calcium from the arteries and open them up.*

Karl consulted me about this method, and I advised him against it. One of the risks is that the drugs can decrease the coagulating ability of the blood, which can cause bleeding or even a stroke in some patients.

Karl went ahead with the treatments anyway. Then, sadly, four days after his first treatment he had a stroke. He was taken to the hospital nearest his home. I never heard from him afterwards.

—⟋⟋—

Ultimately, people make their own medical treatment decisions. These are not always the correct ones. That's why they consult with a physician. The same can be said of physicians' decisions at times, too, however. These are often just educated guesses.

The better the physician knows the patient and incorporates the personal element of care, the more educated the guess. That is one reason medicine is still referred to as "the practice of medicine."

In the final analysis, the decision and recommendations should involve both patient and physician, after the issues have been fully discussed, and a mutual understanding has been reached.

CHAPTER 19

Don't Let Them Get Me!

When I started my career in Kansas City, I made house calls, a practice still common in those days. After I relocated to Philadelphia, I continued this practice for a long time.

The home visit primarily provided urgent care. Incidentally, it also helped the physician to learn about a patient's living situation. Visiting the home and family provided an instant snapshot of the patient's background, which often helped to explain his or her illness.

Some patients in the Kansas City area were amused by the house calls made by a particular internist who was highly regarded. He reportedly would charge through the house under the pretext of looking for items he needed for examination or treatment. He didn't miss a room or even a closet.

One of my first acquisitions as an intern in Kansas City was a "little black bag," the standard requirement for making house calls. Actually, most doctor's bags were not little, as they contained many vials of pills and injectable drugs, along with the necessary needles, syringes, first-aid equipment, dressings, equipment for washing out the stomach, examining equipment, and anything else the doctor favored. As a doctor became more experienced, he carried less and less in his bag. Some ultimately reduced it to the size of a shaving kit.

—∽—

While I was a resident at Research Hospital, Dr. Claude Farley, a general practitioner, had me cover for him upon occasion on house calls. As a resident, I didn't have a state license to practice medicine. Instead, I just had a training certificate that permitted me to practice under a licensed doctor—but only in the hospital.

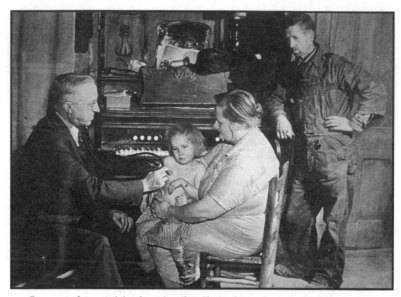

Country doctor visits farming family in Scott County, Missouri, 1942
(b/w photo) by American Photographer (20th century);
Private Collection/ Peter Newark American Pictures/ The Bridgeman Art Library
Nationality / Copyright Status: American / Copyright Unknown

On one occasion, Claude got a call from the wife of a man who was having severe chest pain. Claude was on another house call, so he sent me out.

Immediately upon my arrival, it was obvious that the man was having a heart attack, a myocardial infarction. I called an ambulance. Even though it arrived quickly, the man had died by the time that the ambulance got there.

Naturally, I called Claude to let him know.

"What do you want me to do about it?" He said, a little annoyed.

This startled me. Obviously, since I had no medical license, I couldn't be responsible for treating a patient who died in my care at home. I couldn't sign the death certificate. I reminded him of this. Of course, he signed it.

—⁂—

One of the first patients I visited at home was a very young woman with cramping abdominal pain. Her abdomen was soft when pressed. This indicated that inflammation was not the cause. Bowel spasm was the likely cause.

I had no narcotics with me nor could I inject other drugs that could relieve bowel pain. Pills indicated for this are too slow in acting. She needed rapid relief. I did have nitroglycerine tablets which are indicated for the heart pain of angina pectoris. When placed under the tongue, pain relief occurs in minutes. Nitroglycerine can also ease the spasm of bowel muscle if not severe.

As I had nothing else I could give her, I placed a nitroglycerine tablet under her tongue. This began easing the pain in a few minutes and nearly completely relieved it in 10 minutes. I was surprised by the speed of her relief. Much of this may have been from reassurance and the **placebo effect**, *but either way it was gratifyingly impressive.*

—⚏—

Another of my earliest house calls was to see a 60-year-old man named Luke. His wife had called me, saying that he had a cold and wouldn't get out of bed.

I found him lying on a cot. He was facing the wall. Luke rolled toward me just enough to allow me to examine him, then rolled right back onto his side.

I could find nothing wrong with him, but he did complain of hearing voices for the past 17 years in the generators at the power plant where he had worked for more than 20 years.

Still in bed for my second visit a few days later, Luke rolled over a little more this time. Then he suddenly pleaded with me. "Doc, don't let them get me!"

I suggested that he see a neurologist for his hearing problem. Luke shook his head vehemently.

I said, "See? They're trying to get you now. They're keeping you from seeing the doctor who can help you."

With that, Luke leapt out of bed and started to dress.

Kansas City had some physicians who were Board-certified in both psychiatry and in neurology. I persuaded one located very nearby to see him within the hour.

Luke went, but unfortunately, he refused to go again.

His wife was alone in trying to get some help for him, and her phone calls to me became very furtive. Although he had several brothers in the area, they were in denial of the fact that he needed psychiatric help and were unsupportive of her efforts to get Luke help for his apparent **schizophrenia.**

He never came to see me, and I never did find out what became of him.

—⚏—

One of the home visits I made was through the Jackson County Medical Society's house-call service. It was in a tenement in Kansas City, Kansas, across the river from Kansas City, Missouri.

There, I found three children with sore throats, two of which were **membranous** and suggested **diphtheria**, a condition to which I had been alerted through a newspaper article. I sent the three to Children's Mercy Hospital.

All three children had diphtheria. One developed **myocarditis,** an inflammation of the heart muscle, which is a well-known complication of diphtheria. Fortunately, the children eventually recovered. The epidemic amounted to nine documented cases in the area.

Some of the calls I made at the time were to care for my patients who were confined to nursing homes. These were generally pretty dismal in the 1950s. I came to regard nursing homes of that era as the socially acceptable form of **euthanasia.** One of the best criteria for judging a home can be made immediately on walking through the front door. If the air smells bad, the care is substandard.

—⚏—

During my two months locum tenens in Baron, Wisconsin, I made several house calls. This was an area with many farms, and after a heavy snow, a doctor would need to leave his or her car at the edge of the road by the lane to the house. The farmer would then pick you up with his tractor and chauffeur you to the house and back. The brother of Dr. Stacey Long, one of my co-interns at Research Hospital, was a general practitioner in Ft. Smith, Arkansas. One November, Stacey went with his brother on a house call. It was some distance from town, up a mountain to the end of the road, where they were picked up by a tractor and taken to a cabin near the top.

Stacey's brother found that the grandmother had pneumonia. He gave her a shot of penicillin and some pills for her cough. During the winter, the family usually didn't come down from the mountain to go into town. His brother said he wouldn't find out before spring whether the grandmother had lived or died.

—∿—

On one of our vacation trips in 1951, after going through the Cumberland Gap in the Appalachian Mountains, Dorothy and I stopped to visit our friends Jim and Alma Jones in Harlan County, Kentucky. Jim had interned at Kansas City General Hospital in 1949 to 1950, and Alma had worked as a nurse at Research Hospital with Dorothy.

Today, the doctor's house call, once such an
important facet of personal care,
is practically extinct.

Harlan County is in the mountains at the extreme southeastern end of Kentucky. Born and raised there, Jim was working as a doctor for a coal-mining company located halfway between the towns of Harlan and Evarts. Evarts was notorious as the town in which nine sheriffs had been shot over several preceding years.

Jim and Alma lived in a large, yellow, two-story house, which was dingy from coal dust. This dingy appearance from the coal dust was the same as all of the company executives' homes and other buildings located across the creek.

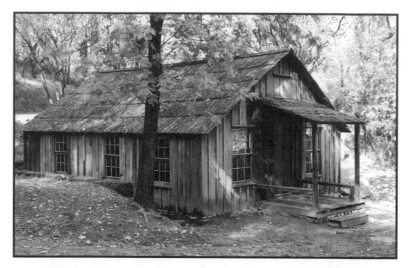

While we were there, I went on a house call with Jim. He drove his jeep up the mountain, along a creek that was lined with shacks. Halfway up the mountain, the road ended, but the shacks continued. We then drove up the center of the stream.

We passed a knoll that was well up the mountainside. Jim's great granddaddy "B'ar" Jones was buried there. He was the first one to climb over the ridge from Virginia and settle in the valley.

We finally reached a shack three quarters of the way up the mountain where Jim made his house call. Although we didn't go further that day, there were even more shacks beyond that point, extending to the top of the mountain ridge. Driving up the mountain and through the stream to get to these shacks makes one realize just how far removed some people are from the safety, convenience, and social support found in more populated communities.

—m—

The house calls I made in Philadelphia weren't emergencies or even urgent. Most were prearranged, and usually follow-ups to hospital care.

Sixty-year-old Gertrude was unable to come into my office, so I arranged to see her in her South Philadelphia home once monthly.

She had heart failure from severe valve damage. I would visit on Saturday afternoons, after I'd made rounds at the hospital.

One day, after I examined her, she asked, "Could you also see my son?"

"Of course."

Every month thereafter, I saw several unscheduled people—a sister who happened to drop by, a neighbor, another neighbor, and so on.

After I finished holding these home clinics, Gertrude would invite me back into her large kitchen where the table was set for five. The food was fabulous.

—⟶⟶—

Elderly Mary was also unable to get into the office, even though her house was nearby. She lived with her husband and a grown son in a row house, and said she missed her many children. She was unhappy and suffering more from mild depression than from her high blood pressure. She needed cheering up more than medicine.

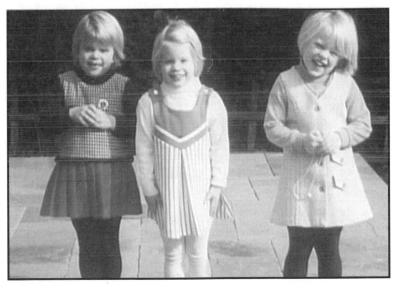

Norman Makous' three daughters, Ginnie, Meg, and Doll in Sunday best

While "off duty," I went to visit her on a Sunday afternoon. I brought along my three daughters, Ginny, Doll, and Meg, who were all under the age of six. The girls were dressed in their Sunday best.

Mary was delighted. Both her husband and son were home when we arrived. After I talked to her a bit and checked her blood pressure, we sat and chatted. I learned that after her husband had lost his job during the Great Depression, he had traded or sold homemade wine to South Philadelphia merchants, in order to care for the family.

After a while, the son brought up a bottle of wine from the basement. It was 35-years-old and heavenly, one of their last eight bottles from that era.

—ᴠᴠ—

My home visits were cheaper than office visits. They saved patients the expense of parking or cab fare. Some patients who were able to come to the office took advantage of this. I could conduct a better examination at the office, and wanted to encourage visits there rather than at the home. I raised my fees for house calls so that it exceeded the charge for an office visit, plus the cab fare in both directions.

Through the 1950s and 1960s, the number of house calls made by doctors in general steadily declined. This happened as a result of a number of reasons.

Often, one could tell from the nature of the complaint if the patient needed the special diagnostic services only a hospital could provide. I'd tell patients that I'd make a house call, but only if they wanted to settle for second-rate medical care. They usually chose to go to an emergency room. If they could get to Pennsylvania Hospital, I would meet them there. If not, I awaited the call from an emergency department physician of the hospital of their choice.

Today, the doctor's house call, once such an important facet of personal care, is practically extinct.

CHAPTER 20

No Appointment Needed

The first emergency hospital in the Milwaukee area was built in the early 1930s. At the time, most hospitals did not have emergency rooms. When my brother was born in 1934, my father and I went to visit my mother in the hospital. We couldn't get in the front door, as it was locked after 8:00 p.m. We had to go through the employee's entrance, which was a small, single door off of the alley. There was no emergency room. This hadn't improved much as of 1942.

When I was home from college in December, a group of us went tobogganing. One of the girls was thrown from the back of the toboggan and struck her hip against a tree trunk. We feared that her hip was broken. Since there was no hospital emergency room nearby, we took her back to my friend's house, and his folks called their family doctor.

The doctor was there in half-an-hour. After a quick exam of the patient's injury, the doctor made a phone call, and a half-an-hour later, a radiologist arrived. He took an x-ray with what I suspected was the type of portable unit newly developed for the Army's use on the battlefield.

Two hours after arriving at my friend's house with the patient, we learned that she did not have a fracture.

—⚬—

At Pennsylvania Hospital in Philadelphia, the emergency room was referred to as the "receiving ward." By the 1970s, when emergency medicine became a subspecialty, they were called "emergency departments."

Once emergency room facilities caught on, large urban medical centers began to provide their own ambulance services. Many of these operated until the early 1950s. General Hospital in Kansas City operated the only public ambulance service in town. Interns took their turn riding in the ambulances. I rode with my ex-roommate from medical school once, to standby at an athletic event.

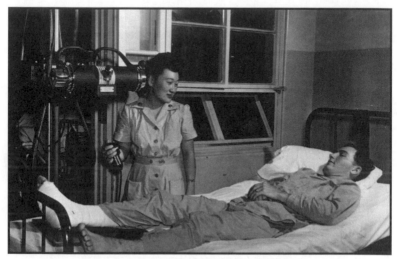

*A technician uses the US Army's portable field x-ray machine
on a soldier's broken foot in a World War II hospital*
Image provided by the U.S National Library of Medicine

These ambulance services were discontinued by hospitals for economic and safety reasons. Sirened vehicles frequently collided at intersections, neither able to hear the other. In Kansas City, an ambulance, police car, and fire engine collided at one intersection, hastening the demise of the public ambulance service.

In Philadelphia in 1961, the new chief of cardiology at Pennsylvania Hospital ran an ambulance service dedicated to acute cardiac care. It operated out of the coronary care unit. When the federal government funded community emergency services in 1964, the fire department took over the ambulance coverage for the entire city of Philadelphia.

—๛—

For years, the triage function of separating cases based on the need for immediate and intensive treatment was delegated to some of the least experienced doctors: the interns and the medical students. Emergency care is among the most demanding in that it requires rapid decision-making, and therefore experienced personnel.

Back in the 1960s, only 70 percent of the people who presented themselves to an emergency room were in need of emergency care. This hasn't changed in more than 40 years. People who have no insurance or no doctor use emergency rooms for their initial medical contact. Some people don't want their freedom restricted by setting a specific day and a time to see a doctor. This is a restriction that many primary-care doctors began to place on patients several decades ago. Before this, many did not work by appointment.

CHAPTER 21

I'll Celebrate Your 90ᵗʰ Birthday

Cancer is almost as common as heart disease, and therefore I saw a good deal of it throughout my career. As with many diseases, cancer frequently presents in unusual ways, and its course can be unpredictable. The standards provide general guidelines to care for most of the afflicted, but adjustment to the unique aspects of each individual may be necessary. Likewise, the anxiety in patient and family requires that the care be personal.

Most patients accept the recommended surgery, radiation treatment, or chemotherapy, but some reject it out of hand. They fear getting trapped in a treatment regimen that might make them feel far worse, due to the side effects of drugs or radiation.

Chemotherapy is the most dreaded. Most agree to try it when reassured that they may find that the therapy is tolerable, that they might be one of the fortunate who not only benefit from it, but are cured by it. They finally are convinced when reassured that they may stop taking it any time that they choose. Few of those who accepted this rationale and began treatment, found it necessary to stop early.

Katherine, an 84-year-old, had been having bloody diarrhea for 11 months before her daughter finally prevailed upon her to see a doctor. Neither one of them liked doctors, so neither had a personal physician. They came to see me.

I found that, until this problem arose, Katherine's health had been good. Now she tired easily. The explanation was obvious when I examined her. In her right lower abdomen, she had a firm non-tender mass the size of a lemon. This was clearly a cancer of the bowel, until proven otherwise.

The laboratory tests explained her fatigue. She was severely anemic due to bleeding from the cancer. Her hemoglobin of 5.0 grams was 40 percent of the normal level.

Katherine needed a barium enema x-ray examination to establish that the mass was within the bowel, as **colonoscopy** *examinations were not yet available at that time. She and her daughter, however, were reluctant to follow through with the diagnostic barium enema.*

Finally, she did have the procedure. It confirmed that the mass was in the bowel and almost certainly was cancer. Still, Katherine would not see a surgeon. She didn't think she could survive the surgery.

They did return to see me the following week. She was in good health generally and should have no problem from the surgery, although they were still reluctant. As my last argument, I assured her that, "If you have the surgery, I'll celebrate your 90th birthday with you." She and her daughter finally agreed.

Katherine went through the surgery without incident. After one follow-up visit, she didn't come back to the office.

I didn't hear from them again until six years later. I got a card in the mail inviting me to one of the historic houses in Philadelphia's Society Hill. This was for a celebration of Katherine's 90th birthday.

As promised, I attended. She'd had no illness since her surgery, and I found her perky and well.

Some people have multiple cancers. Despite this, some may be cured of all of them. They not only survive, but are among the hardy survivors.

—m—

Rose was a patient under my care for 20 years. She had high blood pressure, heart disease, and obesity. When she first came to see me at age 68, she had a hernia the size of a softball in an old scar from gallbladder surgery. She had so much discomfort from the hernia, that both of us thought the surgery was worth the risk. But the chief of surgery wouldn't perform the procedure because of the potential complications from her heart disease. Four years later, an intrepid younger member of the surgical department corrected the hernia without incident, and the problem never recurred.

Three years after that, Rose became progressively short of breath. She had only a minimal response to treatment for congestive heart failure, with a loss of only five pounds of weight from the extra fluid in her system. She was admitted to Pennsylvania Hospital with acute shortness of breath. With the hospital treatment and bed rest, Rose lost 35 pounds of extra fluid in a less than a week.

Three years later, she had a total mastectomy for cancer of the left breast. Nine months after that, she had a total mastectomy of her right breast for a different type of cancer. Seven months later, she developed a mass in her right lung. The right lower lobe of this lung was resected. The mass was not from a cancer that had come from her breasts as expected. It was a primary cancer that had arisen in the lung.

Rose underwent surgery for three different types of cancers in 16 months. She'd never had a cancer before these three, and lived for five years after the last surgery without recurrence or new cancer. At the age of 86, she died of a stroke.

Some people have multiple cancers. Despite this, some may be cured of all of them. They not only survive, but are among the hardy survivors.

—w—

Some people have cancers that are not treated for various reasons. Despite this, some may live as long or longer than expected with treatment.

*Nathan, a 76-year-old, unmarried baker, was sent to me by an ophthalmologist whom Nathan had consulted because of the onset of double vision. An **MRI** showed a small mass behind the* *right eye. A chest x-ray revealed a mass in the top of the left lung. This proved to be a cancer, although he had no symptoms from this second mass.*

Six months earlier, Nathan had a chest x-ray before prostate surgery at another hospital. This also showed the mass in his left lung. Actually, the mass had been reported 18 months before that time, at the same hospital. No one followed up on it nor mentioned it to him or his family on either occasion.

Since the cancer was difficult to treat at this advanced stage, his family did not want Nathan told about it, nor did they want him treated. Nathan never asked questions, but I suspected he knew.

He had no chest symptoms and continued to work daily as a baker. Interestingly, the mass behind his eye causing his visual disturbance—which we thought was a result of the spread of his lung cancer—cleared spontaneously and permanently.

Except for ongoing cold-like symptoms, Nathan remained asymptomatic for nearly five years. He finally stopped working because of discomfort during the last four or five months before he died.

—∞—

These anecdotes are the exceptions that prove the rule. They demonstrate the need to not only individualize the use of standardized treatments, but also to personalize its use dependent upon unique aspects of each person.

A patient named Mike came in to see me with chest pain. He was 56-years old with heart disease from hardening of the arteries. Based on an **echocardiogram**, *we thought Mike might have a* **dissecting aneurysm of the aorta**, *a condition in which the aorta splits without rupturing. Ten percent of patients with this condition heal* *spontaneously without surgical treatment. I treated mike for coronary heart disease.*

Eight years later, Mike was diagnosed with colon cancer and had surgery, which was successful. Except for the symptoms from his heart disease, he had no symptoms and required no further treatment for his cancer. Eight years after that, he developed congestive heart failure. This responded to treatment.

*One day, Mike came to see me because he had **hemoptysis**, that is, he was spitting up blood. Additionally, the blood was uncharacteristically darker than that which is usually seen with heart failure.*

*A lung x-ray was negative as was the MRI. The MRI of the chest incidentally included the kidneys. This showed a number of abnormalities in both kidneys. A needle **biopsy** of one of these defects showed cancer. It could not be determined whether the cancer had originated from the kidneys or from the bowel. Mike had no symptoms from the cancer and he didn't need nor did he receive any treatment for it.*

The cancer never spread to the lungs. A year after the onset of the hemoptysis, it stopped. He explained that he was crossing the street one day and just decided that he would not cough up blood anymore. He didn't. Four years later, Mike died of heart disease without any evidence that his cancer had progressed.

These anecdotes are the exceptions that prove the rule. They demonstrate the need to not only individualize the use of standardized treatments, but also to personalize its use dependent upon unique aspects of each person.

CHAPTER 22

I Don't Wanna Go Yet

Many young people may not express their bias, but feel that elderly people with disabling conditions should be ready to die. Old people make some of the young uncomfortable. The attitude might be characterized as, "They've had a good life, they've lived long enough, and they should be ready to give up living."

Some young physicians even feel this way. They haven't had the experience to learn otherwise. Some of this age bias is medically induced. Advanced age is used as a risk factor for susceptibility to many diseases, in the absence of significant findings caused by disease. Used in the absence of any other fact, this perception alone becomes discriminatory and can lead to underestimation of the prospects for survival of an aged person.

One week, while I was a cardiology fellow at Pennsylvania Hospital, an 84-year-old man named Harry was assigned to see me in the medical clinic. Clearly, Harry had seen better times.

According to his chart, he was partially blind in one eye. He had emphysema from smoking, high blood pressure, and arthritis. He had had several heart attacks and a stroke. His cataracts had been removed. He'd had surgery for a cancer of the tongue. Also, he'd had surgery on his stomach, gallbladder, bowel, and prostate.

Harry slowly dragged himself across the room, and sat down.

After he caught his breath, he rasped, "Doc, I know I'm old and I got a lot of things wrong with me, but I don't wanna go yet."

Harry was the most vocal of the elderly patients I'd cared for whose survival instinct—which many of the young regard as their entitlement alone—persisted so vigorously.

The following week, 82-year-old Mabel came to the clinic. I'd never seen her before. She had suffered a mild heart attack and was being treated for high blood pressure. She didn't have much else wrong with her and didn't have any symptoms.

Her opening observation complemented Harry's comment.

After she pertly crossed the examining room and sat down, she hastily gave me this advice. "Now, Doctor, if you're going to be old, be rich."

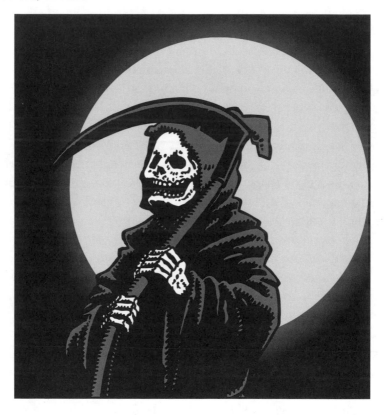

Like Harry and Mabel, most older people have a desire to survive. A few near the end stage of a long, chronic, incurable illness accept the inevitable and are ready to pass on. But the rest are usually fighters.

Esther was one of them. As a slender, 55-year-old African American school teacher, Esther first came to see me because of pain in her legs. She felt this whenever she walked a block or two, and couldn't shop in town anymore. This had gotten worse since an injury to her ankle four years earlier. Inexplicably, it was followed by a temporary right-hand paralysis. Her legs were cold, with no pulses at the knees or in the feet.

Following that time, she had numerous hospitalizations for kidney infections, abdominal pain, skin grafts, thrombophlebitis, and nerve surgery to improve leg circulation.

Her legs had actually begun troubling her at the age of 38. Since then, she was treated for many leg complications. These stopped her from playing golf and tennis.

Esther hadn't been well since infancy. "I caught everything that came around," she explained. Other conditions included facial spasms and paralysis, severe scarlet fever at age 12, and then a year of total unexplained blindness. She suffered from frequent colds, thyroid enlargement, and abdominal pains. Esther had gallbladder surgery, ovarian cyst removal, and abdominal surgery for **adhesions**.

Along with these troubles were back injuries from a car accident. This terminated a four-year teaching career. She then became a tailor.

Esther married at age 27 but left after 13 years. "I was tired to death." All three of her pregnancies had ended with spontaneous abortions.

She visited me monthly. We tried several medical therapies, as well as further surgery, but her leg complaints were unchanged.

Finally, I told Esther that I couldn't help her. "Nothing can be done for your leg pain." But I told her that I'd continue to monitor it.

She agreed that we would no longer discuss her legs. Thereafter, Esther continued to come in monthly. She had complaints, but for different problems.

First, she complained of lower back pain. After three to four visits, the treatment helped. Then she developed headaches, which I "cured" after three or four visits. After that, she complained of abdominal pain. This, too, responded to treatment over several months. This was all followed by her complaining of a backache again, and the cycle repeated.

This cycle of back, head, and abdominal discomfort went on for many years. During that time, Esther never complained about her legs again, and her legs seemed no worse.

*She was one who felt that she needed numerous medications, usually 10 or more over-the-counter drugs. These were in addition to several prescription drugs. During some of her hospitalizations, I was able to reduce her medications to three. Then, every time she came in for her monthly visit after her discharge from the hospital, she would have added a few more new pills, until she was back on her usual 14 medications. She was addicted to **polypharmacy**.*

She eventually developed heart problems from high blood pressure. Also, her lungs were causing progressive limitation from the smoking, which she continued over many years. She was seen by many consultants during this time, but none of them were able to significantly alter her medical course.

Esther lived in a two-story house. It never had a bathroom or a commode on the first floor. For years, she went up and down the stairs in a sitting position, step-by-step. At one point, after a surgical procedure, she went into a nursing-care facility for recovery. They would not let her return to her home, since the plumbing there was not working properly. This was complicated by the fact that Esther wouldn't trust anybody with the key, and the plumber couldn't get into the house to make repairs.

Finally, Esther had enough of the nursing home. She signed herself out against medical advice and went home.

She phoned me after that time, but never was able to come into my office to see me. Visiting nurses saw to her medical care. She did have the plumbing fixed, and lived there until she died several years later at age 83.

I cared for Esther for more than 30 years. She was non-demanding and appreciated my efforts to help her. I'd had a psychiatrist and a neurologist see her at one time. They felt that *she had an element of **conversion hysteria**, along with her many other medical problems.*

While medical science can individualize much of one's care, personal attention is an important supplement to the scientific element.

Obviously, Esther was a "tough old bird" with a strong will to live. She is a great example of someone with more than the usual needs. She required a great deal of regular, personalized, medical attention. Even if the medical knowledge that is available today had been available to her then, I don't believe she would have done significantly better nor lived any longer than she did.

The personalized supportive care I provided to Esther over three decades, I believe, was the single most important aspect of care that she received. While medical science can individualize much of one's care, personal attention is an important supplement to the scientific element.

CHAPTER 23

Do What You Think Is Best

Before the 1960s, making a decision concerning the prolongation of life was relatively easy. In a crisis, physicians simply did everything they could and patients either lived or died after a relatively short period. Today, however, the body can be maintained for a very long time with both heart and brain not functioning.

With this development of new life-saving and life-prolonging technology, the physician's burden of care and need for compassion increased greatly.

Comatose patients often died of pneumonia, which some referred to as "the old man's friend." Few became the brain-dead "vegetables" that have been the challenge since that time. Starting in the 1960s, closed-chest cardiac massage and defibrillator technology started to result in the resuscitation of patients, whose lives were also being prolonged by other interventions such as renal **dialysis**, and the respirators that made the "Iron Lung" obsolete. With this development of new life-saving and life-prolonging technology, the physician's burden of care and need for compassion increased greatly.

Advanced directives have been popularized in the 1990s, but have not been very helpful to physicians who have a long-established relationship with a patient. The growing need and call for these reflects the increasing fragmentation of medical care. It also reflects a general lack of understanding of medical care near the end of life.

—ɯ—

I first heard about advanced directives from an activist patient and his family in the early 1960s.

Victor, a librarian, had just retired and moved near Pennsylvania Hospital. He had significant aortic and mitral valvular rheumatic heart disease, but was able to continue working part-time at his occupation of librarian. For nearly eight years, his wife and daughter regularly reminded me that they wanted no extraordinary life-saving medical measures at the end.

*After four or five years, Victor finally developed chronic heart irregularity from **atrial fibrillation**. At that time, the treatment standard was that long-term anticoagulation therapy was not started until after the first **embolic** event, which usually was a small stroke. Victor's first episode, however, resulted in a rather extensive, crippling, left-sided paralysis that involved the left chest, confining him to a wheelchair.*

Over the next four to five years, he suffered about one acute medical event per year that would have killed him, had the advanced directives been followed as requested by the family. Yet Victor found his limitations tolerable.

On one early occasion, the advanced directives produced a startling result. Victor had a myocardial infarction shortly after I left town for the weekend, and he was under the care of a colleague. I returned three days later to find him in intensive care with nasal oxygen; intravenous drugs to keep his heart regular, maintain his blood pressure, and deliver antibiotics; as well as a urethral catheter in his bladder. His blood pressure was very low, even while on the medication. His condition was clearly grave.

Following the advanced directive wishes of the family, I promptly stopped the blood pressure medication and nasal oxygen. His blood pressure went up. I stopped the intravenous anti-arrhythmic drug. His blood pressure went up further and no heart irregularity developed. I stopped the other medications and he continued to get better. Victor returned home in as stable and active a condition as he had been prior to the attack.

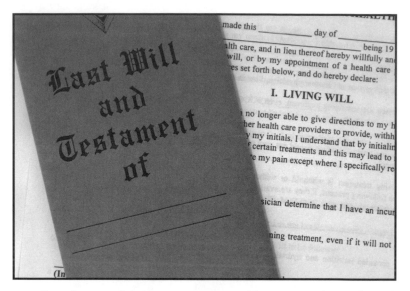

On three subsequent occasions, he was admitted with pulmonary complications. One was for **inhalation pneumonia**, after his daytime attendant had deliberately, for unknown reasons, set Victor's shawl on fire. This resulted in the hospitalization of both of them with smoke inhalation. On two other occasions, he was admitted for pneumonia.

Each of the three times, Victor was resuscitated after respiratory and cardiac arrest, and he ended up with a tube through his mouth and into his trachea to assist his breathing. On the first two occasions, he was **extubated** successfully. That is, the tube assisting his respiration was removed from his trachea and he was able to breathe on his own without assistance. Both times, Victor returned home to resume his prior level of existence, which he still found acceptable, though far from desirable.

The third hospitalization requiring **intubation** occurred five years after the first complication of his stroke. Every time Victor was extubated and the assisted respiration was stopped, he would develop another episode of respiratory and cardiac arrest. This usually occurred during the night when his regular, house-staff *physicians were off duty, and the covering physicians either were unaware of the "do not resuscitate" instructions, or could not bring themselves to allow him to die.*

Finally, after the fourth failed attempt to remove the tube, it was apparent that with his generally weakened condition, he no longer would be able to overcome the complete paralysis of his left chest in order to keep his lungs and throat clear of fluid. Victor would need to remain on a respirator for the rest of his shortening life.

After this, I told his wife that I didn't think we'd ever be able to get the tube out of his lungs. "Do you want me to stop the respirator, as per your instructions?"

She threw up her hands and said, "You do what you think is best."

Of course, I couldn't pull the plug of the device administering the assisted breathing. Then I went to his bedside.

Knowing that Victor was unable to speak with a tube in his throat, I asked him if he understood.

He nodded in the affirmative.

*I told him of my misgivings. I explained that I didn't think he would be able to breathe without the respiratory assistance, but that we could remove the tube from his mouth and throat and place it through his neck into his **trachea**, if he wanted this.*

After a pause of about a minute, he slowly began to shake his head.

I interpreted this as an indication that he understood and rejected that option. I did nothing at that moment.

That night, Victor died for no obvious reason. He was still on the respirator. I wondered if he had willed his death.

Rigid adherence to advance-directive orders that are too specific can result in the undesirable and unnecessarily premature ending of a life. Occasionally, however, patients and families become trapped by the circumstances, as in Victor's situation. Another reason for the physician to be wary is when there are no advance directives, and when family motivations are uncertain.

This is especially true after a cardiac arrest from unknown cause. Patients may remain unconscious for hours after resuscitation and still recover. I've had family members want the respirator stopped after an hour or so, out of fear that the brain damage may be permanent, initiating a chronic, vegetative state. Motives unknown to the physician also may come into to play, requiring some caution in complying with family requests.

—⚭—

Patients react differently to a diagnosis and the realization that they have developed a serious illness. As in bereavement, five different stages may be recognized.

A vigorous, middle-aged man who has never been ill and has been struck down with a heart attack may deny that he could have had one. Patients who have suffered a stroke often ignore the paralyzed side of the body, in denial. Anger is followed by bargaining for a cure or recovery, looking to make an agreement with a higher power.

This is often followed by depression. It occurs in as many as 75 percent of patients with strokes, and may be nearly as high in those with myocardial infarctions. In some of the heart patients, I have suspected that the depression was already present and may actually have triggered the infarction.

Finally, the illness, limitation, or required treatment is accepted, and a period of relative tranquility develops. Some patients may choose to refuse further treatment when the quality of life is low, when living with treatments becomes unacceptably burdensome, and when death within six months is expected.

Patients with intolerable pain who require constant medication for relief—such as those with chronic lung problems or on long-term dialysis—may choose hospice care. Hospice care provides terminally ill patients with palliative treatment, given primarily to keep the patient comfortable. Taking place at one's home or in a hospice facility, hospice care also includes support for both the patient and his or her family.

Ultimately, people should determine their own fate and make their own end-of-life decisions. This should be done after a discussion with the doctor. These decisions are best made if the patient and the doctor have had a long-standing relationship, which leads to mutual understanding and trust. A list of instructions on a piece of paper, which is necessary when medical care is impersonal, is a poor substitute.

—◊◊◊—

Jim was an 82-year-old retired policeman who had had two previous heart attacks. He had a great Irish wit, and a sense of humor about everything in life, including his health conditions.

Thirteen years earlier, following his second heart attack, Jim underwent coronary artery **bypass surgery**, *with the excision of a bulging scar in his heart. He did fairly well over the next 10 years. Even though he had heart pain, it was stable and controlled, and he and his wife would go out dancing every Friday night.*

Jim also had **arthralgia**, *which is a condition that causes painful joints, and he had been on steroid therapy for 25 years. The joint pain bothered him more than his heart condition, and it gradually became worse.*

Jim had to give up dancing and was having trouble moving around the house. His knees degenerated to such a limiting state, that despite his deteriorating heart, he was desperate enough to risk knee-replacement surgery.

One cause of the worsening joint pain was the muscle weakness from his progressive heart failure. The week before the planned surgery, his angina flared up. When I finally was asked to clear Jim pre-operatively in the hospital, I advised against the surgery. I had misgivings about the wisdom of the decision from the outset, especially considering his weakened heart.

The following year was like the trials of Job for Jim, as a result of several losses in his family. During these tragic events, he kept asking, "Why them? Why not me?"

Eventually, Jim was nearly bedfast from his worsening heart failure. He was developing liver failure, and he had constant nausea, as well as intermittent, lower abdominal pain. He finally accepted hospice care at his home.

Jim's mind remained keen and his wit intact, despite all of these hardships. One morning, after two weeks of hospice care at home, Jim called his wife to his bedside, as well as the one of his two daughters who was with them at the time.

He told them, "Today is the day." He was sure he was going to die.

They held hands and told each other what a wonderful life they had had together.

An hour later, the scene was repeated, but now with both daughters present.

In the midst of the loving goodbyes, Jim suddenly looked up and said, "This is just like in the movies. The sick person's head suddenly drops, his eyes close, and he's gone." Suddenly his head dropped, and his eyes closed.

A few moments later, he opened his eyes again.

Everyone laughed. Not only had his mind remained keen to the end, but amazingly, so did his Irish wit.

Several hours later, after a final goodbye, Jim fell into a peaceful sleep and died uneventfully.

Ultimately, people should determine their own fate and make their own end-of-life decisions. This should be done after a discussion with the doctor. These decisions are best made if the patient and the doctor have had a long-standing relationship, which leads to mutual understanding and trust. A list of instructions on a piece of paper, which is necessary when medical care is impersonal, is a poor substitute.

PART III

Life-Saving Technology

CHAPTER 24

I Feel Much Better After That Treatment

After World War II, personal medical care changed dramatically. With the rapid introduction of new technology, expectations rose, along with its real and perceived benefits. Our culture changed and the cost of care rose accordingly. Some money was saved by the new technology, but the net effect of prolonging lives while easing pain and suffering has resulted in a significant increase in the overall cost of care.

Over time, personal medical care—the direct attention given by doctors to patients whom they know well—began to suffer. Tests started to assume large portions of treatment time as well as the costs of care. As the reimbursement for time-consuming personal care was reduced, physicians could not afford to spend as much time with the patients.

Upgrades in technology usually increase the cost of medical care. A more expensive new test, often replaces a perfectly adequate older and much less expensive test. The new method generally provides more and better information, but frequently it is more comprehensive than is needed for the patient at the time. The discovery of an unknown condition through testing is unusual.

The same mandate holds true for drug therapies. More expensive new drugs replace much less expensive older drugs, yet many older therapies are frequently just as effective for most patients.

The interplay among these factors has been particularly evident in the field of cardiology. One good example is related to chest x-ray technology.

As of the early 1960s, many physicians had fluoroscopic units in their offices. This x-ray technique produces a transient image on a fluorescent screen. Cardiologists would trace an outline of the heart and other aspects of the image on the screen, and then transfer the tracings to paper. Certain types of heart disease change the outline of the heart in characteristic ways. For example, collections of fluid seen in and around the lungs are abnormal, and fluoroscopy reveals these changes.

The fluoroscopy was not a substitute for an initial chest x-ray. It was, however, a convenient method for following the effect of treatment.

Patients were told the purpose of the fluoroscopy exam. Despite this, an occasional unsophisticated patient believed that they had just had some sort of therapy.

"Hey, Doc. I feel much better after that treatment!"

The incidental noise and the smell of ozone produced by some of the old fluoroscopic machines gave the impression that there had been some sort of intervention.

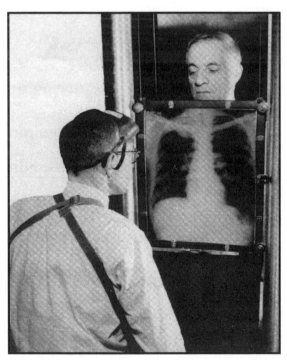

Doctor fluoroscoping patient, 1966

—✕✕—

After fluoroscopy had been broadly adopted, radiologists expressed concern about possible radiation overexposure by radiologically untrained physicians. A few physicians were unnecessarily fluoroscoping every patient every time he or she walked into the office. Also, insurers like Blue Shield expressed concerns about the cost.

By the late 1970s, the licensing of this procedure in medical offices was discontinued by the State Department of Health in Pennsylvania. A chest x-ray was the substitute.

What was intended to be a cost-saving, mandated upgrade in technology, actually had the effect of increasing the cost of care. An x-ray generally had to be done at a hospital and the cost was six to seven times as much as a fluoroscopy performed by physicians in their offices.

Chest x-rays provide much more information than fluoroscopy. Most of this information, however, was superfluous for most patients. Usually, all I needed to know was whether the heart had changed in size. Also, since the information from the chest x-ray was not immediately available, it increased the inconvenience to the patient and delayed any required adjustment in treatment.

A change that was intended to reduce the risk to the patient, ultimately increased the risk, as a result of the delay in new or altered treatment. It also required the expenditure of more time by both the patient and the physician, in place of a procedure that was of no significant danger to either one, when properly used.

This is just one minor example of a mandated technology upgrade that provided the same medical information, while increasing both the costs and the risks to most patients.

CHAPTER 25

Cell Doctors

After World War II, the new molecular and genetic paradigms of medical science rapidly encroached upon and replaced the traditional anatomical models. This fueled a fervor for laboratory science and increased the demand for research funding.

Prior to the 1940s, funding for research was largely non-governmental, provided through nonprofit organizations and foundations. In 1948, the American Heart Association broadened its membership base to include non-physicians, in order to improve its capacity for raising research funds. In the late 1940s, universities started to reject government support because of the belief that the required US loyalty oath compromised academic freedom.

One often got the feeling that many of these subspecialty physicians were better doctors of cells than doctors of patients. Their students then derived this message of reductionism from their academic role models, thus propagating this worldview.

The National Institutes of Health (NIH), which was established by Congress in 1945, provided funding that did not require a loyalty oath. Funding from the NIH for medical research grew rapidly, and by the 1960s, the majority of medical research funding was obtained from the NIH. Every year between 1946 until 1964, congress allocated more money for research than the NIH requested.

One of the consequences was that some medical schools became largely dependent upon these funds for operating expenses. By 1960, 84 percent of one southwest medical school's budget was derived from research funds, according to an NIH staff member. Even hospitals were pursuing this income source. As of the early 1960s, 15 percent of Pennsylvania Hospital's income came from research. It became big business.

In this environment, the more successful research fundraisers, the grants men, rose to higher positions as section and department heads in medical schools. The ample governmental funding of research thus introduced a technological bias into medical school faculties and the education of medical students.

Molecular biology became preeminent in researching disease mechanisms and treatment, with less emphasis placed on direct patient care. Since publish or perish was the academic mantra, time constraints drove many in academia to regard patient care and teaching clinical medicine as too easy and not worthy of their time. They had to stay in the laboratory.

One often got the feeling that many of these subspecialty physicians were better doctors of cells than doctors of patients. Their students then derived this message of reductionism from their academic role models, thus propagating this worldview.

Professors, consumed with career-advancing research, relegated teaching to their residents and fellows. Compared to senior physicians, residents have relatively little experience in patient care. They know many facts, but need to turn to the latest medical journals as their authorities. The teaching presentations consisted largely of the science, to the exclusion of the art of medicine, and its personal-care component.

Teaching rounds were no longer made at the bedside. They were held in conference rooms without the presence of the patient, or even without a prior examination by the attending physician.

Obtaining a history and performing a physical examination rapidly became lost arts. Technological testing took their place.

More than 100 tests were done daily on some patients at the Hospital of the University of Pennsylvania. Trainees' skills in examining patients were not properly developed or assessed.

Twenty years ago, a colleague of mine conducting patient rounds asked an intern, "Is the patient's liver enlarged?"

"I don't know. I haven't done a liver scan yet," the intern said.

My colleague and I would laugh about this response. It's just like asking the intern, "What's the patient's heart rate?" And the intern saying, "I don't know. I haven't done an electrocardiogram yet."

Both findings are readily assessable by basic physical examination. Special tests are unnecessary. Whole generations of doctors were being trained to use technology in place of direct patient examination, rather than as a supplement to it.

CHAPTER 26

See One, Do One, Teach One

Pennsylvania Hospital had always been a teaching affiliate of the University of Pennsylvania Medical School. It became a primary affiliate in the late 1950s, and eventually, in the late 1990s, the University acquired the Hospital. The teaching was practice-oriented more than academically oriented. In medicine, we taught physical diagnosis and hypertension, among other courses.

Many students at Penn Medical School as well as other medical schools in the area took their electives, including those in cardiology, at Pennsylvania Hospital. We had 10 staff cardiologists, all of whom did the teaching. We had no residents or fellows.

Physicians at teaching hospitals are, by and large, specialists. They focus on medical conditions in the area of their expertise, such as nose and throat, lungs, heart, or kidneys, to the exclusion of the rest of the body. They are apt to start a patient's evaluations with testing, rather than a basic physical exam.

Unfortunately, students learn this bias. The history and physical examination involving the rest of the body is delegated to trainees and may be overlooked. In this setting, many of these specialists have found that the history and physical examinations prove of little help in arriving at a diagnosis. This is particularly true in the case of the patient who is referred because a diagnosis cannot be made.

Prior to the referral of a case that is a diagnostic challenge, the patient has been seen by one or more specialists. By the time he or she is referred to a medical center, the history and physical examination may have little to offer and are all but ignored. But the history can prove to be critical. When ignored, significant conditions can be overlooked. This occurs even when the referring physician notes a problem that needs attention, and particularly when it is in another specialty area.

—⟋⟍—

John came to see me in the office for a check-up at the urging of his regular tennis partner. John hadn't been playing as well as usual. He had a heart condition, which was stable. He had no specific complaint, and his examination was not helpful.

A blood test showed that John was very anemic. He had a microscopic amount of blood in his urine. This might have been the cause of the anemia, but anemia of this degree without symptoms is more likely to have come from the bowel. A barium enema x-ray of the colon showed a mass in the right colon. It was a cancer.

John was referred to a specialist at a medical school hospital that he chose. The surgery was uncomplicated. The history of blood in his urine was ignored. They were about to discharge him, but John insisted that they evaluate the urine problem. They found that he had cancer of the prostate. Four months later, this too was surgically removed without complication.

Several years later, John had uncomplicated knee replacements. After the knee surgery, he gave up tennis and played golf. Despite his serious heart problem, he lived cancer-free, for 17 years after his first cancer surgery, until age 84.

But the history can prove to be critical. When ignored, significant conditions can be overlooked. This occurs even when the referring physician notes a problem that needs attention, and particularly when it is in another specialty area.

—⟋⟍—

In addition to having their histories ignored, another problem for hospital patients is that frequently, no one follows-up on test results. For instance, I've seen a large mass in the lung reported by a radiologist, but ignored by the urologist, during two hospitalizations over a two-year period at another hospital. It was a cancer. This patient is not alone;

studies have determined that physicians do not follow-up on most of the tests done before patients are discharged from the hospital.

On the other extreme, unnecessary testing is also a hazard in teaching hospitals. In the early 1960s, during his oral cardiology board examination, a medical school expert insisted that every patient with high blood pressure should have an **aortogram**. With later procedures, less-invasive catheters are threaded into an artery through a limb. These were not available at the time, so the procedure required the injection of an x-ray-opaque dye directly into the aorta through a needle stuck in the back. It had risks that far exceeded the hoped-for benefit of finding a curable condition. The expert did not pass the boards, according to one of the examiners.

Nonetheless, this type of thinking—favoring a risky new test over a patient's best interests—was becoming widespread in teaching facilities. The risk of performing any test should be less than the risk of not performing it.

In time, the testing procedures usually improve and the risk decreases. Then it is applied to more and more patients in search of an uncommon curable condition. The benefit then becomes less and less. As a result, the overall cost to medical care rises without proportional benefit.

As Sir Osler said, medicine is an art based on science. And as noted earlier, medicine is still referred to as the "practice of medicine," and it is delivered by "practitioners." It is not called the "science of medicine" or the "technology of medical care," nor is it delivered by "medical care scientists."

All of the available tests cannot be done on every patient. We do not have a "Star Trek" type of total body scanner that automatically makes a diagnosis of all of the conditions in a particular person. To determine which complaints by a particular person are important and which are not, requires a practitioner with many years of intense training and experience. Physicians must possess years of supervised devotion to learning not only how to care for each patient, but how to meet his or her personal and individual needs as well. As of the middle of the last century, this clinical-training structure was still in place.

"Since that time, the medical internship has changed significantly, bearing almost no resemblance to the one I did," says Herbert L. Fred, MD, MACP of the University Of Texas Health Science Center in a 2007 article in the *Texas Heart Institute Journal*. "Given the ever-increasing emphasis on sophisticated technology, the shrinking of government funding for medical services, and the devastating impact of managed care, clinical teaching has suffered a serious blow. In addition, medical schools are so strapped for money these days, that they force the clinical faculty to spend more and more time caring for paying patients, while spending less and less time caring for medical students and house officers."

Clinical research devoted to patient care has suffered. Physicians in medical schools cannot devote the time to research. By the 1970s, limited research funds were captured by an increasing number of non-physician doctors doing research.

Add to this the pressure among recent medical school graduates to pay off their several-hundred-thousand dollars in education bills, and there is less incentive from both sides to add years of non-income-producing clinical learning.

The teaching of young house officers has customarily been conducted by those with only a few more years of experience. The traditional teaching dictum has been: "See one. Do one. Teach one." As of the middle of the last century, this was performed under closer supervision by experienced staff physicians than it has been in the recent past in many hospitals.

The fair and accurate measurement of a physician's competence to practice is a challenge. It should not be limited to knowledge of the latest facts, but should also include an evaluation of skill in conducting a physical exam and the ability to make decisions in light of the patient's individual needs.

States determine clinical competence to practice medicine according to the applicant's amount of training along with a written examination of the applicant. The written National Board examinations, required after completion of medical school, are accepted by all states as satisfaction of the training requirement for a license to practice. Most states also require a minimum of at least one year of post-graduate training as an intern before a physician can practice medicine.

> *The risk of performing any test should be less than the risk of not performing it.*

Until the 1960s, the Internal Medicine Board requirements for certification as a specialist were three years of special training at an approved hospital, after which a written examination was required. In that era, an oral examination after two years of practice was also required. After passing the Internal Medicine Board examination, the additional requirements for certification in the cardiovascular disease subspecialty was another oral examination.

The oral examinations provided a very helpful mechanism for face-to-face assessment of examination proficiency, problem-solving abilities, and medical judgment. But they also introduced a personal bias that was hard to avoid.

— ɯɯ —

Milton Peterson, the head of anesthesiology at Research Hospital in Kansas City, had arrived from Boston several years before I got there in 1947. He was on the National Board of Anesthesiologists. This group tried to eliminate the examiners' bias by giving the oral examinations to candidates identified only by a number. The candidates and their training institution were unidentified.

Soon, too many candidates from leading programs of some of the more prestigious National Board members were failing. A greater number of candidates from second-tier institutional programs were passing. The blind exam policy was rescinded.

Oral board examinations were finally abandoned in all subspecialties. Cost was cited as a factor, but the unconscious and conscious biases of the examiners had become unacceptable.

Written board examinations accurately evaluate technical knowledge, but they do not evaluate whether the physician knows how to obtain adequate information from the patient, nor whether he or she can conduct a competent examination. Judgment in how to approach problems is difficult to assess in a written examination.

The physician must be conscientious and willing to not only observe but to listen to and learn from patients. They are not simply subjects for technology, like cars that come off an assembly line.

Some consider physicians "good" if they keep up with the cutting edge of technology and the standards of care, and written tests can evaluate these competencies. Others want physicians who are sensitive to the personal and unique needs of each patient. Written tests do not evaluate this.

—⁓—

Patients themselves are among the best instructors. Even patients with no money have often paid for their medical care in other ways. Those in charity hospitals or on charity services of General Hospitals paid for their care by offering themselves for the training of young physicians.

The physician must be conscientious and willing to not only observe but to listen to and learn from patients. They are not simply subjects for technology, like cars that come off an assembly line. Nor are they merely a member of a herd to whom general treatments are applied. Rather, they are unique individuals for whom the care must be individualized and personalized.

Training has been another area in which technology has taken preeminence over patient care. For decades, new physicians have been trained for technical competence, more than for the thoughtful care of patients. The focus must return to personal medical care. This type of care can limit unnecessary testing and the cost of medical care.

CHAPTER 27

The March of Technology

Technological innovations that came into use in the decades following my entry into medicine also, of course, had many profound and positive impacts on medical care. Advances in the field of cardiology in diagnostics, surgery, and medical therapies provide a good example of the influence of technology on medical practice. My career paralleled many of these advances, allowing me to try innovative methods as they were available, and apply them to the benefit of my own patients.

As of 1950, medications available for heart treatment were few and their mechanisms of action were not understood. Surgery was limited to procedures that did not directly involve the heart. And the only useful diagnostic techniques available in heart care were electrocardiology and radiology, both of which had been introduced in the latter part of the 19th century.

When I entered the profession, most diagnostic techniques were difficult to use and did not provide very useful information. **Phonocardiography**, which recorded heart sounds and murmurs, was more useful as a teaching tool than as a clinical one. An **apex cardiogram** recorded the motion which the heart imparts to the chest wall. This information was too indirect with too many variables to be generally useful. The **ballistocardiogram** recorded total body motion imparted by the heart through the body to a table. This was too imprecise, subjective, and indirect to prove useful.

Flicker fusion was a measurement of how fast a light has to flicker in order to appear steady. This rate was supposed to be related to the amount of arterial disease from atherosclerosis or hardening of the arteries in the head, but it was not clinically useful.

The traditional electrocardiogram was hard to obtain and

depended on photographic recordings. These required a dark-room for development of the tracings.

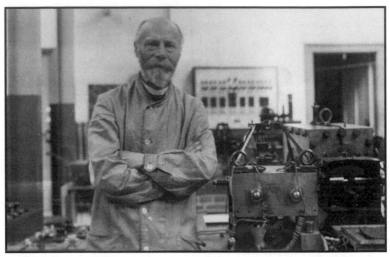

Professor Willem Einthoven in Leiden, Germany, with his string galvanometer, which he invented in 1903, the first to measure the electrical impulses of the human heart
Image provided by the U.S National Library of Medicine

Given the shortcomings of the earlier technology, three new diagnostic techniques—the direct-recording electrocardiograph, echocardiography, and cardiac catheterization—were developed and became standard in time. The electrocardiogram and echocardiogram quickly became part of routine evaluations.

The direct-recording **electrocardiograph**, which used a hot stylus on heat-sensitive waxed paper, became available in the early 1950s. It provided instant information, allowing for more rapid decision-making, and replaced the photographic recording that required time for developing in the dark room.

As a result of this convenience, the twelve-lead electrocardiogram became the standard. The leads on the arms, the legs, and locations on the chest, provide several different views of the heart's electrical field. This provides better insight into how the various diseases may be affecting the heart muscle.

A second new technique, **echocardiography**, uses ultrasound waves to visualize the heart walls and valves through the chest, much like sonar is used to visualize fish and submarines under water. While available in industry by the early 1950s, it wasn't introduced into medicine until the mid-1960s.

When echocardiography first became available, many radiologists—the interpreters of x-rays and other photographic recordings—didn't want anything to do with it. They had not been trained in this new method. They had a change of heart once they realized it could produce income for the department. The cardiology service, however, retained the control of echocardiography in most hospitals.

In 1965 at Pennsylvania Hospital, echocardiography was being evaluated in neurology for determination of a shift in the brain caused by blood clots or tumors. In cardiology, we started using this apparatus primarily to determine whether narrowing of the mitral valve was present. Usually, detection and confirmation of this required an invasive heart catheterization.

Cardiac catheterization was the third new diagnostic method that was becoming standard at the time. At first, the technique was limited to threading catheters through a vein, usually in the arm, and into the right side of the heart. Catheterization of the left side of the heart through an artery didn't become routine until the 1960s.

Cardiac catheterization labs would soon become a requirement for approved cardiology residency programs. As of the 1950s, however, catheterization labs were just starting to be installed in some hospitals throughout the country. As noted in the next chapter, this significantly affected my selection of career opportunities at the time.

CHAPTER 28

Treat the Dogs Like People

In 1955, after my cardiology fellowship ended, the decision as to where to move for my first career job was made for me when I was offered the chance to set up and run a cardiac catheterization laboratory at General Hospital in Kansas City. The Memorial Diagnostic Heart Service Association (MDHSA) was started in 1952 by two thoracic surgeons, John Mayer and Hector Benoit; along with Martin Mueller and Edward Fisher, both internists; and a pediatrician, John Sealy. This facility and the catheterization laboratory at the University of Kansas in Kansas City, were the only two in the area.

Before I started in January of 1955, heart catheterizations at General Hospital in Kansas City, Missouri, were done in the radiology department run by John Barry. The MDHSA office occupied a long, narrow, dark room. Several months after I started, the new facility for the catheterization laboratory was completed in the hospital basement. The facility consisted of four very large rooms.

That spring, I spent several days at the Mayo Clinic in Rochester, Minnesota, observing the catheterization procedures of Earl Wood. He was a renowned physiologist there, who had done work with human centrifuges for the Air Force in the 1940s. He also supervised Mayo's use of the heart-lung machine developed by John Gibbon at Thomas Jefferson University. Wood was measuring 36 variable functions in open-heart surgery patients during their operations at the clinic.

Earl Wood had two large rooms adjacent to the operating room, each with its walls covered by banks of recording-string galvanometers. He didn't consider electronic equipment reliable, so he used this much older technology, which measures electric currents based on shifts in fixed magnetic fields.

We were going to use new equipment made by the Hathaway Company of Denver, which created multi-channel photographic recordings of a light beam reflected by small mirrors on string galvanometers, thus measuring tiny shifts in electrical current. Initially, I spent several days in Denver learning to troubleshoot and repair our equipment.

Later, I was astounded to find that at this same time, Steve Langfeld at Pennsylvania Hospital was using electronic equipment from a company named, "Electronics for Medicine." This equipment was hardy and trouble-free for as long as 10 years, even when taken out to the hospital wards for use at the bedside.

We had weekly conferences at the MDHSA. The data from the catheterizations of the preceding week were presented to the group. I then discussed the new patients, whom I had already examined, and then these cases were reviewed by the group. Together, we made decisions concerning catheterization. Initially, we catheterized two patients per week.

The arrangement was unique. Private patients could be admitted to General Hospital only in an emergency. So patients were transferred by ambulance from the other hospitals in Missouri. If they were not already in a hospital, they were catheterized as outpatients. This was considered daring at the time and regarded by some as an unnecessarily dangerous practice.

Catheterizations were of the right heart only, usually by way of a vein in the arm. While an arm vein was used most of the time, occasionally the stiff catheters could not be maneuvered behind the collarbone into the chest and heart. In those cases, the femoral vein in the groin was used. Left-heart catheterizations, which require the puncture of an artery, were not done until the 1960s.

We were faced with several types of problems while conducting these early cardiac catheterizations. The accurate measurement of the oxygen content of blood samples drawn from various locations in the heart was very important. Contamination of the blood sample from air leaks in the metal stopcocks, the valves that controlled the flow of blood through the catheter, was a constant problem that I found very frustrating.

Also, the catheters had to be reused. Flushing and sterilizing them by heating under pressure in an **autoclave** prevented infections, but up to 10 percent of the reused catheters caused high, transient fevers. Trace amounts of residual blood contaminants in the catheters were the cause of the fevers, not infection.

Once we eliminated the catheter contamination problem, we had few serious complications. In more than 900 catheterizations at MDHSA during the next four years, we lost three patients, about average for the times.

One of these may have been because the procedure was done on an outpatient. The 45-year-old man had a large, **atrial-septal defect** and developed angina pectoris, heart pain. The pain only occurred when the catheter entered his left ventricle through the defect. Several hours after the catheterization and while in stable condition, the patient was dressing to go home when his heart developed the fatal chaotic heart arrhythmia of ventricular fibrillation. The open chest cardiac resuscitation attempt, standard for the time, failed to resuscitate him.

A 9-month-old baby died the night of the procedure after he was transferred back to St. Mary's Hospital. The baby had arrived at the catheterization lab in severe congestive heart failure from a very tight **pulmonary valve stenosis**.

The third death was a 4-year-old girl whose heart wall was punctured by the stiff catheter. The team was too inexperienced to recognize this curable complication in time to save her life.

—∿∿—

In 1958, the MDHSA surgery team started going to a veterinary facility in Kansas City, Kansas, once weekly. This was to gain experience with the use of the new heart-lung machine during open-heart surgery on dogs, prior to working with patients.

We couldn't keep the dogs alive. They all developed tremendously high fevers after the procedure and died of shock within several hours.

Other groups around the country also had trouble keeping the dogs alive. Some advised not to spend too much time with dogs. They said that it was much easier to keep people alive.

To maintain the circulation while the dog's heart was stopped, blood from donor dogs was needed to prime an artificial lung and heart pump. We found that the veterinary technician had been collecting the blood in a dirty pail. After we started using sterile procedures in collecting the blood for priming the pump, essentially treating the dogs like people, this complication was no longer a problem. Ultimately, the team not only successfully operated on dogs, but successfully performed heart surgery on human patients.

I ran the cardiac catheterization laboratory for 18 months. I remained a member of the team for three more years. Before I left the Kansas City area, in recognition of my time spent working in the lab, the team gave me a dinner and presented me with a gold-plated stopcock, a symbol of the challenges I had faced with the early laboratory.

This time with the lab, introducing cutting-edge technology into medical practice, provided experience with medical innovation that would prove very helpful for my entire career.

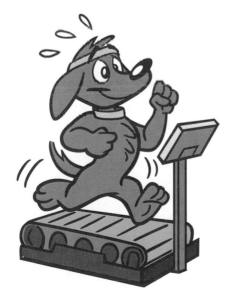

CHAPTER 29

Leveling the Playing Field

In the cardiac catheterization laboratory at Kansas City General Hospital, 40 percent of the catheterizations were performed on children. Most of these young patients were from Children's Mercy Hospital. Throughout my private practice tenure in the Kansas City area, I did some pediatric cardiology, along with my other specialties in adult cardiology and internal medicine. I continued with pediatric cardiology in Philadelphia until the mid-1960s.

At Mercy Hospital I was appointed to the staff. I did consultations and worked in the cardiac clinic. I was also appointed to the staff of the Children's Cardiac Center. It was not part of any hospital. This facility was for the treatment of children with rheumatic fever complicated by heart disease. Some with severe congenital heart disease were also treated there.

In 1959, I became head of cardiology at both Mercy Hospital and the Cardiac Center. As a consequence, I was asked to see infants and children at other hospitals and in time, at my office practice. Until I left the Kansas City area later in 1959, I was the only pediatric cardiologist in that region of Missouri.

—ɱ—

Many of the most dramatic illustrations of the impact of innovative diagnosis and therapy in this era were exemplified in the treatment of congenital heart diseases, those conditions present at birth. **Patent ductus arteriosus** is one of the most common congenital malformations. This connection between the aorta and the pulmonary arteries is necessary before birth. The connection normally closes spontaneously at birth, but at times it fails to close, which can cause complications.

Some pediatric cardiologists by the late 1950s were advocating surgery based entirely on clinical diagnosis. Echocardiography was not introduced as yet.

A 9-month-old baby referred to me had the distinctive continuous murmur, the so-called "machinery murmur," characteristic of patent ductus arteriosus. There was no other abnormality of any kind. I saw the baby on two separate occasions before allowing surgery to proceed. It was a simple, uncomplicated abnormality and the surgery was successful.

—m—

Children live in a world of inequality and often learn to accept their limitations as a fact of life. While these medical interventions are life-saving and extend lives, the successful treatment of children also has a wonderfully positive impact on their entire outlook for the future. Seeing these results, which level the playing field for many children, was a particularly rewarding application of these new methods of diagnosis and treatment.

The social deprivation of the sick child with severe heart disease may be strikingly revealed by heart surgery.

Greta was 14-years old with very severe congestive heart failure from extreme narrowing of her pulmonary valve. This valve prevents blood which is ejected into the lungs from flowing back into the heart. Greta was very reticent and shy as a result of her disabling condition.

Through very attentive and protective care by her parents, she managed to graduate from high school. They drove her back and forth to school daily.

Greta was 24-years old when she had surgery for the abnormal valve. After surgery, her shyness disappeared. Her demeanor and behavior became that of a young teenager, a period of normal development of which she had been deprived by her disease.

—ᴡᴡ—

At Children's Mercy Hospital, I followed 9-year-old Emily. She had severe narrowing of the mitral valve. Her activity was so limited that she was almost bedfast. She was very shy and reluctant to talk.

Several visits after her corrective surgery, I said to her, "Emily, you know you didn't talk much before your surgery. You wouldn't even answer my questions. And now you like to talk a lot. What happened?"

"I didn't know anything was really wrong with me. I just thought I didn't know how I should feel or what I was supposed to say. I thought I was just shy. Now that I feel better and can do the things that everyone else does, I talk a lot more!"

Emily had turned into one of the brightest, most outgoing, responsive, and communicative children of that age that I've known before or since. She hadn't realized how limited she had been. She thought her disabilities were simply normal differences that might be expected between her and other kids.

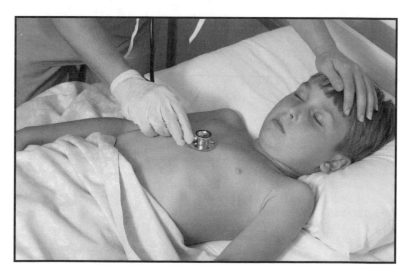

—〰—

Prior to 1950, rheumatic heart disease was the predominant heart condition diagnosed in children. Today, it is less prevalent than congenital heart disease. A near doubling in the reported frequency of congenital heart disease is actually the result of improved diagnostic capability provided by echocardiography.

Some forms of congenital heart disease are quite rare. For example, over the years, I've seen eight cases of the uncommon **Ebstein's anomaly**, a condition in which the **tricuspid valve** develops and functions abnormally. Six were in children but two were in older adults.

*Ralph was 6-years old when I first started following him in 1961. He had a **Tetralogy of Fallot**, a congenital defect of the ventricles and pulmonary valve.*

Starting at age 6 and then over the next 15 years, he had four corrective surgical procedures. I followed him off and on for more than 45 years.

As of the last update, Ralph was in his 50s and doing well, despite residual abnormalities. I lost contact with him after that.

—〰—

Aortic coarctation is a birth defect that consists of a ring-like constriction in the aorta that usually occurs just beyond the branch of the brachial artery into the left arm. When blood from the heart is ejected into the aorta for distribution throughout the body, the constriction elevates the blood pressure in the arms and lowers it in the legs.

The most remarkable instance of coarctation I saw was at Kansas City General Hospital in a 14-year-old girl who was pregnant. She had absolutely no palpable pulse or blood pressure in her legs. Ordinarily, the pulses in the abdomen and legs are reduced in coarctation but not absent.

She was kept in the hospital at bed rest for the last three months of her pregnancy and delivered uneventfully. Several months later, she underwent successful surgical correction for the most minimal constriction of the aorta I've seen.

The constriction was located in the **descending aorta**, just above the diaphragm, which is a very unusual location for it. Instead of the usual constriction with 80-percent obstruction, her constriction was less than 20 percent. After surgery, the pulses in her legs could be felt. The unusual location of the constriction caused the pulsations from blood ejected from the heart to be canceled out by the prior pulsations bouncing back from the peripheral tissues.

In the late 1960s, at Children's Hospital of Philadelphia, Dr. Rashkin developed a minimally invasive technique for treatment of a defect in the wall separating the **atria**. Various devices for the correction of such defects were threaded through the veins and arteries, a procedure which avoided the discomfort and risks of chest surgery.

Children live in a world of inequality and often learn to accept their limitations as a fact of life. While these medical interventions are life-saving and extend lives, the successful treatment of children also has a wonderfully positive impact on their entire outlook for the future. Seeing these results, which level the playing field for many children, was a particularly rewarding application of these new methods of diagnosis and treatment.

CHAPTER 30

Doc, Can I Stop? I Need a Drink of Water.

When I returned to Pennsylvania Hospital, I was able to devote more time to research, most of which was in exercise physiology and clinical diagnosis. Shortly after I started, I was recruited by a committee of the Philadelphia Medical Society to determine the best way to use electrocardiograms to screen for heart disease.

The committee had obtained permission to use subjects from among the 4,800 men, ages 50 to 81 years, who were being screened for lung cancer in the **Pulmonary Neoplasm** Research Project (PNRP). This project was supported by the Heart Association, the Heart And Lung Association, and the Philadelphia and State Health Departments.

The subjects were receiving photo-fluorograms of the chest at six-month intervals. The expectation was that early detection of cancer of the lung would lead to a greater number of surgical cures. It didn't then, and a recent study, 50-years later, has arrived at the same conclusion. Survival is better today, but it's due to improved non-surgical therapy rather than earlier detection.

In order to conduct my research, I first had to obtain permission from the participants' personal physicians to examine the men in the PNRP. I was able to examine 885 of the men. At each visit, I had them fill out a questionnaire. My technician took their blood pressure and an electrocardiogram. I evaluated the heart on the chest x-ray, as did a radiologist.

The main finding was that, for a group of people, a greater number of abnormal electrocardiograms could be found using a format with a limited number of leads compared to the standard clinical format. The reason is that the limited electrocardiogram is faster to obtain and more people can be screened. Five times as many people can be tested in a given period of time. The subject doesn't have to partially disrobe, as is necessary for the standard electrocardiogram. I subsequently verified this from multi-phasic screening of nearly 5,000 people at seven health fairs in the Greater Philadelphia area.

—⟋⟍—

Over the years, most of my clinical research projects were devoted to exercise physiology, particularly the responses in recovery after various types of exercise. This interest started with the requests from life insurance companies that exercise testing be part of the heart examination for determining the underwriting of policies.

The insurers didn't specify the type or amount of exercise, so most doctors simply had candidates do a couple of sit-ups on the examining table. In time, candidates were supposed to hop on one foot for half-a-minute. Both of these exercises inadequately exert the heart, and therefore don't help at all in revealing underlying disease that is not evident on physical examination at rest.

The only standardized exercise test in usage as of the late 1940s was the Master's "two-step" test. This test was done to determine the effects of exertion as revealed by an electrocardiogram. A "one-way trip" consisted of climbing up two stairs, each eight-inches high, and then down two stairs on the other side. About 18 one-way trips in one-and-a-half minutes was average.

A chart showed the number of trips required for a given weight. Based on this chart, I found that lightweight people were taking too many trips and were over-exerted and obese people were taking too few trips and were therefore under-exerted.

An electrocardiogram taken during the test was difficult to interpret due to body motion interference, so it was taken after completion of the trips. Changes in the electrocardiogram revealed potential disease. I would explain to patients that a stress test was similar to taking a motor vehicle out for a road test.

—⟋⟍—

When I first started practice in Kansas City, another young internist,

George, opened his first office in the same building. Morrie, a radiologist in our building, made George a gift of the Master's two-step equipment. Ironically, Morrie was soon victimized by his own gift.

Morrie had applied for a very large insurance policy. The company required a "double" two-step exercise test, which required 36 one-way trips in three minutes. Morrie asked George to do the test. George had never conducted a double two-step test. He thought a trip over and back was a one-way trip. He therefore had Morrie take 36 of these, or what was actually 72 one-way trips, in three minutes. That was equivalent to running up and back down about eight stories in three minutes.

The insurance company considered Morrie's electrocardiographic changes abnormal for his age and level of exercise, so they gave Morrie a very high rating on the policy. I couldn't convince the company that the electrocardiographic readings were normal for that level of exercise. I did convince another company, however. It awarded Morrie his large policy, unrated.

—⁂—

In time, I developed my own office tool for evaluating exercise tolerance. I used the eight-inch step stool that people used to climb up onto my examining table. They stepped up and down for one minute at their own speed, thus avoiding any possible charge that I had exercised them excessively if they claimed an adverse reaction.

Most young and active people were able to step up and down 20 to 25 times in one minute. Even those with advanced disease could usually do six to 12 trips per minute. Some feigned great exhaustion after going up and down only one or two times.

The six-minute walk, in which a patient walks around the physician's offices, is unnecessarily time-consuming and disruptive. The doctor has little time left to examine the patient and to evaluate its effects. For this reason, most physicians have an assistant conduct the test, and in doing so, information of importance that might be observed by the physician during the evaluation, may easily go undetected.

The stationary bicycle and the treadmill were found to be more useful as tests, since the electrocardiogram can be recorded while testing. During the 1950s and 1960s, these two replaced the Master's two-step as standard tests.

Most stress tests are done in order to determine the effects of exertion on the electrocardiogram or on an echocardiogram of the heart. Others are done to measure the heart's uptake of a radioactive material that indirectly measures the circulation to the heart muscle.

If stress tests are left to technicians, the physician loses or ignores a tremendous amount of useful clinical information. I found that this information, which may only occur during the test, to be of more help in the care of many patients than the tests' technical results.

—⚏—

Al was a patient of mine who experienced chest pain with exertion. This was most apt to appear in the morning after getting off a commuter train in Center City Philadelphia and climbing the stairs to the street level. I gave him a treadmill test.

After seven minutes on the treadmill, Al suddenly said, "Hey Doc! Can I stop? I need a drink of water."

He had a dry mouth and throat, and he was beginning to develop the chest pain.

*After this, I noted that other patients developed throat dryness or thirst, known as **xerostomia,** suddenly during exercise testing, but without chest pain. I called this "exertional xerostomia." I wondered whether this was a heart-pain equivalent, similar to* *how some people may experience pain in their arm, stomach, or neck from heart problems, rather than in their chest.*

After studying some 300 patients, I found that if dry mouth occurred, the heart's work was nearing 85 percent of its maximum function. It was not a heart-pain equivalent.

—∿∿—

I conducted a great deal of physiologic testing of volunteer subjects over the years using the two-step test, the stationary bicycle, or the treadmill. I took an electrocardiographic recording each minute during exercise and for at least 10 minutes afterwards. Other measurements included the **intra-arterial blood pressure**, heart-blood output using **dye-dilution curves**, and total body-oxygen consumption.

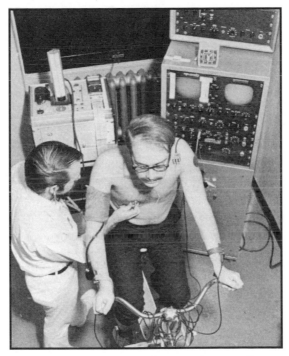

A doctor administers an exercycle stress electrocardiogram test

One of the most fascinating and unexpected findings in all of my physiological studies was a phenomenon that occurred during the first two minutes after exercise ended. The circulatory changes were counter-intuitive. The stress on the heart actually becomes greater at that time than during the exercise in some patients. I found that this was due to the dynamic shifts of function within the heart triggered by termination of exercise. This explains in part why nearly 5 percent of those who develop heart pain, do so not during exercise, but after exertion has stopped.

—⋙—

Exercise testing can reveal many other physical abnormalities and conditions, too.

Ed, a physician colleague of mine, had scheduled a treadmill test with me. He was nearing middle age and he was concerned because his father had died of a myocardial infarction.

As I always did, if I had not seen a patient previously, I took a brief history and examined him. Ed was active and well. But upon examining him, I was surprised by the large liver I was able to feel in his abdomen. I didn't say anything then so as not to alarm him before the test.

He did well on the test. No heart or circulatory abnormalities. However, his liver enlargement had all but disappeared.

He had seen the look of concern that I had when examining him before the test and asked about it.

I told him what I had found. "I have no other explanation for your enlarged liver except that it must have some vascular element," I said. "That's the only thing that would explain the sudden disappearance of your liver enlargement. Marked circulatory changes can develop from exercise."

I have never had this experience before or since, nor have I read of it.

Ed had an arteriogram that evening at another hospital. This procedure consists of injecting a special dye into the bloodstream that is then visible on x-ray.

The x-rays showed that he had collections of enlarged blood vessels throughout his liver, possibly from an automobile accident injury some five years earlier. Some were on the surface of the liver and in danger of rupturing. He had them removed surgically.

—⁓—

Physical examination during the actual testing itself, though limited, can be very revealing. In some 6,000 stress tests I've conducted over 55 years, I've found this simple clinical information during the test to be very valuable. Today, however, most doctors leave the execution of exercise tests to technicians.

If stress tests are left to technicians, the physician loses or ignores a tremendous amount of useful clinical information. I found that this information, which may only occur during the test, to be of more help in the care of many patients than the tests' technical results.

CHAPTER 31

Anyone Who Would Lie Down

on the Operating Table

When I entered the profession, heart surgery was on the verge of a huge revolution. At that time, heart surgery was performed on a beating heart. Due to the high risk, it was done only when worsening symptoms indicated the heart function was deteriorating. Prior to that, most of the surgery was performed on the aorta and large pulmonary arteries next to the heart.

Dilatation of the narrowed mitral valve, which is in the left side of the heart between the atrium and ventricle, was the most common open-heart surgery at the time. The surgeon made a slit in the atrium, inserted his finger or a tool and widened the valve by stretching, tearing, or cutting the scar tissue. Similarly, narrowed aortic and pulmonary valve defects were corrected. Several techniques allowed the blind repair of a defect in the wall separating the right and left atria of the heart.

Confirmation of abnormal conditions in valves in the left heart was imperfect at the time. Heart catheterization studies were limited to the right side by way of the veins. On the occasion that it was absolutely essential to know whether a narrow valve had built up pressure in the heart, a needle six-inches long was inserted into the back through the skin, chest wall, and lung, into the left atrium or ventricle. The risk of this procedure was reduced in the 1960s with the introduction of left-heart catheterization. The surgeon could then thread the tube into the **femoral artery** in the groin, up through the aorta, and into the left ventricle.

—⟋⟍—

Dr. Charles Bailey, one of the foremost cardiac surgeons of the time, traveled throughout the country and beyond, performing heart surgery. When I was an intern at Research Hospital in Kansas City in 1948, he visited to remove a simple cyst involving the pericardial sac around the heart. He left immediately after the surgery was completed. The patient died that night.

Some years later, when asked what criteria he used to decide whether someone required heart surgery, he replied that he would operate on "anyone who would lie down on the operating table."

This seemed like an outrageous statement at the time. Soon, however, I realized that patients who know the huge risks of open-heart surgery and remain willing must be desperate. They would rather die trying something very risky than continue the crippled life they are living.

Dr. Bailey was very innovative. One of his approaches for treating the pain from blocked circulation to the heart muscle was to connect the aorta to the large vein of the heart. This was not physiologically correct, but it seemed to work for him. He reported that in one instance, six weeks after surgery, a patient was able to run around the block without stopping and without pain. However, he soon abandoned the approach, due to the amount of risk involved with this unorthodox procedure.

— ww—

Dr. John Heysham Gibbon of Thomas Jefferson University in Philadelphia developed the heart-lung machine in 1952. Its first successful clinical use was for repair of an atrial wall defect in a young woman at Jefferson Hospital, in May of 1953.

*However, its first use on a patient was in march of 1952 at Pennsylvania Hospital. "P.D." Was a 41-year-old man with severe congestive heart failure. Serial x-rays were taken of his heart after the injection of an x-ray-opaque dye. This **angiocardiogram** revealed a filling defect in the right atrium. A number of cardiologists agreed that this dark mass on the x-rays was a tumor. However, Dr. Vander Veer, my fellowship sponsor, didn't accept this theory. He thought* *that this heart problem was the result of a weakened heart muscle, caused by inflammation in and around the heart.*

P.D.'s condition was quickly deteriorating, so he couldn't be moved safely. Therefore, Dr. Gibbon transported his heart-lung machine from Jefferson to Pennsylvania Hospital. The pump-oxygenator functioned well for the 44 minutes of its use.

As it turned out, Dr. Vander Veer was right. There was no tumor. The apparent filling defect in the right atrium appearing on the angiocardiogram was from the backwash of blood containing no dye. Blood without the dye had leaked back into the atrium through the tricuspid valve from the right ventricle, which was weakened by inflammation. The mass of die-free blood looked the same as a solid tumor on the x-rays.

About ten years later, I had a similar finding in a man at Bryn Mawr Hospital. A dark defect appeared on the patient's angiocardiogram, which I assumed—based on the prior experience—to be caused by a leakage of blood without dye; not a tumor. This too was an error, but for the opposite reason, and it had tragic consequences. Eight months later, the man died elsewhere of a **myxosarcoma**, a malignant tumor, that arose from the wall of the right atrium, extended through his right ventricle, and into his lung. This time it actually was what it looked like in the x-rays—a tumor.

—⁂—

The heart-lung bypass machine completely revolutionized open-heart surgery. It made many new techniques possible. By the 1960s, artificial valves were available to replace various damaged valves. Congenital heart defects could be corrected or alleviated. Patches were used to cover the abnormal holes within the heart.

Over the past 40 years, surgeons have devised many clever procedures for the correction of numerous, complicated congenital and acquired heart abnormalities. Now many defects can be repaired without opening the chest or the heart. These repairs are made using catheters threaded into the heart from a vein or artery in the groin.

During this time of rapid innovation in surgical procedures, there was an ongoing debate about the most ethical way to introduce new, unproven, high-risk surgical procedures into patients. One position was that innovative risky procedures should be used only on terminally ill patients in attempts to save their lives. They would die shortly if not helped. The other view was that the extremely high risk in these patients was unacceptable and that less critically ill patients should be the initial subjects.

In the early 1960s, these two opposite approaches to the use of the still relatively new heart-lung bypass machine were illustrated in the surgery programs at the University of Kansas and the University of Missouri. The University of Kansas adopted the rationale that the repair of congenital heart defects that required the use of the heart-lung machine should be used only as a salvage procedure in very critically ill children about to die.

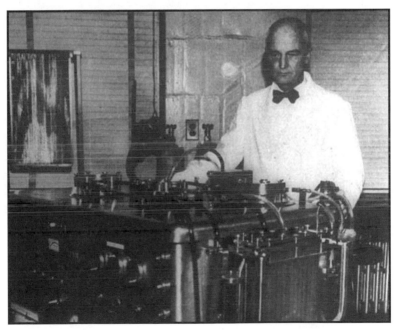

Dr. John Heysham Gibbon with his heart lung bypass machine, 1952

Nine of the first 10 cases at the University of Kansas were for repair of a **ventricular septal defect**, a hole in the wall between the right and left ventricles, in children who were experiencing life-threatening heart failure. All nine of these died. The sole survivor, the 10th child, represented the one exception to their rationale. The child was operated on for an atrial septal defect, a less serious condition for which a safer, established surgical procedure was already available.

Today, heart transplants are an accepted method for the treatment of end-stage heart disease. Patients can be expected to survive for more than 10 years, and some are doing so for twice as long.

Conversely, the program at the University of Missouri adopted the opposite approach. They used the heart-lung machine for surgery on patients who had a condition for which other proven procedures had been established. Nine of the first 10 children on whom they operated were for repair of atrial septal defects in patients who were not as severely ill, and they all survived. The one child they lost had a ventricular septal defect.

The rationale of the University of Missouri's approach could be faulted as there were several proven and safer procedures for the closure of atrial defects. Their approach exposed these children to the added risk of the new procedure. Ironically, the high mortality rate at the University of Kansas, using an approach that many considered more ethical, set its open-heart cardiac surgery program back several years.

In 1966, the leading cause of death in children in Ohio was surgical correction of ventricular septal defects. By the 1970s, it finally became evident that most ventricular septal defects closed spontaneously and needed no surgery.

—w—

The most common use of the heart-lung bypass machine upon its introduction was for surgical repair of **stenotic**, or narrowed, valves. More of these were caused by rheumatic heart disease than congenital heart disease. As the following story illustrates, people with narrowed valves can still have remarkable exercise tolerance.

In the mid-1950s, we studied George, who was 18-years old. He had a very severe narrowing of his pulmonary valve, which regulates blood flow from the heart to the lungs.

A constricted pulmonary valve increases the pressure in the right ventricle, which usually rises to double or triple the normal level. George's pressure was 200 millimeters of mercury, about seven-times the normal reading. He underwent surgical treatment of the valve without benefit of the heart-lung machine.

Several months later during a follow-up examination, I asked him, "Can you exercise any more now than you could before surgery?"

"Oh, yea."

"How so?"

"Before surgery, I could only run up six flights of stairs at the power and light building. Now I can run up fourteen flights."

"Without stopping?"

"Without stopping."

Considering the severity of his valve abnormality, his preoperative exercise tolerance was as astounding as was his improvement after surgery.

—ɷ—

I also found unusually high exercise tolerance in most patients with significant, even severe, mitral valve stenosis, which is a narrowing of the valve between the left atrium and ventricle.

Since this condition often does not become clinically evident until middle age, patients assume their reduction in exercise tolerance is the natural effect of aging or related changes such as weight gain. Only after corrective surgery do they realize how much their exercise capacity had been reduced before surgery.

Some heart surgery is curative. This is particularly true of certain congenital conditions. Most surgery, however, is ameliorative. It improves heart function and the quality of life. When the end stage of heart disease is reached, replacement is the only answer. This is accomplished by transplantation of a heart from a person who has just died, or by replacement with an artificial heart.

The first human heart transplantation was performed in 1967 by Dr. Christian Barnard. For many years, the rejection by the body of the transplanted heart was a major problem severely limiting survival. The body is intolerant to foreign substances introduced into it, especially proteins. This reaction protects the body from infection, but it causes serious difficulties when organs are transplanted. At first, survival after transplantation was measured in months.

The post-war technical revolution in heart surgery has provided incalculable relief and saved many lives. The soaring expense of applying the new technologies in surgery, however, raises the issue of its economic limitations in society. As costs increase, rationing of these expensive, high-tech healthcare procedures will become more and more prevalent.

It wasn't until the early 1980s that effective immunosuppressive drugs were developed to minimize the problems of transplanted organ rejection. Today, heart transplants are an accepted method for the treatment of end-stage heart disease. Patients can be expected to survive for more than 10 years, and some are doing so for twice as long.

As with many organ transplant procedures, however, the demand continues to grow much more rapidly than the supply. The percentage of hearts available from the potential donor pool has not increased in the past 25 years. Also, the cost of each procedure and the management after surgery is astronomical.

Some see the artificial heart as a solution to the shortage of available organs. These devices have many unsolved problems and are still experimental. Among the long-term technical problems is a reliable, self-contained power supply. Complications from infections, bleeding, blood clots, and organ failure remain to be solved. Patients survive with an artificial heart for only a matter of months. The primary application therefore has been as a temporary life-supporting bridge until a transplant is available.

In 1964, Congress approved the allocation of funds for research on an artificial heart. The National Heart, Lung, and Blood Institute has supported the research annually since then. A panel there has arrived at the conclusion that the device is life-saving and feasible.

If permanent, artificial hearts ever become practical for widespread use, the cost of implantation, maintenance, and treatment of complications would be phenomenally high. The cost per unit would fall, but its widespread use could consume a major portion of the gross national product. Its use would have to be rationed.

—⁊⁊⁊—

Surgery today is a very labor-intensive process. Some surgeons of an earlier era thought of themselves and their skills as the sole determinant of the success of a surgery, like a "hot dog" solo fighter pilot. Actually, the surgeon relies heavily upon special nurses, anesthesiologists, house staff, technicians, and numerous others to insure the success of the surgery. They are more akin to bomber pilots that have a large trained crew behind them.

At Pennsylvania Hospital in the 1960s, I counted at least 26 different disciplines that were involved in the care of a heart-surgery patient. Thirty years later, a **Medicare** study reported that there was an average of 33 disciplines involved in heart surgery, with many represented by more than one person.

The post-War technical revolution in heart surgery has provided incalculable relief and saved many lives. The soaring expense of applying the new technologies in surgery, however, raises the issue of its economic limitations in society. As costs increase, rationing of these expensive, high-tech healthcare procedures will become more and more prevalent.

CHAPTER 32

Special Care Units

In addition to the installation of emergency departments and the improvements in surgical procedures, the availability of new technologies affected hospital care in a number of other ways, too. In the 1960s, hospitals began to create intensive care units for the more efficient management of critically ill surgical and non-surgical patients.

The first intensive care units, or ICUs, were created by the installation of various instruments that made it possible to continuously monitor each patient's condition. Special nurses were trained for this duty. This increased the cost of care for each patient.

The Pennsylvania Hospital ICU Committee was created in the mid-1960s and assigned the task of designing the Hospital's first intensive care unit. I was the cardiologist appointed to the Committee, which included medical staff from other departments and a bioengineering consultant. We decided to acquire equipment to monitor each patient's electrocardiogram, blood pressure, respiration, and temperature. We also evaluated the various alternatives.

At first, the bioengineer recommended specifications that called for equipment that was so accurate it could make measurements to a tiny fraction of a unit. The bioengineering field was just coming into its own, so most engineers in this field were trained in other areas of engineering and expected the same degree of accuracy prevalent in those areas. Such a degree of precision is meaningless in clinical medicine. I told the engineers that I often have to work with a 20-percent error. The Committee changed the specifications for the equipment so that it was only as precise as needed for clinical use.

Another decision the Committee was asked to make was to determine the daily charge for ICU patients. It was unusual to assign this type of management decision to a medical-staff committee. At the time, the hospital charges were not based on cost-accounting studies. The charge for regular hospital care was set at $65 per day. The suggestion from Committee members for the ICU charges ranged from $100 to $200 per day. The administration settled on $130 per day, twice the usual rate.

One of the other key changes in hospital care in the 1960s was the introduction of Coronary Care Units, CCUs, for the treatment of acute myocardial infarction. In time, they were used to treat other types of acute cardiac cases, too. At Pennsylvania Hospital in the late 1960s, cardiology was able to get only a "quasi-CCU," which had three beds set aside in separate rooms in the ICU. They were under the care of the ICU nurses.

This incident is a microcosm of the political, economic, and administrative dilemmas surrounding decisions to adopt new technologies in healthcare facilities. The costs are significant, but the needs of patients and the physicians caring for them cannot be denied. Meeting those needs by adopting life-saving technologies and procedures is inevitable.

A separate CCU did not become a reality at the hospital until 1970, and its creation became a political football. The increased cost of such a unit was a concern of the Hospital administration and they wanted proof of its benefit.

The proof arrived in the summer of 1969 when disaster struck both the ICU and the quasi-CCU. Visitors discovered several ICU patients dead in their beds. One of the patients was a staff doctor's cook of some 30 years, who was discovered by the doctor's family member. This patient was in an area of the ICU that was not visible to the nursing staff at all times. Also, the electrocardiogram monitor alarms were either not working, were turned off, or were ignored. This was common in many early ICUs because of the disruption caused by the high frequency of false alarms. Poor skin contact for the electrocardiogram wires attached to the patient resulted in numerous false alarms.

Shortly after this, one of my patients in the CCU was found in fatal ventricular fibrillation by the sole CCU nurse who had just returned from lunch. During her absence, the patient had been under the care of an ICU nurse who had duties attending surgical and other patients requiring more than surveillance care. At the time, the CCU had its own nurses only part of the time. Again, the alarm failed to go off.

My patient was converted to normal rhythm immediately, but did not regain consciousness. She had had the fibrillation for more than five minutes and, sadly, was brain dead.

As a result, the cardiology staff began pushing hard for a CCU with completely separate staffing 24 hours-a-day. The September ICU Committee meeting attracted, among others, the chief of surgery and a number of high-powered Hospital administrators. The administration was running scared.

The chief of anesthesiology was the Committee chairman. Meetings were held every two weeks until December. At the first meeting, the consensus was that a problem existed.

When we attempted to address the problem at the subsequent meeting, however, the Hospital administrators' responses were, "What problem?"

The Committee would plow through it again, agree that there was a problem, only to have the scenario repeated at the next meeting.

At the January 1970 meeting, I pointed out that this was a medical-staff committee meeting, that we should start keeping minutes, and that only the physicians on the medical staff could vote. Finally, we started to make progress. At the May meeting, we got a vote for a new and separate CCU.

Nothing happened for several days afterwards, so I called the chief of medicine and told him the results of the vote. You'd have thought I had handed him a glowing coal. So I contacted the Committee chairman, and told him what I thought were the consequences of the vote—that a separate CCU was mandated. He leapt at it. He was in the middle of negotiating a new contract with the hospital, so he thought this gave him more leverage.

I made these calls on a Thursday. The following Monday, a high-level Hospital administration meeting was held. The decision was that something would be done, but it couldn't be started until the new chief of cardiology arrived several months later. This was a good example of the deleterious effect of the "wait until the new management" syndrome.

Even after the new head of cardiology arrived, the separate CCU took a year to complete. Fortunately, however, no more deaths occurred from neglect in the interim, and there have been none since.

This incident is a microcosm of the political, economic, and administrative dilemmas surrounding decisions to adopt new technologies in healthcare facilities. The costs are significant, but the needs of patients and the physicians caring for them cannot be denied. Meeting those needs by adopting life-saving technologies and procedures is inevitable.

CHAPTER 33

Let's Not Take Sudden Death Away from the People

The death of a patient is not only devastating to the family and to loved ones, but also to the physician caring for the patient. It is a personal loss to both the family and the physician, but to the physician, it is also a professional failure.

"Could I have prevented it?" The doctor wonders. "What did I miss? What could I have done better?"

I first had this experience in medical school with my patient Charles, after he received that first dose of digitalis. After he died later that same day, I examined and re-examined my treatment, and found that I had followed all of the standards at the time. The treatment could not be faulted, but I still felt defeated.

Sudden death is defined as death within 1 to 24 hours of the onset of symptoms. Instantaneous death occurs within 15 minutes. Heart-rhythm disturbances are the most common cause of sudden or instantaneous death.

Prior to the 1960s, it was particularly frustrating and depressing for medical professionals when a patient died of a heart-rhythm disturbance with "a heart too good to die." Outside of an operating room setting, nothing could be done. In the 1960s, three new procedures became widely available and dramatically changed everything. These procedures were **closed-chest manual cardiopulmonary resuscitation**; **electro-cardioversion** for the electrical restoration of the chaotic heart beat to a normal rhythm; and the **implantable pacemakers** that provide electrical control and pacing of the heartbeat.

Ventricular fibrillation is a fatal heart-rhythm irregularity that is the most common cause of instantaneous death. It is caused by conversion of the heartbeat from a normal "**sinus rhythm**," to a chaotic, fast beat. The uncoordinated contraction of the heart muscles from the fast rhythm fails to pump the blood, and death of the brain occurs within minutes.

A number of possible causes can lead to irregular ventricular rhythm. The most common cause is poor circulation due to hardening of the arteries. Occasionally, sudden or instantaneous death is caused by progressive slowing of the heartbeat until it either comes to a standstill or ventricular fibrillation develops. Approximately half of all deaths from hardening of the arteries occur suddenly. In 20 percent, death is the very first, and last, manifestation of heart disease.

—⟋⟍⟍⟋—

The death of a patient is not only devastating to the family and to loved ones, but also to the physician caring for the patient. It is a personal loss to both the family and the physician, but to the physician, it is also a professional failure.

In the 1950s, open-chest cardiac massage and resuscitation were advocated, but resuscitation was rarely successful outside of the operating room. In some places, surgical residents were going about, on and off duty, with a sterile scalpel and a few other instruments in a pocket in case they heard the thud of somebody hitting the floor in cardiac arrest. The chest was opened, the heart exposed, and the circulation maintained by manually massaging the heart until an electrical defibrillator could be obtained.

I never personally knew of a successful in-house resuscitation in the 1950s. I arrived at least at one attempt on a Pennsylvania Hospital medical ward where the heart was being massaged, but nobody was ventilating the lungs.

The first instance of a successful resuscitation outside

the hospital received some notoriety. A doctor had just had an electrocardiogram at Cleveland University Hospital because of chest pain. The results would be available the following day. He collapsed in the parking lot. He was taken immediately to the emergency room, his chest was opened, his heart was massaged, and the usually fatal heart irregularity converted to normal rhythm by an electric shock. He had had a heart attack, an acute myocardial infarction.

In San Francisco, where armed services personnel were collapsing from pulmonary emboli, a complication of blood clotting after a long flight from Korea, there was some success in saving lives. Emergency surgical teams were set up at the site to restore the heart rhythm and to remove the blood clots from the pulmonary arteries.

Starting in the 1960s, some success was achieved in cardiac resuscitation outside of the operating room. In 1961, closed-chest massage was found to be effective in maintaining circulation. External **electro-cardioversion** became available in 1962. This procedure consists of administering an electric shock to the heart through the chest wall, using paddles.

Hospitals set up resuscitation teams. At Pennsylvania Hospital, it was called the CRT for Cardiac Resuscitation Team. In 1965, Joel Nobel, a surgical resident at the Hospital, introduced "Max" to the hospital. Max was a self-contained mobile resuscitation cart on which the unconscious patient was placed. It had an electric defibrillator which was used to shock the heart back into a normal rhythm.

Heart massage was administered by a pump with a rubber-cushioned plunger at the end. It extended down from an arm which swiveled on a post built into the cart. The plunger could be positioned over the lower sternum and the heart. The rate and the depth for compression of the chest were adjustable. It was powered by a tank of compressed oxygen. We irreverently referred to this contraption as "The Bottle Capper."

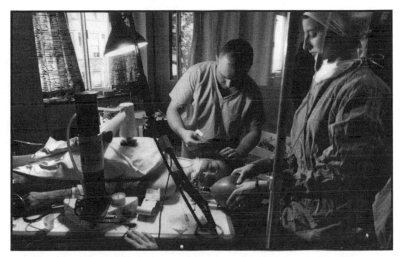

In 1965, Dr. Joel Nobel with his invention "Max," a mobile
resuscitation cart with an electric shock cardioverter
and pump for chest compression
Photograph by I C Rapoport

Max also had equipment for controlled lung ventilation procedures. This included materials for intubation of the trachea, a breathing bag for assisting ventilation, and oxygen. These procedures maintained the patient's circulation and breathing before and after resuscitation. There were also a number of drawers for medications.

The Hospital was eventually organized to an extent that even the elevators could be controlled by the CRT, which became the code for a cardiac arrest announced over the loud speakers. I was one of the team leaders for a large part of the first several years. It took nearly a year-and-a-half before we had our first successful resuscitation followed by complete recovery.

We quickly found that early detection of the arrest was the most important element in successful resuscitation. I often wondered whether the weakest link might be the ever-present housekeeping personnel. Did cleaning people, upon entering a room where the patient "just didn't look right," leave for another room without alerting the nurses—for fear of embarrassment of being accused of unnecessarily crying wolf over a sleeping patient?

—∿∿—

House doctors often wasted a great deal of time obtaining an electrocardiogram first to verify the rhythm before administering the electric shock to the chest wall. The longer it takes to return the heart to normal rhythm, the greater the deterioration of the heart and circulation, and the more resistant the heart becomes to restoration of its rhythm.

At the time, there was some discussion as to the advisability of lay personnel performing resuscitation procedures, especially electro-cardioversion. One of the concerns was that the electric shock might trigger a potentially fatal ventricular fibrillation in a person who had only fainted. I felt that this was an unnecessary concern. If a person who had only fainted was given an electric shock that caused an arrhythmia, a second shock could be applied immediately to correct it. In recent years, this concern has been addressed by the invention of a defibrillator that won't work when it detects a normal rhythm. These are increasingly available for use in public places.

Not until 2005 were the resuscitation standards updated to recommend that chest compressions be restarted immediately, even after a successful defibrillation shock that had restored a normal rhythm. The standard recommends that compressions be continued for at least two minutes. This is important because the heart is dilated and still very weak from the low oxygen it had been receiving during the arrest period.

As early as the 1960s, I found that it was important to continue the compressions for as long as five minutes or more after a regular heart rhythm had been restored. When compressions were discontinued too soon, the rhythm rapidly deteriorated and ventricular fibrillation often recurred.

Restarting the compressions would frequently reverse the deterioration of the rhythm and help maintain the heart in normal rhythm. This was more successful if we continued the heart massage until we were sure the pulses as well as circulation were adequate, and the heartbeat became strong enough to maintain blood pressure on its own.

The importance of restarting compressions had become evident from my fellowship days, working in the lab on resuscitation of **hypoxic rat** hearts at the University of Vermont. My findings were reinforced during my time spent monitoring the electrocardiograms during heart surgery at Kansas City General Hospital in the 1950s.

I would be impressed with the regular rhythm on a nearly normal electrocardiogram. Then the surgeon would have me come over and look at the heart in the open chest. It would be blue instead of pink, greatly dilated, with ineffectual twitches instead of contractions. It obviously required continued mechanical support during this early recovery phase, even when the electrocardiogram appeared normal.

Over the past 40 years, the most permanent change in the resuscitation guidelines has been the increase in the rate of compressions and the reduction in the rate of ventilation. The initial recommendations were to apply the heart compressions at a rate of at 40-to-60 per minute.

Then, it was instructive to observe a patient who had regained consciousness with the initiation of heart compressions by a wiry young nurse who was compressing the chest at a fast rate. Unconsciousness would recur when a hefty intern relieved her and exerted slower, deeper chest compressions. Today, the standard for rate of compression has increased to more than 100 per minute.

The early guidelines for the resuscitation efforts, especially for those outside of the hospital, were that the chest compressions be interrupted at intervals to administer several breaths mouth-to-mouth. Recent survival data suggest that this interruption may be detrimental if done by an inexperienced person, because of the loss of time taken from the chest compressions.

As an intern, I learned of another reason why respiratory support may not be required immediately. I was asked by the neurosurgeon to shut off an iron lung respirator that was keeping a 16-year-old girl alive. This was several days after she'd had brain surgery for a fast growing, malignant brain tumor, a **glioblastoma multiforme**. She had not regained consciousness or spontaneous breathing. Even if she had recovered, she would have had only six months to live.

After discontinuation of the respirator, her heart continued to beat strongly and did not stop for 15 minutes. I noticed that the strong beating of the heart shook her chest quite vigorously and may have moved some air with oxygen in her bronchial tubes deeper into her lungs. Similarly, I would speculate that the resuscitation effort of chest compression partly mixes some air in the lungs, making the mouth-to-mouth efforts less critical.

—m—

One of the most distressing consequences of resuscitation attempts occurs when the blood flow to the brain is restored, along with the patient's consciousness, but the heartbeat cannot be restored. This tragic outcome first happened to me with a vigorous young man in his 30s in the Hospital's ICU in the late 1960s.

The second time occurred a few years later. During a foundation's board meeting, the chairman, a well-known "Mr. Philadelphia," collapsed, his head falling on the table. We were attempting to restore a normal heartbeat in the Hospital's receiving ward when he awoke and comprehended what we were saying to him.

Despite everything we tried, we couldn't get his heart to start, so we were faced with a very difficult dilemma. Do we tell him about the problem? Do we ask him what his final wishes are? Do we keep him alert and call in his family from the waiting room to say goodbye?

*After agonizing over the dilemma, we concluded that any of these would be inhumane. We decided to heavily sedate him to unconsciousness with intravenous **Valium**. But how long should we* *continue trying to resuscitate the heart? At this point, the attending physician, anesthesiologist, nurse, and I agreed that all treatment decisions must be unanimous. We continued the resuscitation efforts on Mr. Philadelphia for an hour-and-a-half. Sadly, despite everything we tried, we were still unable to get his heart going. Finally, we all agreed we had to abandon the effort.*

I thought that supporting his circulation for several days on a heart-lung pump while the heart healed would have worked in this situation and might be feasible some day. A number of years later, this was reported for the first time.

One life-threatening rhythm disturbance, **ventricular tachycardia**, is a rapid heartbeat that originates abnormally in a ventricle instead of the atria. This condition may complicate an acute myocardial infarction, as well as other types of heart disease. **Tachycardia** makes the heart much less effective in its pumping action, causing **hypoxia** and blood clotting. Ultimately, ventricular fibrillation develops and is the usual cause of death.

Prior to the 1960s, a diagnosis of ventricular tachycardia meant almost certain death. In the 1950s, Dr. Vander Veer admitted a middle-aged man with ventricular tachycardia into the hospital. The condition continued for 46 days, before he died from the usual complications of heart failure and blood clots to the lungs and brain. At that time, only two patients reported in the literature had lasted longer. The patient who lived the longest was from Argentina, who went on for 123 days.

In the 1960s, with the availability of electro-cardioversion methods, ventricular tachycardia could be restored to normal rhythm. A man reported in the literature had ventricular tachycardia for 74 days. Although many attempts at electro-cardioversion had failed, a normal rhythm was eventually restored. Ironically, this appeared spontaneously without electro-cardioversion.

—m—

In the 1970s, and nearly five years after her last visit, a 72-year-old patient named Alma came in to see me. Once again, her complaint was of palpitations. She was the last survivor in her family, all of whom had died suddenly in their 50s.

*During this exam, as she had in previous exams, Alma demonstrated a large number of abnormal **ectopic beats** originating in the ventricle. She had many more of these than normal **sinus beats**. This can be a precursor of ventricular fibrillation or other serious arrhythmias.*

I called Alma's personal physician, Dr. Hipple, who was 76 years old herself.

Dr. Hipple's first comment was, "Is that old biddy still living?"

I related my concern about Alma's arrhythmias. "She needs treatment," I said. "She's at high risk of succumbing to the family affliction of sudden death."

There was a pause on the other end of the line, followed by Dr. Hipple's slowly enunciated admonition. "Now, let's not take sudden death away from the people."

I assumed she was referring to the advantages of a painless, sudden death over the possible prolonged agony for the patient and the family of a slow, painful death.

Several years later, Dr. Hipple retired. About a year after that, she was in the admissions office of a suburban hospital for cataract surgery, which was still done in the hospital at that time. She collapsed there, and despite the office's location close to the emergency room, she could not be resuscitated by the highly trained personnel so immediately available.

Dr. Hipple might be pleased to know that, even today, we still haven't taken sudden death away from the people.

CHAPTER 34

Struck in the Chest with a Fist

Atrial fibrillation is the most common, serious heart-rhythm disturbance. The chaotic beating of atrial fibrillation is limited to the atria, the upper chambers that receive blood from the lungs and the rest of the body, before it flows into the **ventricular pumps**. It is not fatal. It reduces the efficiency of the heart, but does not prevent the ventricles from pumping blood to the rest of the body, as does ventricular fibrillation.

Atrial fibrillation is usually a manifestation of heart disease, but it can occur in people without heart disease as a self-limited response to certain kinds of stress. A few may experience it with anxiety—such as an appearance before a large audience. It is more common with the various excesses around holiday times, especially increased alcohol consumption. This is referred to as a "holiday heart."

The thyroid hormone stimulates metabolism. An excess of hormone from an **overactive thyroid gland** over-stimulates the heart and can cause atrial fibrillation. This cause can be corrected.

Measurement of the hormone level became possible in the early 1950s. A number of hospital heart clinics found that about 5 percent of the patients with atrial fibrillation had overactive thyroid glands. These, if known, could have been treated with the drugs available at the time.

The longer the duration of atrial fibrillation, the more likely it is to persist. On occasion, it develops in hearts that are otherwise normal. Doctors suspect that atrial fibrillation is not always just a complication of heart disease already present, but that it can actually cause heart disease. Until recent years, the appearance of this condition was regarded as an indication for hospitalization, so that the drugs used at the time could be monitored in order to prevent complications.

In 1954, we found that even when atrial fibrillation had been present for more than three months, it reverted to normal rhythm in one out of 10 people after hospitalization and before any treatment with drugs, other than digitalis. Some people with atrial fibrillation and without known heart disease have a naturally **high heart block**, which means that the ventricles beat many times slower than the atria. This keeps the actual heart rate under control, even during vigorous exercise. Patients with this condition usually do not need treatment.

Prior to 1962, the only methods for treatment of atrial fibrillation required the use of drugs. The therapy was directed first to slowing the heart rate with digitalis. This was followed by the use of **quinidine** or **procainamide** to convert the fibrillation back to a normal rhythm. Drug conversion of the arrhythmia in those with heart disease was effective only about two-thirds of the time.

Blood clots have a tendency to form in the heart during atrial fibrillation. These tend to break loose and float, or **embolize**, to a distant part of the body, causing harm such as a stroke. Therefore, treatment with drugs to prevent the formation of clots is important. Coumadin, a pill taken by mouth, or **heparin**, given by an injection, are common anticoagulants, or "blood thinners," used to prevent blood clots.

People under the age of 65 years are not prone to develop clots if they have no known heart disease. They need no anticoagulant therapy. Those over age 65 are prone to develop clots in the heart with fibrillation, even if they have no known heart disease. They need to be on anticoagulants to reduce the risk of embolic complications.

—◊—

In 1962, Bernard Lown introduced a convenient and safe way to administer an electric shock through the intact chest wall to a heart beating abnormally fast. No longer did the shock need to be delivered directly to the heart after the chest had been opened and the heart exposed surgically. With this new technology, the likelihood of successfully converting a heart in atrial fibrillation to a normal rhythm improved greatly.

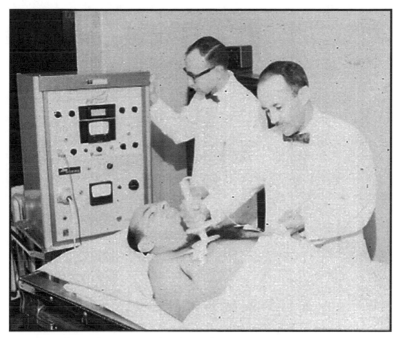

Dr. Joseph Vander Veer applies the paddles in a demonstration of the first electric shock cardioverter machine at Pennsylvania Hospital, 1962

In 1962, the same year that this new technology was intro-duced, a 45-year-old policeman named Vince was referred to Dr. Vander Veer at Pennsylvania Hospital. He'd had a fast, irregular heartbeat due to atrial fibrillation for a matter of weeks. He was in heart failure, which was further complicated by a small stroke and blood clots in his lungs.

*Medication did not work in slowing his heart rate because of **Wolff-Parkinson-White syndrome**, caused by an abnormal short-circuiting electrical connection between the atrium to the ventricles. We gave Vince heroic doses of medication. We administered these in the operating room with surgeons standing by to open the chest* *and massage the heart if ventricular fibrillation developed. The only method of converting the rhythm to normal at the time was by an electric shock applied directly to the heart.*

Vince was in the Hospital for about a week when three of us from cardiology went to the annual conference of the American Society of Clinical Investigation in Atlantic City, New Jersey, which was referred to as the "Young Turks" meeting. Dr. Bernard Lown presented the results of a new technique of external electro-cardioversion administered as an electric shock across the chest wall to the heart.

We immediately recognized that this was the only hope for Vince. Dr. Vander Veer got on the phone and the fourth electro-cardioverter made by this company, and its first commercial sale, went to Pennsylvania Hospital.

*Upon receiving the device, we again gathered in an operating room with a surgeon. The precaution of having a surgeon on hand became obsolete in moments. The result of the electro-cardioversion was spectacular. A normal rhythm was restored by the first electric shock. Vince's heart failure resolved rapidly. The effects of the strokes and **pulmonary embolism** from blood clots cleared.*

Much later, when Vince was in his 80s, I found out that he had come under the care of a colleague of mine. Vince had been doing well for most of the 40 intervening years, without the recurrence of atrial fibrillation or any heart irregularity, and without any specific treatment.

—ᴍ—

For most of the following year after acquiring this life-saving device, I was responsible for delivering this elective procedure at the Hospital. Since it was so new, no guidelines were available. I developed a protocol from an extension of prior experience with atrial fibrillation and its conversion with drugs. Electro-cardioversion proved effective more than 80 percent of the time. After a year, however, only 50 to 60 percent remained in normal rhythm, which was the same rate as after drug conversion.

Fatalities from electro-cardioversion were reported in the

literature, but I never had a fatality. They appeared to occur when conversions were attempted in people with hearts that were very enlarged from advanced disease. I avoided these.

I found that when I attempted electro-cardioversion within the first week of hospitalization, the success rate was low. I suspected that this was due to residual congestive heart failure weakening the heart. The success rate improved for those who had the procedure during the second week, when the congestive heart failure was under more complete control. For those scheduled to have the electro-cardioversion after the second week and for several weeks later, I found that 75 percent converted to a normal rhythm with just the drug therapy alone.

This and similar experiences with my initial use of the electro-cardioversion procedure raised questions about a psychological component in cardiac arrhythmias.

The day before the procedure was scheduled, I would obtain the patient's permission to perform the electro-cardioversion. After getting permission, I saw a high rate of conversion in patients on the medication alone. I wondered whether there was a psychological aspect to the arrhythmia. Did the prospect of the electro-cardioversion "shock" them into a normal rhythm? This possibility again arose during a study to determine how long a normal rhythm would persist after electro-cardioversion.

A study participant by the name of Althea was an excitable 70-year-old woman with mitral and aortic valve abnormalities. She was one of the paired patients selected by chance for electro-cardioversion. Her atrial fibrillation had been documented for more than 10 years. Her equally excitable daughter always faithfully brought her into the cardiac clinic.

I carefully explained the procedure and the plan to Althea and her daughter, with some concern about their reception of the new method.

They received the proposal calmly.

I told them that I didn't need a decision immediately, but asked them to think it over and come back the following week.

They returned as scheduled. To my surprise, they agreed to the procedure.

I then checked Althea's electrocardiogram. Not only was she now in normal sinus rhythm, but she remained in it for one year without any change in her original treatment. After 10 years of fibrillation, this just doesn't happen. But it did.

This and similar experiences with my initial use of the electro-cardioversion procedure raised questions about a psychological component in cardiac arrhythmias.

For patients with significant valve disease, the intervals between the recurrences of atrial fibrillation after successful cardioversion to a normal rhythm became progressively shorter. One man with rheumatic valvular disease first required conversion yearly, then every six months, and eventually at monthly intervals. Finally, when the normal rhythm would last for only one week, I refused to try any more conversions, over his objection. It was no longer worth the risk.

We usually performed the procedure under light anesthesia. At Philadelphia Veterans Hospital, however, electro-cardioversions were being conducted without anesthesia. It was done often enough that a patient who was still in the Hospital would convince the next candidate to have the procedure without anesthetic. Apparently, it was the macho thing to do among these veterans.

One patient of mine agreed to have the procedure without anesthesia.

Afterwards, I asked, "What was it like?"

"Like being struck in the chest with a fist."

"Would you go through it again?"

"Well, maybe," he said hesitantly.

"If you had to, would you?"
"Yes."

Valium became the standard anesthesia used by other doctors for the procedure, but I found that it had serious drawbacks. It required at least 10 minutes to work, and patients were incapacitated for hours before they could leave. I preferred using **Pentothol** intravenously, administered by an anesthetist. The patients were unconscious for only a minute or two, and ready to leave in about an hour.

—⁓—

One of the problems after a successful conversion to normal rhythm is how long to continue the drugs. An anticoagulant prevented clotting and an anti-arrhythmic prevented recurrence of the arrhythmia. Can they be stopped safely at the same time? If not, which one should be stopped first? The risk of clotting and embolization is usually greater than the adverse effects of a recurrent arrhythmia, so I stopped the anti-arrhythmic first and continued the anticoagulant for weeks or even months, until I was certain that the fibrillation would not return anytime soon.

An occasional person tolerates atrial fibrillation for years without symptoms or limitation. No control of the heart rate is necessary. However, the risk of embolization is still significant, and anticoagulation is important.

A number of new electrical and surgical **ablation** techniques have proven to be of value in some patients resistant to conversion. But these are not likely to permanently eliminate the fibrillation. I suspect these patients will require more and more invasive procedures unless fibrillation becomes an accepted condition for them.

Atrial flutter is a rhythm disturbance that is similar to fibrillation but is a fast, regular rhythm, rather than a fast, irregular one. Drugs prove less effective in conversion of flutter, but electrocardioversion is effective 95 percent of the time. Many of those who don't convert to normal rhythm revert to atrial fibrillation and are treatable as such.

The only person in my experience who died during a planned conversion of an abnormal atrial rhythm, did so from the drug given prior to the actual administration of the electric shock—and not from the electro-cardioversion itself. She had a **flutter**. She was middle-aged and had no known heart disease. She was in a cardiac care unit and had been given an intravenous injection of the anti-arrhythmic, **lidocaine**, prior to the planned electro-cardioversion.

Upon administering the drug, her most vital functions instantly stopped, including her heart and breathing; she immediately became unconscious. Her heartbeat and circulation were restored a minute later, but she never regained consciousness. She died within a week. We found that it was the result of a rare type of hypersensitivity to the lidocaine.

After electro-cardioversion caught on, it wasn't long before doctors regarded the treatment issue as a question of drug conversion versus electro-cardioversion. This debate failed to address the main problem. The first thing to determine was whether the benefits from restoring sinus rhythm were worth the risks from attempting any type of cardioversion. If the heart was moderately to markedly enlarged, I would not risk the attempt at cardioversion, either with drugs or electrically.

I would tell patients and teach students that while atrial fibrillation is a second choice, it can be an acceptable choice and an acceptable condition. It has taken 25 years for this to become a standard recommendation supported by a number of studies. Nonetheless, some doctor purists today still do not accept this viewpoint and it remains controversial.

CHAPTER 35

I'd Rather Die than Go Back on It

The third post-World War II technical innovation that saved lives through the correction of heart-rhythm problems was the implantable pacemaker. This device, made available for practical use in the 1960s, provides electrical control and pacing of an abnormally slow heartbeat. Temporary pacing was done via a catheter threaded through a vein and into the heart. By the 1970s, small battery packs implanted under the skin allowed permanent pacing through such a catheter.

As a medical resident in the 1940s, I had patients with no known heart disease whose heart would gradually become very slow but maintain a normal, steady rhythm. The available heart stimulant **epinephrine**, given intravenously, would speed the rate to normal, but this was only temporary. Drug resistance would usually develop. Also, we didn't have equipment that could deliver an intravenous drip of much less than one milliliter at a time. The result was that we delivered too much fluid into the body, overloading the heart and lungs, and in essence, drowning was often the result.

In 1954, an external cardiac pacemaker first became available. It partially helped address the problem of very slow heart rates.

At that time, a middle-aged man named Ralph was sent to Pennsylvania Hospital from Scranton with episodes of a slowing heart rate that occurred constantly, as often as several times per minute. This had been going on for weeks, and it was worsening.

Whenever his heart rate fell below 18 beats per minute, one-fourth of the normal rate, Ralph would lose consciousness. He would regain consciousness after the rate rose spontaneously to more than 18 beats per minute.

"Every time this happens," he said, "I feel like I'm dying."

Ralph's doctors in Scranton had him purchase the first commercially available external pacemaker at a price of $350. This *early device delivered a small electric shock to the heart through the skin of the chest wall. The rate was adjustable. However, no matter where the skin electrode contacts were placed on the chest, the chest muscles would contract painfully. If Ralph needed the pacemaker for any length of time, he would require a narcotic for the pain.*

When he arrived at Pennsylvania Hospital, we asked Ralph, "Did you bring the pacemaker?"

"No!"

"Why not?"

"I'd rather die than go back on it."

And that's what eventually happened.

We tried every accepted drug treatment available to speed up his heart rate. By the end of the first week, after every conventional approach had failed, we were able to convince Ralph to send for the pacemaker. We put it back on him and gave him painkilling medication.

*Knowing he couldn't tolerate lengthy use of the device, we explored other, less conventional approaches. Dr. Sam Bellet, a cardiologist at Graduate and Philadelphia General Hospitals, had found that a **one-molar lactate solution** given intravenously would speed up the heart rate. It did so in Ralph, but only for a few days when he began to require increasingly larger amounts.*

When he became terminal, I began giving him the lactate solution through a needle directly into a heart chamber. This worked for awhile but proved increasingly ineffective. The same thing happened with the increasingly strong injections of epinephrine. During all of this, he was unconscious and under heavy sedation.

Despite all of our efforts over several weeks, Ralph's condition progressively deteriorated. With his heart rate slowing more and more, it finally stopped permanently.

Autopsy failed to reveal the cause of his heart condition. Coronary artery disease was not significant. As no specific cardiac condition could be found, the chances were excellent that, had implantable pacemakers been available, he would have lived for many more years.

—ᴍ—

Rosario became a patient of mine in 1970. At age 72, he reported that his heart rate had been around 40 beats per minute for the past six years.

One summer afternoon, while body surfing the waves of Atlantic City, New Jersey, he rode one in, stood up, and passed out. He then came to and got up, dressed, walked a mile to the bus depot, and rode a bus to Center City, Philadelphia. He walked alone for nearly a mile to Pennsylvania Hospital, without any adverse effects.

Permanent, implantable pacemakers had just become available, and Rosario was a good candidate for one. He accepted this.

The new devices required the passage of a small catheter through a vein into the heart and up against the heart wall. The other end of the catheter was attached to a flat battery pack, and the regular electric impulse stimulated the heart to beat at a predetermined rate. The pack was implanted under the skin and attached to the pectoral muscle under the collar bone.

Heart block is the most common mechanism that causes slow rates. The heart impulses arise normallys, but half or less actually get through from the atrium to stimulate the ventricular pumping chambers. When the blockage is total, it is called complete heart block. The natural rate of the ventricle is under 40 beats per minute.

The cause of heart block is usually not apparent, as only about one in four is associated with arteriosclerosis. Severe, acute rheumatic fever, as well as childhood infectious diseases, can cause heart block. Other infections can also be the cause. I have seen a community epidemic of a viral infection cause severe heart block in three young adults who seemed to only have a mild cold. One died of **myocarditis**, which is an inflammation of the heart muscle, shortly after the onset of the heart block.

A lifelong risk of heart block can result from **diphtheria**. Even though the incidence of diphtheria is low, there are still sporadic cases yearly. For my new patients, I always included a query about diphtheria in my litany of questions concerning past illnesses. As late as the 1980s, four out of five patients I saw with complete heart block said they'd had diphtheria as a child.

One 40-year-old patient named Frances would wake up with no heart block and a normal rhythm. As the day progressed and she became fatigued, however, the heart block would set in and get progressively worse until it became a high, second-degree block with the heart rate at 40 beats per minute.

Frances had a severe case of chicken pox as a child and was in bed for three months. She developed the slow heart rate at age 20. The late-day symptoms of fatigue, chest pain, and shortness of breath began at age 30. Still, she was able to engage in hard physical labor such as building a stone wall without symptoms. She had no coronary artery disease.

In a treadmill test, her ventricular rate and pulse would not increase above 110 beats per minute, while her atrial rate would rise to 180 per minute, due to the block. Frances finally agreed to treatment with a permanent, indwelling, cardiac pacemaker. This cured her progressive late-day fatigue.

—ᴍ—

Heart medications such as digitalis as well as other non-heart medications can cause heart block.

*Luke was 80-years old when he was admitted to the Hospital because of a complaint of shortness-of-breath. This had not changed, despite several weeks of treatment in the Veterans Administration Hospital two months earlier. He had a severely leaking mitral valve, which was from a marked **mitral valve prolapse**.*

Atypically, Luke's shortness-of-breath was present at rest, but not when he climbed a flight of stairs, which he could do without stopping. At rest, his heart rate often fell below 50 beats per minute. His shortness-of-breath improved with activity when his heart rate rose to above 60 per minute.

*Several months prior to Luke's first hospitalization, he'd been placed on **Timoptic eye drops** for his **glaucoma**. This is a **beta blocker** that can slow the heart rate excessively when it is systemically* *absorbed, as it can be in an occasional eye patient. When the eye drops were stopped, his shortness-of-breath at rest disappeared.*

The shortness-of-breath returned, however, about a year later when another ophthalmologist at the Veterans Administration failed to note in his record that the beta blocker eye drops were prohibited. Again, upon changing the eye drops, Luke improved. He continued to do fairly well for about three years, when the shortness-of-breath developed again. This time it appeared upon exertion, not at rest, and was from heart weakness caused by the worsening leaky valve.

Luke was readmitted to the Hospital, where he had a mitral valve replacement. Immediately after the surgery, he developed excessive slowing of his heart rate to 42 beats per minute due to a complete heart block. This time, he was given a permanent pacemaker.

—৩৩—

Implantable pacemakers and other devices for treating rhythm irregularities are very valuable, life-saving innovations. They must, however, be applied only after considering the patient's entire condition. The myopia suffered by some specialists, however, forces them to rigidly apply the rules indicating the use of these devices—without regard for the individual patient. This can lead to unintended and disastrous results.

In addition to helping correct slowed heart rates, the implantable pacemaker proved helpful in treating other types of rhythm disturbances.

In the mid-1960s, Gilbert showed up at the Hospital for evaluation of frequent episodes of rapid heartbeat from ventricular tachycardia, a potentially fatal arrhythmia. The episodes had started at age 35 while playing tennis, and he was now in his early 40s. They always spontaneously reverted to normal.

Gil was quite intense. He played two golf balls in every round, and ran between shots. He carried a golf bag that contained only three clubs so he could run faster. He traveled a great deal on business and, given his condition, was known by the personnel in many emergency rooms around the country.

Gil's heart catheterization showed normal coronary arteries. During treadmill tests, with the increased heart rate, his episodes of tachycardia decreased in frequency. We found that this was also true when a temporary, artificial pacemaker was used to maintain his heartbeat over 70 per minute. Based on this result, we put in a permanent pacemaker.

Over time, Gil was evaluated at many prestigious centers, one of which removed the pacemaker, as it was no longer effective in reducing his tachycardia. Still alive 35 years later, he received a heart transplant and remains very active 10 years after that.

In the intervening decades since the introduction of the first implantable pacemakers, other similar electrical devices for correction of rhythm disturbances have been introduced. Since the mid-1980s, life-threatening arrhythmias have been treatable with the **implanted cardiac defibrillator**. The device is placed under the skin of the chest or abdomen, along with a battery pack. Wires are attached to the inside of the heart by way of the veins. The defibrillator detects serious rhythm irregularities and restores the heart rhythm to normal by delivering an electric shock to the heart.

The defibrillators are placed in individuals with a high propensity for these potentially fatal episodes. Curiously, according to several reports, in the first year and a half of use, no defibrillation shock was triggered by a potentially fatal rhythm disturbance. This again raises the issue of psychological and neurogenic effects on the heart's susceptibility to rhythm disturbances. Subsequently, the defibrillators have proven to be of great value and have prolonged many lives.

Over the years, the entire field of rhythm-disturbance treatment has been too focused on the arrhythmia and the heart alone, without regard for the patient's overall circumstances. This emphasizes the importance of individualizing and personalizing care.

World-class athletes and others in top physical condition are notorious for their slow heart rates, which often are below 50 or even 40 beats per minute at rest. This is not necessarily a manifestation of disease, even though the average normal heart rate is 72 beats per minute.

Some years ago, I was reading the electrocardiograms of Pennsylvania Hospital patients along with a resident. A normal preoperative tracing, which is the printout that shows the electrical activity of the heart, appeared in the pile to be interpreted. The heart rate shown on this tracing was 36 beats per minute.

The resident took one look at it and immediately said, "Should we put in a pacemaker?"

He knew nothing about the patient. Had the resident looked at the name, he would have recognized that it was that of a star on the Philadelphia Flyer's Stanley Cup hockey team. Superstar athletes have super-slow heart rates. The patient continued to play vigorous hockey for many years without requiring a pacemaker.

On the other hand, if the heart rate in a patient with a heart abnormality is below 60 beats per minute and this causes symptoms such as dizziness or fainting, then a treatment to increase the rate to more than 60 beats per minute is indicated. This is best done with an implanted artificial pacemaker.

Implantable pacemakers and other devices for treating rhythm irregularities are very valuable, life-saving innovations. They must, however, be applied only after considering the patient's entire condition. The myopia suffered by some specialists, however, forces them to rigidly apply the rules indicating the use of these devices—without regard for the individual patient. This can lead to unintended and disastrous results.

CHAPTER 36

Overstated Promises

Overall, the many technological improvements in medicine introduced since the middle of the 20th century, have been marvelous in providing greater health and happiness. This includes valuable test methods, life-saving devices, and the science of new drug development.

Certain innovations, however, have been introduced prematurely, and the promise they offer frequently has been overstated and oversold. The data about medical equipment usefulness from the laboratory and sales departments of manufacturers, generally has been overly optimistic for most new medical equipment.

The batteries of the first permanent pacemakers, as one example, were claimed to last six to 12 months. They lasted three months. The next generation of pacemaker batteries was supposed to last 12 to 18 months, but they only lasted six to 12 months. The 18 to 24 month models lasted 18 months. So it has gone with most types of medical equipment over the years.

Also, with medical equipment in general, as it improves, indications for its use broadens. It is used earlier and earlier in the disease on more and more people, many of whom don't need it. The cost per unit may fall, but the overall expenditure in the use of the equipment goes up.

These technical innovations have saved countless lives and have dramatically improved individual quality of life as well as overall life expectancy. But these improvements come with a price tag, and it's important to keep this in mind when evaluating the potential future directions in healthcare.

One of the themes throughout all of these technological improvements has been the shift in emphasis they have created, from the physician's personal care for the patient, to a focus on test results and the use of complex new procedures. The focus should not be on the medical technology itself. Even while implementing new technologies, physicians should apply them and interpret results only in light of individual patient situations. These include personal understanding, expectations, and biases.

PART IV

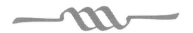

Advances in Art and Science

CHAPTER 37

The Individual versus the Herd

Fifty years ago, heart disease caused more deaths than the next 10 most common causes of death combined. Over the past 30 years, deaths from heart disease have declined, and since 2000, deaths have fallen by 4 percent to 5 percent each year. Nonetheless, heart disease still remains the most common cause of death today.

During the last half century, progress in diagnosis, treatment, and prevention of heart disease illustrates the interplay of new technology and the individualization of care. The resultant medical advances have saved many lives and improved the quality of lives for many others.

The progress comes at a cost, however. The medical community's shift in focus—from personal care to technological applications—has resulted in a decline in the quality of care in many ways.

The changes in care of heart patients during the latter half of the 20th century provides a microcosm of both the positive and negative impacts of technology. In some situations, advances in the science of medicine seriously complicate and challenge the art.

CHAPTER 38

Cholesterol and Clots

Atherosclerosis is a disease that narrows the arteries providing blood to the heart muscle and other organs. Two major theories as to the cause of atherosclerosis originated in the 19th century. One proposed that cholesterol deposits are the major culprits. The other theory was that blood clotting caused the vessel damage. Both are true, and the two theories were combined toward the end of the 20th century.

Atherosclerosis starts with inflammation of the artery lining. The blockage of the arteries, which can happen suddenly or over time, impairs the function of various organs and parts of the body. In the brain, this causes strokes. In the toes and feet, it can cause **gangrene**.

A blockage of the coronary arteries in the heart is the most common cause of heart disease. The heart may react so as to cause six different clinical manifestations, called "syndromes."

First, **angina pectoris**, or chest pain, and its equivalents are caused by gradual, incomplete blockages of the coronary arteries.

Second, **acute myocardial infarction**, or "heart attack," occurs when the flow in a coronary artery is completely blocked and the tissues nourished by that artery die. Myocardial infarction is the most common cause of death from atherosclerosis. The sudden onset of persistent chest pain is the most readily recognized and dreaded symptom of an acute myocardial infarction. When the damaged tissue heals, a scar forms.

Third, the **acute coronary syndrome** can be caused by the sudden episodic partial or complete closure of an artery, with or without muscle death.

Fourth, **congestive heart failure** eventually results from the heart muscle weakening over time.

Fifth, **heart enlargement** is caused by the gradual weakening of the heart muscle.

Sixth, **arrhythmias**, or irregularity of the heartbeat, can complicate any of these conditions. If this arrhythmia is ventricular fibrillation and is not immediately treated, it is fatal.

With dramatic advances in the scientific understanding of these and other aspects of heart disease, significant life-saving and life-prolonging treatments, as well as more specialized technical procedures, became possible. While progress in the management of the individual with these diseases improved, reliance on technology was beginning to supplant the all-important personal relationship between the doctor and patient, especially in the realm of chronic disease and prevention.

Chapter 39

The Killer in Disguise

Angina pectoris comes from the temporary reduction of blood flow to the heart muscle, and is a symptom generally thought to be "chest pain." It appears upon excess exertion or with excitement. As one might suspect, this pain can also be the initial symptom of an acute myocardial infarction.

In its classical form, angina pectoris is a severe constricting pain in the area of the breast bone. Unlike the persistent pain of myocardial infarction, the pain of true angina pectoris subsides in minutes. When it doesn't, a nitroglycerine tablet placed under the tongue relieves the pain rapidly. A number of other medications can readily prevent angina pectoris from occurring.

Many other symptoms are equivalent to the pain from angina pectoris. Patients will refer to these as a "squeezing," "pressure," "burning," or "aching" sensation anywhere in the area of the breast bone or on the left side of the chest. Like the pain of angina pectoris, all of these symptoms will end in minutes after stopping the exertion or calming the emotions.

The symptoms from sudden inadequacy of coronary artery blood flow often appear in forms and guises other than the chest pain of typical angina pectoris. It can be different in each individual.

Heart pain can be referred to unusual locations such as the wrists, arms, neck, lower jaw, upper abdomen, or even over the liver. This makes diagnosing any unusual complaints of body pains much more complicated and challenging.

The left arm is notorious as a site to which heart pain is referred. I found this to be true until my last 25 years of practice, when I found that the heart was not the most likely cause of the pain in the left arm. In fact, I had come to find that it was the least frequent cause of pain in that area of the body.

Pain that resembles angina pectoris but arises from parts of the body other than the heart poses a challenge to the examining physician. Spinal and muscular conditions in the left neck and shoulder that have nothing to do with heart disease can be referred to the left chest and arm. In these instances, thumb pressure applied between the vertebrae of the lower neck may elicit the same left-chest pain.

On one occasion, a middle-aged man was brought in by ambulance with sirens screeching and a lot of bustle. He was at a filling station when a high wind blew a light pole down, striking the top of his left shoulder. He was having severe pain over his left chest and was thought to be having a heart attack.

His blood pressure and heart rate were normal, and he had a normal electrocardiogram. He had no broken bones, but the area above his left clavicle was tender. Compression of the spot reproduced his chest pain. It had nothing to do with his heart.

In addition to pain from orthopedic sources, pain in the upper gastrointestinal track can also be referred to the left shoulder and arm. I've been able to reproduce this pain in some patients by abdominal **palpation**. I had one woman with such pain swallow a tube with a balloon at the end, which I positioned in her upper intestine. Its sudden expansion produced pain that spread from the upper abdomen, over the left chest, and into the left arm, reproducing her complaint.

—\\\—

Occasionally, chest-wall sensitivity comes from **hyperventilation** due to lung disease or other condition that is not related to impaired heart-muscle circulation. One middle-aged man, for example, was awakened frequently in the middle of the night by severe pain in the region of his heart. He had a trigger point at the tip of his left shoulder blade that was stimulated by over-breathing when lying flat during sleep. This pain was reproducible by applying thumb pressure over the area. The pain was abolished by injection of a local anesthetic into the tender spot.

On another occasion, I saw a middle-aged woman who had a chronically abnormal electrocardiogram with deeply inverted T-waves in the leads over the heart. Normally, the T-waves are upright. This abnormality is usually a very reliable indication of heart-muscle disease. But she also had a tender spot at the tip of her left shoulder blade. The injection of a local anesthetic in the tender spot normalized her electrocardiogram within 15 minutes. This electrocardiographic response, suggesting a neurological relationship between the chest wall and the heart, was unique in my experience.

—⟋⟋⟋—

Symptoms from other heart conditions are often mistakenly thought to be caused by acute coronary artery insufficiency. For example, pain over the heart can be caused by **pericarditis**, an inflammation of the sac around the heart. This pain can be as severe as that from an acute myocardial infarction. In older individuals who are more apt to have hardening of the arteries, this can present more of a problem in diagnosis than in a young person.

*As a consultant at the Richards-Gebaur Air Force Base near Kansas City, I saw a 20-year-old airman on active duty who had pain over his heart of such severity that his breathing was impaired. He actually turned blue from lack of oxygen. I sprayed **ethylene**, a cooling agent used as a local anesthetic, on the skin over the heart area.*

This relieved his chest pain enough so that he could take deep breaths. Soon, he lost his blue color. This gave us the time needed to inject the area with a longer-acting local anesthetic, which in turn provided relief until anti-inflammation pills for his pericarditis could take effect.

The symptoms from sudden inadequacy of coronary artery blood flow often appear in forms and guises other than the chest pain of typical angina pectoris. It can be different in each individual. Physicians need to be aware of these many variations so as not to be misled. They then can order the required diagnostic testing so an early, potentially life-saving diagnosis of myocardial infarction can be made.

CHAPTER 40

I Went Outside and Ran Around the House

Myocardial infarction is a potentially fatal condition. If diagnosed and treated quickly, death can be prevented and the amount of heart damage limited. If correctly recognized, the treatment is relatively straightforward. In as many as half of all patients, however, the symptoms are not typical. This challenges the physician to recognize and correctly diagnose the potentially fatal condition.

When the physician overlooks the possibility of atypical presentation of symptoms, the risk of death greatly increases. One out of three men with acute myocardial infarctions, and as many as half of all women with this condition, go undiagnosed.

Until the 1960s, the diagnosis of myocardial infarction was based on the combination of symptoms, electrocardiographic changes, and non-specific blood tests indicating the appearance of inflammation from the death of heart muscle.

A large proportion of myocardial infarctions, however, do not result in any changes in the electrocardiograms. In the latter half of the 1950s, of the 100 successive acute myocardial infarction patients who were autopsied at Pennsylvania Hospital, only 62 had new electrocardiographic changes of any type. This included all of those with even slight and nonspecific abnormalities. Only 33 had electrocardiographic changes typical of recent heart-muscle damage. And only 25 of these 33 had developed new Q-waves, which is the classic diagnostic change.

The blood tests available at the time to determine whether recent heart muscle damage had occurred were nonspecific. A rising abnormal **red-blood cell sedimentation rate** and an increasing **white-blood cell count**, which are nonspecific measures of inflammation in the body, were of some assistance.

Since the end of the 1950s, blood tests have been developed for muscle enzymes leaking from newly damaged heart muscle. In time, these tests became increasingly more specific for heart-muscle death from myocardial infarction.

For any of these new tests to be helpful, a high index of suspicion for recent heart damage was required, so that the proper diagnostic tests could be performed. The following two cases illustrate some of the problems presented when a diagnosis had to be based upon clinical symptoms and physical findings alone.

—ɯ—

During my medical school preceptorship, Paul was admitted to Sacred Heart Hospital. He was middle-aged, complaining of the sudden onset of severe chest pain. We thought the pain was from a myocardial infarction. The chest pain eased, then began to recur intermittently, gradually shifting from the chest to the upper abdomen. Paul's electrocardiogram was abnormal but not diagnostic of an infarction. The physical examination did not change.

A week later, Paul died suddenly. His autopsy revealed a ruptured dissecting aneurysm. The inner layer of the aorta had broken open and split the vessel into two tubes, one inside the other. Then, as is usual with this condition, the aneurysm had ruptured into the chest cavity. He immediately bled to death.

An early diagnosis would not have helped Paul, as no treatment was available for an aneurysm at that time. Today, when properly diagnosed, aneurysms can be cured by surgery, but the diagnosis is often missed because atypical features are common.

A year later, during my internship, I had a similar but even more confounding experience. Quentin was middle-aged when he was admitted to Research Hospital with severe chest pain suspected to be a heart attack. The electrocardiogram was abnormal, but once again it was not that of a typical heart attack.

Over the following week, Quentin had recurrent chest pain, then abdominal pain. When the pulses in his groin disappeared and then reappeared in several days, while maintaining normal blood pressure, we were sure that he had an aneurysm that was dissecting the aorta from his chest to his groin.

Quentin died suddenly the second week. To our surprise, the autopsy revealed that he had no dissecting aneurysm. Instead, he had experienced an extensive myocardial infarction.

Newer technology would have allowed a precise diagnosis to be made, but even today, the diagnostic possibility must be considered so that the appropriate tests are conducted.

When the physician overlooks the possibility of atypical presentation of symptoms, the risk of death greatly increases. One out of three men with acute myocardial infarctions, and as many as half of all women with this condition, go undiagnosed.

—ᴠᴠ—

Not only do physical manifestations of acute myocardial infarction vary greatly among patients, but so do the patients' reactions to the symptoms. Some walk through it, barely noticing it, and others are sick for weeks or months. The patient's reaction to the symptoms can affect the outcome of the condition, too.

In 1952, Bjorn came to see me during my temporary practice in Baron, Wisconsin. He was having a myocardial infarction. He refused to go to the hospital and insisted on going back home to his farm, which was a short distance out of town. He promised to stay in bed.

I visited Bjorn at his home a few days later. He was up, dressed, and moving about. My examination revealed no complication, but again I urged Bjorn to stay in bed. I'm sure he didn't follow these directions, as two days later he died suddenly at home.

—ᴠᴠ—

At that time, about half of the patients with heart attacks were not hospitalized. The frequent failure to reduce activity at home was one reason patients were encouraged to stay in a hospital bed until healing could take place.

A few years later, the dire results of the refusal to follow directions was again vividly demonstrated by George, whom I saw in the Medical Clinic at Pennsylvania Hospital. His symptoms and tests were diagnostic of an acute myocardial infarction. Despite urging by a number of staff physicians, nurses, and administrators, he was adamant in his refusal to come into the hospital. He said he would do anything else I asked.

He lived a block away, so I asked that he stay in his apartment and come in to see me at the hospital daily. I thought he might soon accept hospital admission.

He came in daily. First, his heart became progressively larger. Then it became weaker and weaker. Gradually, despite treatment, excess fluid from heart failure was retained by his body. Then, his heart rhythm became irregular. Despite these accumulating complications, he still refused hospitalization.

A week after his heart attack, the police found him dead on the sidewalk in Washington Square. He was found on a route going away from his home, in a direction that was opposite that of the Hospital—so George was apparently still venturing out to other places despite his serious heart condition.

In the 1950s, nine out of ten patients with a myocardial infarction who were not admitted to the hospital immediately, but were admitted one to two weeks later, died. They had complications of an enlarged heart, very low blood pressure, and heart failure. This figure had not changed by the 1970s despite advances in treatment. Complications, including death, are reduced the earlier people experiencing a heart attack are put to bed. They also do better when they are mobilized early.

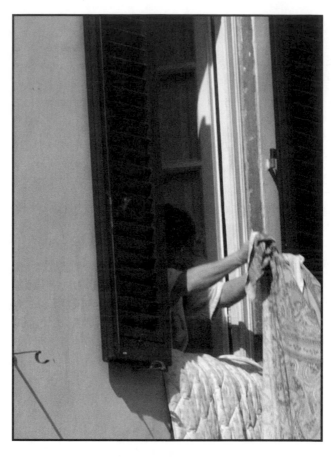

Doris, a 56-year-old Dutch housewife from the Allentown, Pennsylvania area, had another very unusual reaction to a myocardial infarction. Doris was in the hospital because of severe chest pain that she was experiencing for several months. Her problem had started six months earlier when she walked nearly a mile up a slight grade and developed a diffuse ache over her chest and into her arms. The pain disappeared rapidly upon resting. It was typical heart pain. Then it got worse.

"What happened?" I asked.

"I was working hard shaking linens out the window, when it came on," Doris explained. "For two days, I continued to work

hard, and the pain would come and go. Finally, it got so severe that my doctor had to come by and give me a shot."

"Did he send you to the hospital?"

"No."

"What did you do then?"

"After a couple more days, I decided to quit babying myself. I went outside and ran around the house. I then came back in, ran up the stairs, and took a shower. I was suddenly very exhausted."

Since then, she said she had remained exhausted and a different type of chest pain had set in.

Examination of her heart led to an extraordinary finding. At the side of her left chest, between two ribs, a visible bulge appeared with each heart beat. I asked her to take a deep breath and try to expel the air without letting it out, as if lifting something heavy.

Doris did so, and the bulge enlarged alarmingly.

An electrocardiogram showed that Doris had had a severe myocardial infarction. Fluoroscopic examination showed a prominent bulge protruding from the left border of her heart. With each heartbeat, it expanded instead of contracting as is normal.

Doris's heart attack had torn open her heart wall and ruptured the heart. The pericardial sac, a thin wall around the heart, had prevented it from bleeding into her chest cavity and killing her instantly. It was the pain from the irritation of the sac that had caused the new type of pain she experienced later in the episode.

She gradually improved on treatment with medications and had no more chest pain. Finally, more than 10 years later, she agreed to have the aneurismal bulge in her heart surgically corrected. This was done without complication. She not only had a high tolerance for pain, but also for risk. Ironically, during her delay in receiving surgery, the surgical risk had decreased considerably.

CHAPTER 41

I Just Felt Lousy

Heart disease without typical symptoms, combined with symptoms from other illnesses, can cause a myriad of complications that can seem unrelated to the heart. These complexities provide a great challenge to the physician in recognizing a cardiac connection, so that appropriate testing can be performed. Only through practical experience does a physician learn to recognize the many variations that lead to a diagnosis of heart disease versus other illnesses.

Insufficient blood flow to the heart during exertion weakens the heart, which in turn causes reduced blood flow to the various other parts of the body. Pain or other symptoms may appear in that part of the body. Most commonly, these symptoms appear during exertion as dizziness or even fainting, indigestion, cramping in the lower abdomen with an urge to move the bowels, aching in the legs, or pain in the lower back.

In many patients, the onset or worsening of coronary insufficiency or even an acute myocardial infarction goes unrecognized, because the symptoms are so atypical or mild that neither the patient nor the physician thinks they are related to the heart. This problem is part of the explanation for the failure to recognize the one-third to one-half of myocardial infarctions that go undiagnosed.

In the early 1960s, based on my patients, I suspected that thousands of teeth throughout the country were mistakenly removed annually because of heart pain referred to the lower jaw. Gall bladder disease has been one of the more notorious misdiagnoses of heart disease. "It's just indigestion from something I ate," I would hear. Over the years in the Philadelphia region, I have found that the most common misdiagnosis of heart disease was a "chest cold" or "the flu."

On occasion, I've examined a new patient with an electrocardiogram showing the typical pattern of a healed scar on the heart, and the patient denies that he or she has ever had a myocardial infarction. In most of these cases, detailed questioning would elicit an account of some other illness, which the individual usually regarded as a cold or the flu. Sometimes the patient would have had gallbladder surgery or some other major medical intervention.

These were actually the accounts of the acute infarction episodes. The episodes were atypical in that they were more severe and it took longer for them to recover. Coincidence was unlikely. I was never able to get this type of history from patients with other types of new electrocardiogram abnormalities, confirming the connection between the other reported illnesses and the acute infarctions indicated on the electrocardiograms.

One such case came under my care when a colleague referred a 68-year-old attorney to my office for an electrocardiogram as part of a check-up. Steve's electrocardiogram showed that he was recovering from a fairly recent myocardial infarction, which had occurred just a few weeks earlier.

"Do you recall any pain or discomfort in the chest or stomach recently?" I asked him.

Steve shook his head. "No."

The physician's personal knowledge of a patient helps in the recognition of atypical illnesses that may not be what they seem. The advantages offered by technology cannot be properly utilized without this type of personal insight. The alternative of applying batteries of unnecessary tests to all patients is not only prohibitively expensive, but also leads to diagnoses that may be premature and may therefore result in unnecessary treatments.

"Any grabbing in your chest? Dizziness?"

"I don't remember anything like that," he said.

I couldn't determine exactly when his attack had happened. He did recall a cold about three months earlier and a sore throat about nine months before, both too long ago to have been the infarction episode.

As his myocardial infarction was uncomplicated and was healing, hospitalization was not necessary. I asked him to come back a week later.

During that second visit, he said he had recalled an unusual weekend about six weeks earlier. "I felt lousy," he said.

"How so?"

"I just felt lousy. I spent the entire weekend in bed."

This was completely out of character for him, he admitted. In fact, he said, the following Monday morning, he felt so bad that he took his first day off from work in many years.

Steve was a bachelor who lived with his elderly mother. His room was on the second floor and it had a separate entrance in the rear of the house. So as not to alarm his mother, he woke up that Monday morning and got ready for work as usual. He went downstairs, bid his mother goodbye, and went out the front door. He then sneaked around to the rear entrance, where he went up to his room and back to bed.

"The next morning," he said, "I awoke feeling great and went to work as usual. I feel great now."

Sudden, extreme fatigue is one way a myocardial infarction presents in some patients. Even though he did not admit any heart pain, I put him on a long-acting oral nitroglycerin medication.

A month later, Steve returned.

"How are you feeling?" I asked him.

"A lot better."

"But you said you were feeling great a month ago, too, even before I gave you the pills."

"Yes, but I feel even better since I'm on them."

"How is that?"

He waved his hands fleetingly across the front of his chest. Finally, he admitted, "I just feel lighter."

Steve did well for four months after I first saw him. He then came in for another visit.

"I don't feel well," he complained.

Knowing of his high tolerance to severe illness, I took this very seriously. Again, he had no specific pain or cardio-respiratory symptoms.

His physical examination did not reveal anything abnormal. His electrocardiogram had not changed. But blood tests showed that his creatinine was more than 4.0 milligrams per deciliter. Normal is less than 1.4 milligrams per deciliter. He was in kidney failure.

I hospitalized him.

Pursuit of his history in greater depth revealed that every morning he would awaken at about 5:00 a.m. with an urgent need to move his bowels, which he did at least a half-dozen times over the next hour. The stools were profuse and watery. Diarrhea is dehydrating and can deplete blood volume, which in turn can cause kidney failure.

Further probing revealed that his lady friend to whom he had been engaged for 15 years was pressuring him to get married now. He said he was depressed about this. Early awakening can be a symptom of depression.

So I prescribed a bedtime antidepressant. This cured his depression, which in turn ended the daily bouts of diarrhea and corrected his kidney failure.

—w—

A large number of my patients had an element of depression as the primary or a contributory cause of symptoms. As mentioned earlier, during one period of my practice, I actually found that I was helping more people with antidepressant medications than with cardiac medications.

The patient who presents with a new set of symptoms or abnormalities may readily suggest what he or she thinks is the cause. Often this is not the actual problem. As the old saying goes, "Things are not always what they seem."

To be most competent, the physician needs to maintain what we refer to as a "high index of suspicion," so that proper testing and diagnosis can be made. Finding the proper treatment depends upon this.

The physician's personal knowledge of a patient helps in the recognition of atypical illnesses that may not be what they seem. The advantages offered by technology cannot be properly utilized without this type of personal insight. The alternative of applying batteries of unnecessary tests to all patients is not only prohibitively expensive, but also leads to diagnoses that may be premature and may therefore result in unnecessary treatments.

CHAPTER 42

Ice Cream at Bedtime

Prior to 1950, a greater number of acute myocardial infarctions went unrecognized compared to today. Many people from these earlier years who were suffering from a heart attack never went to a hospital or saw a physician.

Part of the problem, even today, is that less than half of patients having a myocardial infarction experience pain. They feel "a pressure," "an ache," "a burning," "a shortness of breath," or they use terms other than the word "pain." Some seem to believe that if it's not pain, it must not be related to the heart.

As of the 1940s, only those diagnosed with acute myocardial infarction with more severe pain were admitted to the hospital. The standard treatment was three to four weeks of bed rest during a five to six-week total stay at a hospital. It was believed that the lengthy rest period was necessary for the heart muscle to heal.

One problem with prolonged bed rest is that it also promotes the development of blood clots in leg veins. These tend to break off and float to the lungs as **emboli**, causing severe complications or death.

In the late 1940s, Irving Wright directed an uncontrolled, multiple-hospital study in which Pennsylvania Hospital participated. The study demonstrated that dicumarol, an oral anticoagulant or "blood thinner," reduced hospital mortality after myocardial infarction from 28 percent to 22 percent. The use of an oral anticoagulant requires daily monitoring because of the risk of bleeding. At the time, it was not known whether anticoagulants prevent only the leg-vein clotting, or whether they also help to reduce the clots in coronary arteries of the heart. Today, we know that anticoagulants are effective for both conditions.

At the time, many patients were being admitted to hospitals for the preventive treatment of blood clots that developed largely because they were in the hospital. This unappreciated paradox resulted in a greater number of hospitalizations and an increase in the cost of medical care over many decades.

Nitroglycerine was the most common treatment to relieve the pain of angina pectoris, but at that time it was contraindicated during and immediately after a myocardial infarction. In a few patients, it caused an excessive fall in blood pressure, which in turn created a risk of serious complications. Once the pharmacology of nitroglycerine and its use was better understood, and the drug was carefully administered and monitored, nitroglycerine was found to be more beneficial than harmful in the treatment of myocardial infarction.

—◊◊◊—

Many patients of that era required **narcotics** in high doses for several days.

In one case, a middle-aged man named Buerger suffered an acute myocardial infarction. Ironically, Mr. Buerger had **Buerger's disease***, a rare inflammatory condition of the arteries, yet the disease was not named for him.*

Mr. Buerger had pain that was so severe, he would keep scooting up in bed until he was sitting on top of the headboard. This seemed to be an attempt to rise above the pain.

Mr. Buerger received 20-times the usual dose of morphine intravenously. Still, it did not relieve the pain. He required large doses for days. Surprisingly, he did not become addicted.

Patients being treated with narcotics for heart pain over several weeks did run the risk of becoming addicted. This occurred with several of my patients when treated with the **opiate Pantopon** over a four-week period. In one patient, stopping the narcotic resulted in a full-blown withdrawal syndrome, which he survived.

—◊◊◊—

In many patients at that time, the failure to receive hospital care for an acute myocardial infarction was fatal. This was particularly true for those whose acute myocardial infarction was complicated by heart failure or very low blood pressure, and who were not admitted to the hospital until a week or more after the initial event.

As I would tell patients, "It's not a cure. It simply gives you a second chance to clean up your act." Permanent lifestyle changes are basic to the success of any treatment.

In part because of this type of experience, some doctors were fearful of letting a patient exert in any manner for several weeks after an acute myocardial infarction. Their patients weren't allowed to feed themselves. They weren't even allowed to hold a book to read.

Bowel management during this bed-rest period was a big issue. Patients had to use a bedpan. The theory was that it was less demanding on the heart than using a commode at the bedside. Later, tests showed that using a bedpan actually is more demanding and strenuous than using a bedside commode.

One doctor at Research Hospital in 1947 wouldn't even allow his patients to use a bedpan. They were supposed to have their bowel movements on newspapers slipped under their buttocks in bed. Neither the unaesthetic aspects nor the threat of complicating fecal impactions due to constipation seemed to bother the doctor at all.

—ᴍ—

In the late 1940s and early 1950s, the renowned Boston cardiologist Samuel Levin began treating selected patients by helping them out of the hospital bed and into a chair, shortly after acute myocardial infarction. They were not permitted to ambulate until sometime later.

By the late 1950s, bed rest and hospital time had been reduced by half in the Western US, compared to treatment in the Eastern US.

I defended the old, Eastern practice to my friend, Hal Braun, who was then practicing in Missoula, Montana. I pointed out that there was actually an increase in deaths after five to six weeks of hospital care, when patients were finally ambulated, according to the Irving Wright study and my own experience.

Hal's rejoinder was, "You're boring your patients to death by keeping them in bed so long!"

—⁂—

In the early 1960s, I studied **intravascular dynamics** on patients immediately after an acute infarction. It was evident that the cardio-circulatory function was maximally depressed 24 to 48 hours after the onset, but would improve by the end of the week.

Then, after the first week, the heart functions gradually deteriorated. This was caused by the prolonged bed rest, just as had been found in healthy people subjected to prolonged bed rest. The ongoing deterioration was not from the damage to the heart, unless the damage was extensive. These studies justified the shortening of the periods of bed rest. Today, patients with uncomplicated myocardial infarctions often are hospitalized for less than a week.

—⁂—

At the Kodak plant in Rochester, New York, under the supervision of Dr. Arthur Moss, the thousands of workers throughout the plant were trained to treat cardiac arrest. Sufferers were treated immediately and given bed rest early. Dr. Moss lamented that it did not reduce the overall incidence of sudden death there, given the many other causes. However, no employee died of acute infarction.

I suspect that they had been educated enough about the condition, so that even when away from work, they had learned to recognize and respond early to the manifestations of the onset of an acute myocardial infarction.

The conclusions that could be drawn from these experiences were supported by the accumulating medical evidence over the years. The sooner patients suffering an acute myocardial infarction are given treatment and bed rest, and the sooner they are mobilized and ambulated afterwards, the better they do.

—∾—

Changes in lifestyle to reduce risk factors are key to long-term success and for prevention of future illness, whether before or after a myocardial infarction or bypass surgery.

In the 1970s, coronary artery bypass surgery became widely available. In this procedure, the part of the artery clogged by atherosclerotic disease is bypassed by a blood vessel transplanted from another part of the body. The transplanted vessel connects the aorta to the coronary artery beyond the point of blockage. At first, a vein from the leg was used, then studies found that an artery from the wrist lasted longer.

Bypass surgery greatly improves heart symptoms, but does not treat the underlying causes of the atherosclerosis. In its early years, bypass surgery did not improve longevity over medical therapy alone, and it did not extend the 10-year time frame to recurrence of serious complications.

As I would tell patients, "It's not a cure. It simply gives you a second chance to clean up your act." Permanent lifestyle changes are basic to the success of any treatment.

By the 1980s, some studies demonstrated the benefits of surgery beyond mere symptomatic improvement, but this remained controversial. There has been a similar controversy in **angioplastic surgery** of the coronary arteries, which involves widening of an obstructed artery using a catheter. This device is threaded into the vessel through a femoral artery in the groin. The question remains whether it provides anything more than symptomatic relief.

One key reason for a failure in long-term improvement after bypass surgery or **angioplasty** is that most patients undergoing the surgery are after a "quick fix." They lose their symptomatic motivation to change their lifestyle, even though they may have received instructions on reducing the risk factors of the disease. When patients change their lifestyle after they have had coronary artery surgery, they do better in the long run than those who change their lifestyle with medical therapy alone and no surgery.

Before recommending patients for surgery, I insisted that they participate in their own care and change their living habits. I urged them to increase their activity levels, improve their diets, lose weight, and help manage their blood pressure, cholesterol, and blood sugar levels. And when they were smokers, they had to stop.

For those who participated in this type of regimen and also received medical therapy, the symptoms were greatly reduced. And for some, intensive medical therapy has actually been shown to reduce the degree of coronary artery blockage, which by-pass surgery cannot do.

In time, many patients would need surgery, but I found that for those who improved their lifestyle, this did not become necessary for 10, 15, or 20 years, or longer, even if their initial manifestation had been a myocardial infarction.

The elimination of symptoms, whether by surgery or medical therapy, often leads to complacency in adhering to the necessary risk-factor control measures. Some patients on medical therapy without a surgical procedure have a recurrence of angina after it has disappeared on treatment. Their bad habits return after they lose their symptomatic motivation.

Gerald's story is a good example of this. He came to see me with a recent onset of angina pectoris. I put him on medication, with some benefit. His main dietary indiscretion was eating a dish of ice cream at bedtime every night. After he stopped this, his angina pectoris disappeared within several months.

Two years later, Gerald's pain returned.

"Have you been taking your medicine regularly?"

"Yes."

"You haven't gone back to eating ice cream at bedtime, have you?"

"Well, yes. Sometimes," Gerald sheepishly admitted.

Adhering to lifestyle changes, especially those relating to diet and exercise, can be very difficult. Many patients have a hard time giving up what seem like harmless little pleasures, yet that can be the key to a healthy lifestyle.

The treatment of atherosclerotic heart disease varies according to each individual situation. And the physician needs to understand the patient and motivate him or her to participate in his or her own care. Changes in lifestyle to reduce risk factors are key to long-term success and for prevention of future illness, whether before or after a myocardial infarction or bypass surgery.

CHAPTER 43

A Choice or a Disease?

Risk factors for coronary heart disease are features that directly or indirectly cause or are related to the underlying atherosclerosis. Several risk factors cannot be changed, but most are controllable. Those that are not modifiable include age, sex, and genetic factors that may be reflected in family history.

Abnormal blood fats and cholesterol, **diabetes mellitus**, and hypertension are risk factors that can be genetic, but these can be aggravated by the secondary risk factors of excessive body weight and poor diet, both of which are controllable. These are now grouped together under the name of "**Metabolic Syndrome**."

Among the more important controllable risk factors are tobacco use and sedentarism. Exercise level, which is considered a tertiary risk factor, can help control many primary and secondary risk factors.

Most other risk factors are essentially minor. Many, such as the **C-reactive protein**, are determined by special blood tests only.

If the heart condition for which the lifestyle change is undertaken has improved, then there's the gradual tendency to resume the old bad habits instead of making the changes permanent. It seems that only a fortunate few are successful in permanently changing their habits.

Lifestyle changes are required to address the modifiable risk factors. When a physician regards the factors of a patient's lifestyle as a disease that requires specific treatment, the chance of controlling it is reduced to less than 10 percent. By regarding the lifestyle factors of smoking, sedentarism, diet, and weight mismanagement as controllable habits, the physician shifts the responsibility for treatment away from the physician back to the patient.

Patients want to believe that, "It's a genetic defect," "It's not my fault," and, "There must be a pill for it." This places the responsibility back onto the medical profession, and away from the patient.

Motivation to change one's lifestyle is generally weak until a life-altering event or a threatening complication develops. Even when a risk factor is modified, the change is difficult to maintain. If the heart condition for which the lifestyle change is undertaken has improved, then there's the gradual tendency to resume the old bad habits instead of making the changes permanent. It seems that only a fortunate few are successful in permanently changing their habits.

CHAPTER 44

Only Six Eggs a Day

Weight management is required for the control of obesity, which is second only to smoking as the most modifiable risk factor for atherosclerosis and its complications. Obesity, however, is viewed through a distorted glass, and it's hard for an overweight person to see the real problem clearly.

Because it has complications of medical significance, obesity has been regarded as a medical problem, and the medical field continues to seek solutions. People are only too eager to regard all obesity as a disease. They rationalize that it must be a genetic or metabolic problem that should be curable by a pill or surgery. This is true for some, but not for the majority of obese individuals. The medical model has failed miserably in its attempt to treat obesity primarily as a disease.

Obesity is strongly influenced by lifestyle and cultural factors, in addition to the metabolic factors. Obese friends are more likely to influence a person to become obese than a spouse or family member. Yet even within families, lifestyle and culture are important factors.

—⚭—

Over the years, most patients in my care who were still significantly overweight by age 80 didn't last long. But then there are always the exceptions.

*My last house call was in the early 1990s. Natalie was 90-years old, obese, and in fair health, except for **osteoarthritis**. She would fall down about once a month. She couldn't get up because of pain in her arthritic knees and weak arms.*

Natalie never broke a bone or hurt herself in the fall. She wore a cordless phone on her belt. When she fell, she'd lie on her back

*and call her sons to come and help her up. They worked only a
few minutes away.*

*While waiting for them, Natalie would call friends on the phone
and announce, "Well, I'm down. I'm waiting for the boys."*

—◠◠◠—

By and large, the problem of obesity is mostly one of lifestyle
and habit. Habit is a good term for it, as withdrawal from excess
food is not dissimilar to breaking a narcotic habit. But breaking
the habit is only the beginning, as this only treats a complication,
not the underlying condition. Why was the habit created in the
first place? Emotional issues such as depression often come into
play, as well as other factors, such as lifestyle changes that reduce
exercise and other activities.

A ball game is a good analogy. Just as the ball does not make
the ballplayer, the diet does not make the successful dieter. As in
sport, what makes for success in dieting is the determination in
playing the game.

Weight maintenance depends upon lifestyle and, if obese, a
change in lifestyle often requires as much effort as adapting to the
ways of a new life partner, a spouse. It's less about what you eat,
although this must decrease, than it is about how much you think
you eat.

Presumably, if overweight people eat like they should to
maintain the weight they want for the rest of their lives, they will
automatically reach that goal and stay there. This takes a while,
perhaps a year, even two years for some. Staying the course requires
determination and will power.

If you are completely satiated after a meal, you are probably
overeating. A day of satisfying eating once weekly can help reduce
the boredom of what may be regarded as a stringent diet without
significant damage to the dieting effort. But one must remember
that this style of eating is necessary to maintain the weight-loss.

What people are looking for is a pill that allows us to eat as much
as we want, whatever and whenever, while maintaining excellent

health, with no effort, pain, guilt, or cost. Dream on. While we do have surgical procedures that offer help today, some regard these procedures as mutilation.

—⚹—

In Independence, I had an unusual experience in attempting weight reduction with a drug not indicated for this purpose.

Roberta was a 27-year-old woman who weighed 270 pounds when she was admitted to the hospital under my care. She had collapsed, and proved to be very sick from a pulmonary embolism. This was a blood clot from the veins in her legs that had broken off and floated to the lung. Morbid obesity is a risk factor for this complication, and she had none of the other usual causes.

Atrial fibrillation was complicating her condition, so I gave her digitalis.

Several weeks after her hospital discharge, I saw Roberta in the office and stressed the need to lose weight. I knew that digitalis in excess is known to cause a loss of appetite, followed by nausea and vomiting when accumulating to toxic levels. I had always wondered if this could be used as a weight-loss drug to curb the appetite.

Roberta agreed to give it a try.

Over several weeks, I gradually increased her daily dose until it reached three times the usual dose. She was tolerating it well. After the fourth increase, I asked her to call me in a week to tell me how she was doing on it.

"Are you taking your pill every morning?" I asked.

"Yes, I haven't missed a dose."

"Does it bother you?"

"I do get sick to my stomach and vomit in an hour."

"How is your appetite the rest of the day? Are you eating any less?"

"No, I just vomit and then I go back to eating just as I usually do."

Digitalis is not an effective weigh-reduction treatment.

—⚏—

Another patient in Independence, Millie, came in to see me from a small town some 60 miles away. She was middle aged, 62-inches tall, and weighed 170 pounds. She said that she wanted to lose weight. This was a good opportunity to try another program I'd been thinking about. A high-fat diet suppresses the appetite by making the system acidic. This was a diet still used in the treatment of diabetes by some doctors at the time, for people who were reluctant to take insulin.

The foods of diabetic diets had long been listed by food groups. So I had her use the foods in the fat group with those in the green vegetable list. This would allow her to create a variety of salads to ease the dietary boredom.

Millie came in to see me every two or three weeks and was just melting away. Finally, as she was nearing 140 pounds, I said, "Tell me exactly what you eat every day."

"Well, for breakfast I eat two hard-boiled eggs. For lunch I eat two hard-boiled eggs. And for dinner I eat two hard-boiled eggs."

"Don't you eat anything else?"

"No."

So much for the variety provided by fancy salads, to say nothing of the unhealthful aspects of a diet consisting almost entirely of eggs. However, she suffered no obvious ill consequences from the diet. She undoubtedly was eating some other foods, but she wasn't admitting it.

—⚏—

Throughout my career, people would come into my consultation room, plunk themselves down sideways, wedging one cheek between the arms of the chair, and announce challengingly, "I want you to reduce me, Doctor."

I'd tell them, "I don't reduce you. You do the reducing yourself. But I'll give you all the help I can." I asked them to start keeping a diary of everything they ate.

I didn't care how fast they lost, but they had to weigh less every time they came in, which was monthly at first. If they didn't lose, I'd see them in three weeks, then two weeks, then weekly, and finally daily. They either lost weight or stopped coming to see me, wasting no more of their time or mine.

The classic story is that of the patient who has been placed on a diet but had gained weight with each visit to the office. When finally asked to keep a food diary, the patient says, "Wait, Doc, maybe I'm confused. Do I take my diet before or after I eat my regular meals?" No, I never actually heard a patient say this, but many patients seem to have this sentiment.

People's perception of themselves is what needs changing. When they are motivated and do change, they lose weight.

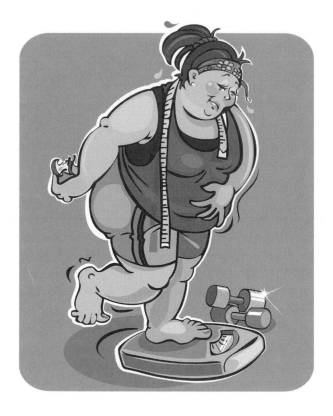

Maintaining weight reduction requires constant, lifelong attention. If you perceive this as "dieting," then dieting is forever. You must diet your whole life. And for most people, initially, if you're not hungry, not suffering, you're not dieting. You're eating too much.

There are certainly metabolic reasons that some people are obese, and there are promising medications in the drug pipeline. But until more is known about ways to modify the **appestat**, which is the internal mechanism that controls eating, there is no easy way. The various types of surgery available today are effective for some , but carry added risk.

People are impatient and easily discouraged. If you need to lose 50 pounds, then eating about 500 calories-a-day less than is required to stay at your current weight, will result in a reduction of approximately one pound per week without officially dieting. It will take one year to reach your goal.

The fast weight-loss that frequently occurs in the first two weeks is due to loss of water weight, or false weight. Actually, with a slow, real weight reduction, fluid retention may actually increase for six to eight weeks, and the scale will show no change or actually show an increase in weight. At that point, a marked loss of weight over two to four days will occur from a sudden loss of large amounts of fluid. The body weight then ends up where it was expected to be by calculation from the calorie deficit.

The failure to lose weight as expected while strictly following a diet can be very discouraging. This is the reason many doctors prescribe a diuretic to be taken during the first several weeks of dieting. This can be satisfying and encouraging, but can also give a false impression of improvement, since most obese people have excess body fluid at the start. After that initial improvement, when weight loss is slow, they become discouraged, frustrated, and are more apt to give up.

Another factor that impedes easy weight reduction is that the calorie deficit that is initially effective becomes less effective after substantial weight loss. With less weight, the body's metabolism becomes more efficient and burns fewer calories.

Each person needs to find his or her own motivators. Drugs are de-motivating. I've noted that an interesting motivator for some is the wedding of an offspring at which the "ex" will be in attendance. Weight Watchers® is successful in part because most people are susceptible to the social pressure.

Some years back, a "fat doctor" in the Philadelphia area had his patients sign a contract regarding how much weight they would lose in a year. They paid up front. If they met the target they would get their money back. If not, he kept it. The doctor retired early and wealthy.

Some of my overweight patients at risk for coronary artery disease complications did manage to lose weight, many only after several years of trying. Unfortunately, a few of them had a heart attack anyway, about six months after their successful weight loss. The incipient symptoms of the impending attack had finally motivated them, and while they worked harder, by then it was too little, too late.

CHAPTER 45

Beyond Fitness

Exercise level is a risk factor for heart disease. High exercise levels improve other risk factors such as weight, cholesterol, hypertension, and inflammation in the blood vessel linings.

Boredom and slight depression are the worst enemies in weight management. People turn to snacking because they mistakenly feel that they are weak from lack of food.

Exercise can also lead to a reduction in smoking. When someone stops smoking without exercise, he or she reduces the risk of atherosclerosis more than exercising with continued smoking. Those who become serious about exercising, however, often stop smoking because it reduces exercise capacity.

The effect of exercise on weight management is not as simple. It's easier to exercise if one is not overweight, and the presence of excessive weight is self-defeating in exercise. The belief that exercise burns off a lot of calories is an effective motivation. After inadequate exercise, however, the appetite is stimulated and many feel they are entitled to eat a little more. The craving for food is controlled best when exercise is vigorous and frequent so that physical stamina is increased.

Boredom and slight depression are the worst enemies in weight management. People turn to snacking because they mistakenly feel that they are weak from lack of food. Exercise is helpful in wiping out boredom and depression, but it has to be long, vigorous, and frequent enough so that good physical conditioning is achieved. This suppresses the urge to eat other than at meal times.

More than 30 years ago, eight severely depressed people who were unresponsive to medication, psychotherapy, or even shock therapy, partook in a very vigorous exercise regimen. Within several weeks, seven of the eight had major improvements in their depression, well beyond anything they had experienced in the past.

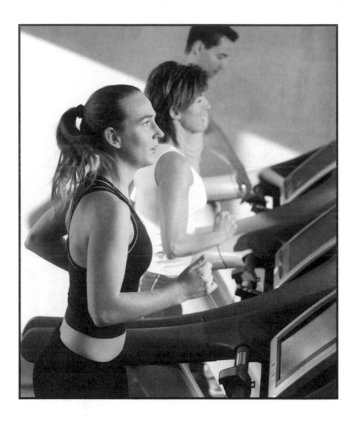

About 15 to 20 years were needed for exercise to gain a toehold in American culture. In the Philadelphia area, a number of exercise facilities that opened up in the late 1960s had to close. Not until well into the 1970s were the new ones able to stay in business, and fitness began to become a way of life for many people.

The obsession with weight management can be motivated from

the enthusiasm of others, as well as from the resultant social pressure one feels to look better. Similarly, exercise also can have a purpose beyond fitness. Many exercise facilities have been successful because they also serve as social clubs.

Most of my patients who resolved to exercise regularly ran outdoors until the winter weather stopped them. Many did not resume in the spring when the weather improved. Getting exercise by participating in a sport activity is one way to relieve the tedium of a regular exercise routine. Many patients successfully take up tennis, swimming, or other active sport, all of which provide cardiovascular benefits. Finding the effective motivation for exercise depends largely on individual interests and preferences.

CHAPTER 46

A Symptomatic Goad

High cholesterol and other lipid abnormalities are risk factors that contribute to accelerated hardening of the arteries from atherosclerosis.

Total cholesterol was one of the blood-chemistry values obtained almost routinely for about 30 years after I started in medicine. The reason for measuring total cholesterol was more or less a mystery, as there was no clear explanation of its value. The vague role of cholesterol in lipid metabolism was controversial and of little practical help at the time. Cholesterol was abnormally low in severe liver disease, which usually was evident through other testing, and very high in some uncommon inherited metabolic diseases.

The "normal" cholesterol level was established for each laboratory by testing a handful of "normal" people who worked in the hospital. As late as 1960, I saw hospital laboratories post normal values as high as 330 milligrams per deciliter, much higher than the mean for the overall population. At the time, the generally accepted normal level was below 300 milligrams.

As a result of clinical studies, the standard gradually fell in the following decades to 280, then 240, and finally to 200 milligrams per deciliter. There is evidence that a value of 150 or lower, closer to that of infants, is desirable, especially if the risk of atherosclerosis is high. By the mid 1970s, the clinical value of breaking out the measurement between the good HDL and the bad LDL cholesterols was becoming apparent.

As of the 1940s, the importance of a fat-restricted diet was already becoming increasingly evident. Convincing patients of its importance, however, was another matter.

In 1992, Angela wanted to know why I had never recommended a low-fat diet. She had been a patient of mine for nearly 20 years.

Upon reviewing her chart, I pointed out to her that I had suggested a low-fat diet in 1977. In fact, my nurse had given her written diet instructions at that time, and had gone over them with her. Her face lit up. "Oh, yes! I remember that now. And I know exactly where I put that diet."

She had begun to feel that it was important after all these years because her friends were now talking a great deal about cholesterol. It was in the news and was becoming part of the popular culture, but like exercise, it had taken decades before people accepted its importance.

—ʍ—

Another group of lipids called triglycerides have some correlation with increased atherosclerosis, but mostly because they relate to the risks from cholesterol. Triglycerides usually are elevated in diabetes mellitus as well as certain kidney or pancreatic diseases, and can also be elevated due to genetic factors.

A triglyceride level below 200 milligrams per deciliter is usually acceptable. I'd seen an occasional patient, usually with diabetes, who had levels as high as 1,400 milligrams.

That was the top of the range I'd seen, until I cared for Doris, the housewife from Allentown mentioned earlier, who came to see me when she'd had her myocardial infarction that tore her heart wall. Doris's cholesterol and triglyceride levels were normal when she had her infarction. Nearly a year later, she had developed burning and shooting pains in her hands and feet.

We drew her blood for testing, and it almost looked like cream. Her cholesterol was 900 milligrams per deciliter and her triglycerides were 8,940 milligrams per deciliter.

Her cholesterol and triglycerides fell to normal after I had her stop her estrogen pills, recently prescribed for hot flashes. These are known to elevate triglycerides in some women. Her cholesterol and triglycerides became a very normal 159 and 110 milligrams per deciliter respectively after eight months of treatment with a triglyceride-lowering medication. One year later, her levels were still normal with no lipid-lowering medication.

Doris had been taking the estrogen preparation off and on for 10 years. These lipid abnormalities from the medicine undoubtedly were the basis for her myocardial infarction.

—⁕—

Trans-fats are a more recent and more precise way of categorizing certain other harmful, partially saturated fats that have been identified in a less precise way for 40 years. Trans-fats are another risk factor for heart disease.

Without a symptomatic goad, people follow a low-lipid diet no more successfully than a weight-reduction diet. I'd put some patients on a low-fat and low-cholesterol diet to determine whether the cholesterol abnormality was dietary or inherent in their systems.

A small cholesterol reduction from 260 to 240 milligrams per deciliter may have been attained after two, three, four, or more months. Then it began to drift upward again, so I would suggest a medication to lower the level.

"No! No! I'll try harder," they would say.

Then the same scenario would repeat itself.

Finally, to save time and before starting new patients on a cholesterol-reducing medication, I urged them to go on a vegetarian diet. We would learn in weeks instead of months, or sometimes more than a year, whether a reduced-fat diet could be effective for them. Provided, of course, they could follow the vegetarian diet.

Most fail on these diets, just as those overweight fail with weight-reduction diets. They prefer medication over a change in dietary habits. That is, they fail until they are motivated by a heart complication.

Diabetes mellitus was known to be associated with a high prevalence of coronary heart disease. After its discovery in 1924, it was controllable by insulin, but as of the 1940s, one of the treatments still being used in order to avoid insulin injections was a high-fat, low-carbohydrate diet.

The argument continued to rage for years thereafter, as to whether keeping diabetics' blood sugar and lipid levels within normal range was necessary to limit the complications from arteriosclerosis. Evidence finally established that it is important to keep blood sugar and lipid levels low, but not too low, as a recent study indicated that this might actually increase cardiovascular complications.

As with so many things, some is good, more is not better.

CHAPTER 47

I Love Licorice!

Hypertension, commonly known as high blood pressure, is a risk factor for the development of cardiovascular complications such as heart attack and stroke.

Blood pressure levels are a continuum. The cut-off between normal and abnormal is derived statistically from measurements among a large number of people. Levels considered abnormally high are determined based upon the probability of cardiovascular complications developing in a large group. The level that is actually dangerous for a specific individual, however, is unknown.

There was some dispute that lasted into the 1960s over what was a normal or acceptable blood pressure level. The standards at the time were derived from blood pressures measured during a large number of insurance company examinations of presumably normal individuals. In general, these were too high.

Systolic pressure, the upper number when measuring one's blood pressure, occurs at the peak of ejection of blood from the heart into the arterial system. Systolic pressures are more variable but are a better reflection of the abnormal state of the arteries due to arteriosclerosis.

Fifty years ago, a systolic pressure reading over 140 millimeters of mercury was considered mildly elevated; over 200, moderately elevated; over 230, severely elevated; and over 280, malignantly elevated. Since then, it has become increasingly obvious that even pressures over 120 are associated with a slightly increased risk of developing heart disease, stroke, and other artery complications.

Diastolic blood pressures are considered more important and more useful than **systolic pressures**. The diastolic pressure is measured between heartbeats. It is the second number, the one below the line, when documenting the blood pressure.

Diastolic pressures are more constant and therefore are the primary basis for classification of severity. A diastolic level over 90 millimeters of mercury is considered mildly elevated; over 104, moderately elevated; over 115, severely elevated; and over 129, urgently elevated.

—⚶—

A great deal of effort has been spent developing stress tests for the diagnosis of various heart conditions. Occasionally overlooked as important in these tests is the stress intrinsic to the examination itself, and this particularly applies to blood pressure tests. Among the many factors affecting blood pressure is emotional stress.

The systolic pressure has been proven to be influenced by emotions induced by the examination itself, or from the sight of the doctor's white coat. The resulting rise in pressure is called the "white coat syndrome."

The importance of this syndrome is suggested by physical examinations of students that most colleges performed upon admission prior to the 1950s. At the University of Minnesota, approximately 30 percent of some 35,000 students who had health examinations upon admission had elevated blood pressures, which dropped to normal with reassurance and rest. Some 35 percent of these individuals developed hypertension within 30 years. While an elevated pressure in young people may not require initial treatment, it is still a risk factor.

—⚶—

Hypertension can be classified as either essential or secondary. **Essential hypertension** indicates that no specific medical cause can be found to explain the condition. Sixty years ago, 80 percent of hypertension was considered essential. Today, it is more than 90 percent.

Secondary hypertension indicates that the high blood pressure is a result of another condition. Kidney disease or infection is the most likely cause. Coarctation of the aorta is an infrequent congenital constriction of the aorta that causes an elevation of the blood pressure. Some glandular diseases such as tumors of the adrenal glands, which are situated above the kidneys, can cause hypertension. While unusual, these tumors can present a dilemma in diagnosis. When present, they change the evaluation and treatment.

—⁓—

A few experts in the late 1940s recommended hospitalization of the hypertensive person for a trial of bed rest. If the blood pressure became normal, it wasn't to be considered important enough to require treatment. This justified not treating the individual.

Until this period, the basic treatment for high blood pressure was a **barbiturate** prescribed for its calming effects. Headaches and some elevations could be controlled with oral **thiocyanates**.

By the late 1940s, it was known that cutting the **sympathetic nerves** along the lower spine was shown to reduce life-threatening complications in urgently severe hypertension. In the 1950s, potent drugs that had an effect similar to the nerve surgery were found to be helpful in treating this hypertension.

A sudden drop in blood pressure, however, was a serious risk with these treatments. Fainting often occurred when these individuals were standing quietly. If this occurred in a tight place such as a phone booth, some people died. The forced standing position prevented restoration of the blood pressure and the blood flow to the brain that occurs when the individual lies down.

After the 1950s, diuretics were shown to reduce fatal complications in the moderately severe hypertensive. Since then, not only has it been shown that mild hypertension can be beneficially treated with diuretics, but also that even those with pressures in the upper normal level may be helped.

—⁓—

Occasionally, the presentation of hypertension is bizarre and a diagnostic challenge.

Theresa was a middle-aged African-American woman with diabetes. She presented to the Pennsylvania Hospital medical clinic in 1954 with the complaint that, "my skin is getting darker."

Upon examination, we found that she was another example of the "220 syndrome." Her weight was 220 pounds, her systolic blood pressure was elevated to 220 millimeters of mercury, and her blood sugar was high at 220 milligrams per deciliter.

*We also found that Theresa had **Addison's Disease**, a condition of adrenal gland hormone insufficiency. The hyper-pigmentation is typical of this disease, but the obesity, diabetes, and hypertension are not. The weight, blood sugar, and blood pressure in this condition are typically very low.*

Despite the fact that she was placed on an appropriate hormone replacement treatment for adrenal insufficiency, Theresa died within several weeks. As is often the case, the autopsy was helpful, but solved only part of the mystery.

The adrenal insufficiency was found to be due to tuberculosis of the adrenal gland, a common cause of this condition. Treatment of the tuberculosis would have made no difference in that short time period, however, and the hormone treatment should have been adequate. The autopsy did not explain her other abnormal symptoms, and did not uncover any other underlying disease that may have caused her death.

—w—

At times, patients with blood pressures under control with treatment present with an unexpected exacerbation that offers a new diagnostic dilemma.

Helen was a patient of mine whom I had been following for 20 years. In one visit when she was in her 70s, Helen presented with a blood pressure that was very high—200 systolic over 100 diastolic millimeters of mercury. Her blood pressure had been unstable for years, and I had started her on a treatment about 10 years earlier. The drug had been very effective until this visit.

Helen had no new symptoms and had not changed her diet or medicine. The only difference in her situation was that her husband was becoming increasingly ill and had been a patient at Pennsylvania Hospital for a number of weeks.

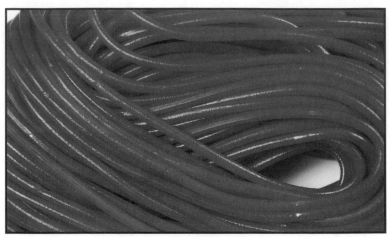

"I love licorice!" she said.

Eventually, I prescribed three new medications in addition to the one she had been taking. Helen's blood pressure improved, but only moderately. It was still marginally elevated. I saw her two to three times at weekly intervals to adjust the dosages with little improvement, and this was somewhat puzzling.

On her last visit, as Helen was walking out of the examination room, I shot a question to her on a hunch. I knew it was a long shot. "Do you like licorice?" I asked.

"I love licorice!" She replied.

*Licorice contains a chemical called **glycyrrhizin**, which acts like **aldosterone**, an adrenal gland hormone that can elevate the blood pressure when excessive. As it turns out, every noon for weeks, Helen had been visiting her husband in the Hospital. On each visit, she bought a package of licorice in the Hospital's gift shop on the way up to his room. During the course of the afternoon, she would eat the entire package of licorice.*

I checked at the gift shop and found that a full package of their licorice contained an amount of glycyrrhizin that was sufficient to elevate the blood pressure. As soon as she ended her licorice addiction, her blood pressure returned to its prior level, successfully controlled by the usual treatment. All of her new medications could be stopped.

Chapter 48

Thinner Blood

Blood clots can cause any number of complications. Clots in the coronary arteries of the heart cause acute myocardial infarction. Clots in brain arteries can cause a stroke. Clots that break loose from the heart during the rhythm disturbance of atrial fibrillation, can go to the brain and also cause a stroke. These floating clots are referred to as emboli.

Conditions such as thrombophlebitis, which is an inflammation of the veins, create the potential for the formation of blood clots. If one of these clots breaks loose and floats to the lung as an embolus, it can be fatal.

Various anticoagulants, commonly referred to as "blood thinners," are used in these conditions to reduce the risk of complications from blood clots. Heparin has been available since early in the 19th century. It is effective only if given by injection.

In the 1940s, a new blood thinner was discovered. Farmers had long been aware that spoiled sweet clover caused bleeding when it was eaten by cattle. In 1941, Dr. Karl Paul Link, professor of biochemistry at the University of Wisconsin Department of Agriculture, decided to tackle the problem. He isolated dicumarol from the spoiled clover. Soon, it became the anticoagulant of choice for patients.

Later, researchers learned that **coumarin**, half of the dicumarol double molecule, was the effective component. It was released as Coumadin, and soon replaced dicumarol as the preferred anticoagulant for patients. Today, Coumadin is still the standard oral anticoagulant therapy.

Professor Link didn't teach at the Medical School, but one evening in the fall of 1944, I heard him lecture on his investigative work. One of his most striking comments was that aspirin and dicumarol had similar chemical structures. In order to determine if aspirin had a similar anticoagulant effect, he personally took 36 tablets of 325 milligram aspirin, about 12-times the maximum recommended adult dose, at one time.

Professor Link found that this dose was effective in prolonging his prothrombin time, the measure of the blood's clotting factor, by about 50 percent. This is within the low end of the therapeutic range for Coumadin.

Since then, aspirin has been found to be effective in preventing the coronary artery clots that cause myocardial infarctions. It can prevent many heart attacks, but in doses so small that it does not prolong the prothrombin time. It is effective for other reasons.

I recalled Dr. Link's lecture when I was an intern treating a patient with acute rheumatic fever. She was a 16-year-old girl who weighed 180 pounds. Aspirin was the standard treatment, but not because of its anti-clotting effect. I gave her the recommended dose for rheumatic fever, which was 36 aspirin over 24 hours. When I measured her prothrombin time, I found that it did increase from 11 seconds to 18 seconds, which was similar to the increase noted by Professor Link.

—m—

Pennsylvania Hospital was one of the 14 hospitals in Irving Wright's study during the 1940s of the effects of anticoagulants in acute myocardial infarction. For 20 years after the end of the study in 1948, the team in the Cardiology Section managed all of the Hospital's oral anticoagulant therapy. At any given time, this responsibility included 20 to 30 ward and private patients, as well as all of the clinic patients on long-term treatment.

Each of us on the team followed many patients at one time. This gave us a good perspective of the wide individual variations in the prolongation of prothrombin time. For example, one patient with prothrombin times within the target range would have complications from bleeding episodes. Another patient with a prothrombin time 20-times normal would not develop any abnormal bleeding.

We were always concerned by the appearance of blood in the urine, which was usually hard to explain, despite further testing. Black stools from gastrointestinal bleeding, on the other hand, were almost always due to a discoverable cause. Peptic ulcers of the stomach or duodenum were the most common cause of intestinal bleeding. Unsuspected cancer of the bowel was the next most common cause.

I used to say, only half-seriously, that anticoagulation therapy was a better screening tool for gastrointestinal cancer than any radiologic study. It would quickly reveal any incipient intestinal bleeding.

We found that Coumadin lengthened the prothrombin or clotting time about twice as rapidly as dicumarol, and therefore variations in dosage carried wider swings. While I could keep the prothrombin time from dicumarol in range 95 percent of the time, I could only keep the shorter acting Coumadin in range 85 percent of the time. Experience may have been a factor, as I had used dicumarol about three to four times more often than Coumadin.

I found that residents in training also had more success maintaining prothrombin time within range with dicumarol than Coumadin. Even though they did appreciably better with dicumarol, however, they felt more comfortable with Coumadin and preferred using it because its more rapid response in the patient made it seem easier to manage.

Many studies in the literature show that with Coumadin, the therapeutic range is maintained only about 50 to 60 percent of the time. The use of very effective oral anticoagulants at that time, among other potent new drugs, added to the growing concerns among physicians about the appropriate use of drugs and the risks to individual patients.

The use of very effective oral anticoagulants at that time, among other potent new drugs, added to the growing concerns among physicians about the appropriate use of drugs and the risks to individual patients.

CHAPTER 49

What Happened to My Legs? They're So Thin!

Congestive heart failure is a very serious complication of heart disease. It is considered a syndrome, which is a combination of similar symptoms and manifestations that may be the result of different diseases or other abnormalities. Two main types of heart failure are recognized, and each of them may be caused by a number of different diseases.

One type of failure develops from heart-muscle weakness, which leads to an insufficient amount of blood being pumped from the heart to meet the body's needs. The other type of failure develops from heart-muscle stiffness, which prevents blood from adequately filling the heart between each heartbeat. Either of these types of congestive heart failure can be caused by hypertension, valve abnormalities, coronary artery disease, or heart-muscle inflammation, also called myocarditis.

Symptoms of congestive heart failure are shortness of breath and fatigue, as well as swelling of the feet and legs from abnormal fluid retention. This also increases body weight.

Different levels of severity may be found with congestive heart failure. Over the past 25 years, I have observed a declining number of patients presenting with excess body fluid, and therefore excess weight. Today, the diagnosis is usually made at an earlier stage of the condition, before fluid retention develops. Excess body fluid can also be masked by the use of the more potent diuretics or "water pills" available today.

Acute pulmonary edema is one of the more dramatic effects of heart failure. In this syndrome, the lungs suddenly fill with fluid, causing shortness of breath with wheezing or noisy breathing. Frothy, blood-tinged liquid may appear in the mouth. The lips and skin become blue, signaling a need for oxygen. This condition is usually due to excess body fluid and sudden weakness of the heart.

In addition to providing oxygen, initial treatment of acute pulmonary edema is directed to procedures that reduce the blood flow back to the chest and heart. A sitting posture is helpful. Tourniquets are applied to three of the limbs and rotated at intervals. A unit of blood may be removed from a vein.

Morphine injected into a vein not only relieves anxiety, but also reduces the load on the heart. The injection of the diuretic **furosemide** into a vein immediately reduces congestion in the lungs to help breathing, before it acts on the kidneys to rid the body of extra fluid. Most other diuretics act primarily through the kidneys, which is not of immediate benefit to the breathing. Other drugs are also helpful.

Some of the earlier treatments for the fluid overload in congestive heart failure have been unusual. In the late 1930s, Dr. Ferdinand R. Schemm of Great Falls, Montana, was one of the first to promote dietary salt restriction as a fundamental part of treatment. He also recommended forcing large amounts of fluids into the patient, rather than restricting fluids, as was considered necessary at that time.

The liquids were taken by mouth and would consist of as much as six, eight, ten, or more quarts of fluid daily. The surprising result was that, if the patients could tolerate this, they would lose more fluid than they had taken.

A net loss of 10 quarts of fluid should produce a loss of about 20 pounds of body weight. A patient whose heart and circulation can handle such large amounts of fluid would need to have fairly good heart function. The heart overload therefore must have been caused by excess salt, water, and activity.

—∾—

Dr. Graham Asher was a cardiologist at Research Hospital in Kansas City when I was on staff there. He had trained at Beth Israel Hospital in Boston. His practice was an example of the changing paradigm of the 1940s, through which **biochemistry** was replacing **pathologic anatomy** as the principle basis of medical practice.

His acute cardiac failure patients were given a concoction we referred to as a "cardiac cocktail." It consisted of 50-percent glucose, combined with digitalis, a diuretic, **thiamine**, and **theophylline**. This last drug stimulates both the heart and kidneys, and improves breathing by strengthening the diaphragm as well as counteracting bronchial spasms in the lungs. The cocktail often resulted in gratifying improvement.

By the late 1940s, a milk diet was advocated by some doctors for hospital patients suffering from acute pulmonary edema. Milk is not an extraordinarily low-salt food. It was effective because most patients had been eating excessive salt, and milk replaced this with reduced salt levels. Also, they were too active physically, given their conditions. Just the simple measures of putting them at bed rest in the hospital, reducing salt intake, and giving them oxygen resulted in a spontaneous loss of excess body fluid without the help of drugs.

*In the early 1950s at Pennsylvania Hospital, Neil, who was only 25-years old, came in with extensive fluid overload of his body, a serious condition called **anasarca**. Neil also had **beriberi heart disease** due to a deficiency of the B vitamin, thiamine, a result of his alcoholism.*

We gave Neil a single injection of a mercurial diuretic. From this single treatment, along with bed rest, no fluid intake, and oxygen, he lost 26 pounds in 24 hours. That's more than three gallons. Neil's heart developed almost every heart irregularity known, except for fatal ventricular fibrillation.

Neil's dramatic physiological response to the diuretic was very unusual.

In later years, after much more potent diuretics had been developed, I had to work to temper interns' impatience in the treatment of heart failure with marked anasarca. Similar excessive responses to potent diuretics are common in patients with a great deal of extra body fluid. Unless enthusiasm for treatment is tempered, a number of preventable complications are apt to occur.

—◊—

As of the middle of the last century, an unresolved debate continued as to whether digitalis was of any value in the treatment of congestive heart failure. The medical profession first discovered digitalis in the late 18th century. William Withering, a botanist in rural England, learned that an elderly woman versed in folk-medicine herbalism was producing an amazing reduction in the leg swelling caused by "**dropsy**," the term in that era for congestive heart failure. She was giving an extract of the plant digitalis purpurea or common foxglove. Withering studied the extract and found that it had interesting effects on the heart.

By the 1940s, many physicians used digitalis only for the control of heart arrhythmias, primarily atrial fibrillation. They weren't using it for leg swelling from heart failure because they found it ineffective most of the time. One reason is that they were using it on all cases of leg swelling, most of which are not caused by heart disease. Swelling from other causes—including varicose veins, kidney disease, liver disease, or an underactive thyroid gland—was twice as common as swelling from heart failure, and these conditions are not affected by digitalis.

—◊—

Heart failure can be resistant to treatment for many reasons.

Scott was 45 when he was admitted under my care at Research Hospital for the treatment of congestive heart failure due to val- vular abnormalities of his heart. He responded well initially and unloaded pounds of fluid.

*After that, he had no extra fluid anywhere in his body, although he still had **rales** in his lungs. Rales are crackling noises heard in the lungs with a stethoscope, indicating the presence of excess fluid. They are classic findings of heart failure. Rales usually go away on continued treatment, but in Scott's case, they were unaffected.*

For the next week, his rales still would not clear. During that time, he complained increasingly of rectal discomfort. I prescribed a hemorrhoid preparation, but he continued to complain.

Finally, when his complaint became more urgent, I did what I should have done in the beginning and performed a digital rectal examination. He had a rather large and firm collection of impacted stool. These frequently don't respond to enemas or laxatives, so I dug it out with my finger.

I was amazed that within 15 minutes, his chest rales completely cleared.

There is a connection between the nerves of the lower spinal cord that go to the rectal area, and those from the upper spinal cord that connect to the respiratory tract. A fecal impaction can affect the lungs through these nerve connections.

The old-time physicians knew of this reflex. One of the feared complications of the old inhaled general anesthetic, ether, was a spasm of the vocal cords, which can prevent air from reaching the lungs. On occasion, a surgical patient suddenly could not breath as a result of such a spasm, and could die. Immediate treatment was imperative. In the setting of kitchen-table surgery in the home, this was particularly challenging.

The surgeon would abruptly stretch the anal muscles. This induces a reflex that overcomes the vocal spasm, causing the patient to gasp and resume breathing. Thus, in addition to the surprise factor, there is also a neurological basis for the gasp reflex from "goosing."

—∿∿—

Some patients with poor arterial circulation to the legs sit constantly to relieve the leg pain. When heart failure is present, this posture further impairs circulation and aggravates the swelling. Constant sitting in and of itself can cause massive swelling of the lower body. This occurred in flagpole sitters who, during the Great Depression, would actually sit in a captain's chair on a flagpole for days at a time as an advertising stunt. They would develop massive swelling, even though they had neither vascular disease of the legs nor heart failure.

Congestive heart failure, when it is present, makes the swelling much worse. The fluid that accumulates in the legs and lower abdomen often cannot be reduced, even with diuretics. In the days before the surgical procedures were available for relieving arterial blockages in the legs, other unusual treatments were used on occasion.

In unresponsive cases, Dr. Garfield Duncan, the chief of medicine at Pennsylvania Hospital, used a treatment that was centuries old. Long needles used for spinal taps were inserted into the legs under the skin. The excess fluid slowly drained off through the needles into a basin. It would then re-accumulate in the legs from the rest of the body, and the drainage would continue. At times, the resulting fluid loss could be an impressive 50 pounds or more over several weeks. More commonly, however, the amount of fluid loss was not very impressive.

As illustrated in my patient Neil's case, as of the 1950s, mercurials were the most potent diuretics available. At the time, these had to be given by injection into a vein or deep into a muscle. This inconvenience was addressed in part by the introduction of **Thiomerin**, a mercurial that could be given under the skin as well. This drug was not very effective when given by mouth.

As a cardiac fellow, I managed a study which determined that Thiomerin was also effective when given as a rectal suppository. That method was very expensive, however, so it wasn't used for very long, and the drug company gave up on its manufacture.

A number of studies in the 1990s verified the value of home management in keeping patients out of the hospital. This was usually accomplished through ongoing contact by visiting nurses. This is another example of the value and effectiveness of ongoing personal care by medical professionals in the prevention and treatment of disease.

By 1958, chlorothiazide was the first effective oral diuretic available. During the early 1960s, a new **thiazide** preparation was introduced almost every six months. In the mid-1960s, **ethacrynic acid** and furosemide, two entirely different and much more potent diuretics were released. At maximum effect, the mercurials and thiazides could cause 25 percent of water entering the kidneys to be excreted as urine. This new generation of drugs could cause 94 percent to be excreted.

The more potent diuretics available today often give doctors a false sense of security in patient treatment. Many patients on long-term hospital treatments, especially pre-terminal ones, are overloaded with fluids intravenously. This can aggravate their condition, despite the use of effective intravenous drugs.

Fluid overload can be detected more readily today by several means, but the tests are not done in patients if they have no recognizable lung or abdominal problem. The hidden fluid collections in the lungs and abdominal cavities used to be discovered upon autopsy. Although it was too late for the deceased patients, this at least made doctors aware of cases in which they were overloading patients with fluids. Today, however, autopsies are not done and doctors are therefore less aware of situations in which they are overloading patients with fluids.

Since about 1970, I have found that in spite of my instructions, at times the house staff would continue to overload some of my patients with intravenous fluids. This would cause continued fluid buildup, despite effective diuretics. I was forced to actually discharge about one patient each year to get him or her out of heart failure. Ironically, I found I could manage the patient better and more safely at his or her home.

—◊◊◊—

Congestive heart failure takes considerable treatment to correct, but much less to prevent. Often, the failure in treatment is a result of poor medical management at home. The key to home management is monitoring the weight daily. I could keep most patients out of the hospital by teaching them how to monitor themselves.

The two state-of-the-art home monitoring instruments needed, even today, are a weight scale and a telephone. When daily changes in weight are excessive, indicating fluid retention, the patient or a member of the family can be taught appropriate modifications in fluid intake and medicine dosage.

Sometimes, cardiac patients receiving care at home do not initially seem to respond to treatment. While they do not appear to be collecting additional fluid in the legs, abdomen, or lungs, their weight doesn't decrease either. They are actually losing weight, but the scale doesn't reflect this, because fluid is replacing the lost fat and muscle.

This happens because the fluid retention from heart failure has been generalized to all of the tissues, where the extra fluid has taken the place of the fat and muscle. These patients gradually develop exertional shortness of breath and fatigue without weight gain. Then, one day, they suddenly become acutely short of breath, go to an emergency room, and are admitted to the hospital. There, they experience a massive **diuresis**, often losing 20 pounds of fluid or more.

"What happened to my legs?" They say. "They're so thin!"

A number of studies in the 1990s verified the value of home management in keeping congestive heart failure patients out of the hospital. This was usually accomplished through ongoing contact by visiting nurses. This is another example of the value and effectiveness of ongoing personal care by medical professionals in the prevention and treatment of disease.

CHAPTER 50

He's Now on a Cruise Around the World

The value of digitalis for the treatment of congestive heart failure continued to be controversial through the 1940s. Then, several purified forms of digitalis began replacing the extract of digitalis leaf. By the 1950s, even though it hadn't yet been proven in evidence-based studies, digitalis was generally accepted as a benefit in the treatment of congestive heart failure.

Pediatricians were less convinced, however. At that time, Tony Diehl, a pediatric cardiologist at the University of Kansas, said that the purified digitalis preparation **digoxin** was about as worthwhile for treating infants and children as "just so much water." Many of us did not concur.

One convincing case for me was that of Andrea, a child of 9 years with a congenital hole in the wall separating the two sides of her heart. She had been in Kansas City Children's Mercy Hospital for several weeks with extensive fluid accumulation from severe congestive heart failure.

Her face was swollen. Rales from extra fluid in her lungs were audible. Andrea had abdominal enlargement from a swollen liver and fluid in her abdomen, and had fluid swelling in her legs.

Ridding the body of this extra fluid with diuretic preparations had not been effective, and the digitalis treatment was not working. It appeared that Andrea would die in the Hospital. Then, suddenly, over a period of about two days, she lost all of the extra fluid through diuresis from the kidneys. All of the swelling went away. She lost more than 15 pounds of fluid weight.

No ready explanation could be given for this astounding improvement. Upon examination of her hospital chart, however, I found that one of the nurses had given the child an adult dose of digitalis by mistake. This was about 10-times the amount recommended for a child. This amount of the drug, considered to be a "toxic" level for a child at the time, resulted in her marked improvement. She went home in several weeks and maintained a stable state.

This would not have been possible had the prior doses at the pediatric levels been continued. In fact, Andrea would have died in the Hospital.

—\\—

Digitalis excess usually becomes evident first as a loss of appetite, then with nausea and vomiting, often accompanied by visual problems. These symptoms may be preceded by excessive slowing of the heart rate. Nurses were taught to check the heart rate before administering a dose of digitalis. If the heart rate was less than 60 per minute, they were instructed to check with a physician before giving the next dose of digitalis.

When a patient already on digitalis was admitted to the hospital with a very slow heart rate, house officers usually withheld digitalis. However, excess digitalis usually presented as an incomplete heart block, not as a slow heart rate. A very slow heart rate and a high degree of heart block occur primarily in those with a structural problem with the heart, such as an abnormal valve or a congenital malformation.

Those without heart disease are more apt to develop complete heart block from excess digitalis. People who do not have heart disease and attempt suicide with a digitalis overdose frequently develop complete heart block. Surprisingly, several of my patients with severe heart disease, who had suffered a myocardial infarction, lost their heart block within hours after treatment with digitalis. Improved heart function or coincidence are possible explanations.

"What instrument do you use to diagnose digitalis intoxication?" Is the question that Francis Woods, chief of internal medicine at the University of Pennsylvania in the 1950s, would pose to students and interns. This was 20 years before it was possible to measure the level of digitalis in the blood.

The answer is illustrated by the following experience.

Jeannie was a 3-year-old patient with a very large heart from Ebstein's anomaly, a congenital heart condition caused by a defective tricuspid valve, the passage between the right atrium and ventricle. It could not be corrected by surgery.

When Jeannie came to the outpatient clinic at Kansas City Children's Mercy Hospital, she had been on a digitalis preparation at the pediatric dose level. It had been started when she'd been a patient in the hospital. I had been following her in the clinic. The digitalis did not seem to be helping her, but I did not stop it.

One day, her mother called me. "Jeannie is flopping around the house all the time," she said.

"What do you mean?"

"Every time she stands up and tries to walk a few steps, she falls down."

"Bring her right into the clinic."

The only change I found upon examination was that Jeannie's pulse was very slow. It was in the range of 40 beats per minute, about one-third to one-half of what it should have been. Her electrocardiogram showed a heart block.

A temporary or permanent pacemaker, the treatment today for a heart block, was not yet available at that time.

"Is Jeannie taking any new medications?" I asked her mother.

"No, but her digitalis prescription was refilled last week."

I called her pharmacist and asked him to check the dose he'd given with the prescription. He checked his records and then admitted that he had misread the prescription. The pharmacist had given her the adult-sized pill, 10-times the dose suitable for children.

Within a few days after stopping the digitalis, Jeannie's heart rhythm returned to normal and she was running and playing like she had been prior to the onset of this episode.

Thus, the correct answer to Dr. Woods' question, "What instrument do you use to diagnose digitalis intoxication?" Was, of course, "The telephone."

—m—

In the late 1940s, when the digitalis leaf extract was being replaced by the purified derivatives, **digitoxin** and digoxin, the proper therapeutic dose had to be **assayed** through the clinical responsiveness of patients. They received an initial larger loading dose, followed by smaller maintenance doses. Physicians monitored heart rhythms and other symptoms.

By 1950, an epidemic of patients who were treated with digitoxin or digoxin in the hospital and discharged, were then readmitted four to six weeks later with bizarre heart-rhythm disturbances. The maintenance dose was too high, and these rhythm disturbances were from the gradual accumulation of the drug to toxic levels. Digoxin was better tolerated than either digitoxin or the older digitalis-leaf treatments, because it didn't remain in the body as long if an overdose had been given.

In that era, the only method available for measurement of drug levels in the blood involved using a duck embryo heart bioassay. This provided an inaccurate estimate which was of little or no clinical value. By the early 1970s, a reliable laboratory assay of the amount of digitalis in the blood was established.

The ultimate test of a drug's usefulness is its proven effectiveness for each individual patient.
The physician needs to be very aware of the differing responses to the same drug among different individuals.

When this new test was applied, the range of digitalis levels found in established patients who had been on digitalis for a long time was astounding. Most patients had blood levels several times the levels now considered toxic. Some had levels that were 10-times the therapeutic level, and without adverse effects.

Soon, we found that the patients who were the most sensitive to the dose level were those with more severe heart disease. In fact, following the same patient over a long period of time often revealed a gradually increasing sensitivity to the same mainte-nance dose. The dose had to be decreased gradually.

Just after drug blood-level measurements became possible, I was asked to see Oliver, a patient who had been admitted to Pennsylvania Hospital from a nursing home. He was middle-aged and had heart disease.

*Over the prior few months, while in the nursing home, Oliver had gradually become bedfast with worsening **dementia**. He was receiving digitalis as prescribed and had none of the usual symptoms of digitalis toxicity.*

Upon examining Oliver, I found nothing very remarkable, except that his digitalis blood level was four-times the highest recommended therapeutic level.

After I stopped the digitalis, he rapidly lost his dementia and returned to the nursing home.

A few months later, I contacted his physician. "How is Oliver getting along?" I asked.

"Just fine," his doctor told me. "In fact, he was doing so well that I discharged him from the nursing home. He's now on a cruise around the world."

Needless to say, I was astounded.

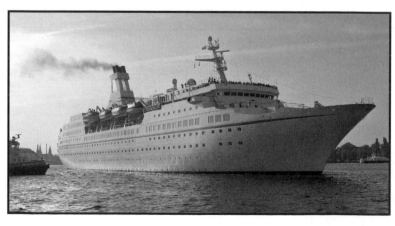

—◊◊◊—

There are a number of types of heart disease for which digitalis is not considered useful. For example, it is not proven to be effective in those with **cor pulmonale**, a heart condition that comes from chronic lung disease. Patients with the advanced form of this disease have fluid retention that is evident through ankle swelling and weight gain. These symptoms can be controlled to some degree through the use of diuretics.

The controversy over the benefits of digitalis continued until its value was definitively established in clinical trials conducted over decades. Early studies found that digitalis was of no benefit in patients with heart disease who did not have congestive heart failure. These trials could be faulted, however, because they only tested the effect of digitalis on cardiac function in patients at rest, when the heart is under less stress.

Later studies have concluded that, for many forms of heart disease, digitalis is effective. It can provide life-saving intervention in critical cases. In disease maintenance, it does not prolong life, but it does improve quality of life.

The ultimate test of a drug's usefulness is its proven effectiveness for each individual patient. The physician needs to be very aware of the differing responses to the same drug among different individuals.

CHAPTER 51

Bad Circulation

Peripheral vascular diseases involve blood vessels outside of the heart. The more common complications of arteriosclerosis are caused by its presence in coronary arteries. The involvement of other arteries throughout the body is less common, but this may be equally devastating.

Atherosclerosis in brain arteries can cause strokes. In the kidneys, its presence may cause high blood pressure. Impaired circulation in the legs causes pain on walking and can cause gangrene.

Disease in the veins is primarily seen in the legs. These veins can become inflamed as **phlebitis**. The most serious complication is **thrombosis**, the formation of blood clots, which, as mentioned earlier, may break loose as thrombo-emboli. They float to the lungs and can cause severe damage. When large, such clots can be fatal.

Dr. Stanley Morest, with whom I started private practice in 1956 in Kansas City, was an internist and cardiologist who was known largely as a peripheral vascular subspecialist. Peripheral vascular disease was an internal medicine subspecialty included in cardiology, but without subspecialty board certification.

Drugs available at that time for the treatment of inadequate arterial circulation were largely ineffective. One procedure, however, did improve circulation to the legs when the vessels were constricted. Surgical excision of the sympathetic nerves along the lower spine increased skin circulation to the legs and feet by eliminating the capacity of the blood vessels to constrict.

Stan had a constant-temperature room installed in Research Hospital, where he could measure relatively small temperature changes in patients' toes and fingers. This test was used to determine whether a patient was a candidate for surgery. One hand or foot would be immersed in ice water or hot water, and the temperature changes in the other extremities would be measured. This tested the arteries located in these other extremities, to see if they had a tendency to contract or dilate sympathetically.

About three percent of the cases treated by **sympathectomy**, as the procedure was called, resulted in severe worsening of the circulation. For these patients, the vessels in the skin stole blood from the deep vessels, which supply blood to the muscles and deep tissues of the limbs. This could result in the loss of toes or a leg by gangrene.

—∿—

*On one occasion while I was in practice with Stan, a man named Mark with atrial fibrillation threw off a blood clot from the heart to the **popliteal artery** behind one knee. Mark's leg, including his foot, was pale and cold below the knee from the impaired circulation. The **embolectomy procedure**, which can remove a clot from an artery, had not been developed as yet. Mark was sure to lose his leg.*

One drug capable of opening blood vessels in the skin is nitroglycerine. In the early 1950s, it was available in an ointment. I had the ointment applied to Mark's entire leg and foot. This improved the circulation enough to make the skin warm and pink all the way to his feet, but it didn't save his leg.

Nitroglycerine ointment also healed many skin ulcers in the legs and feet in those who were not surgical candidates, much to the amazement of the surgeons with whom I worked. The downside to the use of the ointment was that some of those with leg and toe ulcers had intolerable discomfort, which seemed to be similar to the warming of a limb after frostbite. When applied to the chest at times, I found that the skin became fiery red and uncomfortable.

I had also found that nitroglycerine ointment applied to the chest was effective in preventing **nocturnal angina pectoris**. It was the only treatment available at that time that gave patients a longer and better night's sleep. None of the oral medications then available lasted much longer than a few hours.

By 1960, commercial preparations of nitroglycerine ointment were no longer readily available, so I would ask pharmacists to compound some.

—⚭—

Aneurysms are sac-like bulges in blood vessels. They are most frequent in the abdominal aorta of older people, usually without symptoms. They are difficult to detect on physical examination and can rupture without warning. The improvements in their detection and treatment reflect the astounding technological progress of the past 50 years.

As of the 1950s, diagnosis was made through simple x-ray techniques. In time, ultrasound was introduced, followed by the more sophisticated CT scans and MRIs.

At first, to correct the aneurysm, the bulge was surgically excised through an abdominal incision. The aneurysm was replaced with a preserved segment of frozen aorta from a cadaver. A plastic tube was soon used instead of the human tissue.

In time, the aneurysm was left in place and **occluded**. A tube diverted the blood around it to the aorta on either end. Today, an abdominal incision is no longer necessary. The bypass tube is threaded through a femoral artery in the groin, through the aneurysm, and is then connected to the aorta on each side of the aneurysm. Complications of the surgery have been reduced by each new technique.

Pulmonary embolism occurs when the dislodged blood clot floats to the lungs. It is much more common than generally appreciated. When it occurs in people out of the hospital, it can be especially difficult to diagnose. The classic manifestations of chest pain, shortness of breath, and coughing up blood in the **sputum** appear in only 10 percent of those with the condition.

A high index of suspicion is required so that the appropriate diagnostic tests can be ordered. One clue I found helpful is that some patients with pulmonary embolism experience a fainting spell within several days prior to the onset of symptoms. I surmised that this event marked the actual lodging of the clot in the lung, and that it had then taken several days for the lung damage to develop and produce symptoms.

As discussed earlier, embolisms are a particular risk for patients with lengthy hospital stays at bed rest. This has been a serious problem following the types of surgery that limit ambulation. It was therefore of increasing concern to orthopedic surgeons as joint-replacement surgery became more widespread.

When I was practicing at the Independence Sanitarium and Hospital in the late 1950s, I had a rather distressing experience with this complication that was the result of a physical examination.

Several hours after his hip-replacement surgery, I was asked to examine Warren, a middle-aged man who was having a nondescript episode of chest discomfort and shortness of breath.

I immediately went to see him, suspecting a pulmonary embolism. In my usual physical-examination routine, I would start with the head and proceed toward the feet, with emphasis on those portions of the anatomy requiring more attention—as determined by the circumstances. With Warren, however, given my suspicion and the urgency, I started by immediately examining his feet and legs for swelling, tenderness, and unusual cord-like firmness along the blood vessels. These are all findings of a thrombosis, which is a clot in an inflamed vein.

As I proceeded up into the thighs, Warren suddenly had a seizure, and within minutes, died. I surmised that the examination had dislodged a clot in the veins, which then floated to his lung. This led to a reaction that provoked his heart into a fatal rhythm disturbance, causing the seizure. Of course, I'm not sure that this wouldn't have happened had I examined him in the usual head-to-foot sequence.

The main treatment at that time for blood clots in the legs was intravenous heparin, an anticoagulant. Warren had not been given this after his operation. It may or may not have been effective, but this deprived him of at least one more chance of survival.

—⚡︎—

After Medicare was introduced in the late 1960s, with its heightened degree of financial oversight, doctors were forced to reduce the length of hospital stays. As a result, patients did not remain in bed as long, and the risk of thrombo-embolism declined. Today, despite these improvements, it remains a significant, though avoidable, complication of hospitalization and surgery.

Chapter 52

Enough and Not Too Much

The prescribing of medication epitomizes the challenge a physician faces in balancing the treatment of a disease and the need for personal care of the individual patient. This is illustrated in many of the preceding anecdotes.

A drug is any substance that can be used in the prevention, diagnosis, or treatment of illness. Drugs can cure, but most of them simply mitigate the disease or ease symptoms. After the diagnosis is made and the appropriate therapy is selected, the use of the drug requires identification of numerous personal factors that may influence its effectiveness.

The correct dosage of a medication depends upon the weight and age of the patient, associated diseases, and other medications being taken. The frequency with which the dose is taken, relationship to meals, and the time of day also can be important. Whether the drug is provided in a pill, capsule, liquid, or injection form makes a big difference to some people. Ease of swallowing is one factor. The discomfort of administration by injection is another factor that affects a drug's acceptance by some people.

A person's perception of medications and how they work is important. This depends upon their education, work, background, and culture.

Prescribing a drug that a particular patient has never taken before is a trial, an experiment. Its use often requires adjustment. I would explain to patients, "You don't buy the first suit you see on the rack, take it home without trying it on, and then expect it to fit. It often requires alterations." The same is true for medications. They must be tailored to the patient's specific needs.

The proper dosage requires adjustment for the individual. In medical school, the maxim was, "The dose of a drug is enough and not too much." Today, doctors in training are more apt to be advised to, "Start low and go slow."

This approach is particularly important for new drugs. Recommended dosages are based on studies of groups that are considered typical for a specific disease. These groups represent only a small proportion of those who actually suffer from the condition. The studies usually don't address all of the variable factors that affect a drug's effectiveness in a particular patient.

Starting out with the recommended average dosage may result in a side effect. In some instances, an unwanted reaction can be alarming, if not actually dangerous. After such a reaction, many patients are reluctant to try the medication again at a lower dose that may be more tolerable.

Many doctors start with a low, safe dose and gradually increase it until the desired effect occurs, or until unwanted side effects develop. Most patients accept this approach. With some drugs, the desired response may require a larger daily dose initially. Later, this can be reduced to a lower level as an ongoing maintenance dose. On the other hand, for drugs that build tolerance in the patient, the dose may have to increase over time.

Treating a specific individual who is sick involves more than performing a procedure or prescribing a pill that is statistically proven to be effective in most people. Effective and safe treatment must also take into account the multiple factors that make each person unique. The limitation of scientific treatment in drug therapy is a perfect illustration of how personal care must be used to supplement impersonal, statistical applications.

Over the years, the initial recommended dosage upon release has been high for many new drugs, then broad practice over time determines the most effective and tolerable dose, which may be lower. This has been especially true for new cardiovascular drugs. Tablets are grooved so that they can be broken in half more easily for administering smaller doses.

As an example, **hydrochlorothiazide**, also known as HCTZ, is a diuretic still of value in the treatment of hypertension. In the early 1960s, it was released as 50-milligram and 100-milligram scored tablets. In time, 25-milligram tablets became available, and we learned that doses of even half this strength can be effective.

No drug is totally safe for all people. Even substances that are natural to the body and may be classified as drugs—such as hormones, vitamins, and water—can prove to be toxic or even fatal when used in excess. Some drug sensitivities, though rare, can be fatal. For example, an adult who has never before taken aspirin, could die from a single dose—if he or she has a severe allergic reaction to the drug.

—⚈—

Most drugs don't cure. Some alleviate symptoms until natural healing occurs. Even simply controlling symptoms without any cure can help to stabilize the imbalance in body systems and alleviate the disease, so that less treatment is required.

Waiting for symptoms to recur before treating them is like "closing the barn door after the horses are out," as Dr. Long, my internship colleague from Arkansas might say. The delay results in an increase in resistance to correction and alleviation. It's easier to maintain body systems in balance than it is to restore them to balance. As an analogy, it takes much less effort to keep a vertical object in balance than it does to lift it back up once it has tipped over.

The common practice among patients is to take a medication either sporadically or regularly for symptoms from a condition, and then to stop as soon as the symptoms disappear. When practicing in Independence, when all we had for pain relief was aspirin and acetaminophen, I'd insist that arthritics take two tablets four-times daily, and continue even after the pain has stopped. The patients would feel and function better. I quickly became known as an arthritis specialist and was inundated with arthritics.

I would insist that patients with peptic ulcers take their antacid four-times a day, even after they became symptom-free. I was then also regarded as a stomach specialist. The same happened with diabetics as a result of this approach to their treatment.

In order to address the inconvenience of taking a medication regularly, and the human tendency to forget to take a dose that must be taken several times daily, longer-acting preparations were designed. Ironically, however, I discovered that some patients prefer the more frequent dosage. For instance, when feeling "less well," some people want to take some sort of action. It makes them feel more secure when they can take their drug more often than once daily, as though they have more control over their condition. Some people take an extra dose when feeling less well. With a once-a-day-pill, this can result in an over-dosage.

Like these patients, most physicians also prefer the shorter-acting drugs. As mentioned above, doctors prefer to use the shorter-acting anticoagulant, Coumadin, over the longer-acting dicumarol, even though studies show that those doctors don't use it as effectively. Likewise, doctors preferred the shorter-acting digoxin as a cardiac medication over the longer-acting digitoxin.

When in need of a diuretic, both doctors and patients prefer furosemide, a water pill with a startlingly fast effect. It lasts only four to six hours, compared to some that are just as potent, like **Zaroxolyn**, which lasts for a day or more, but without as startling an effect.

With shorter-acting drugs in general, it is easier for the physician to assess the effects and adjust the dosage quickly, as needed. If an over-dosage occurs, the unwanted effects don't last as long. In keeping with the first rule of medical care, "Do no harm," a prescribed treatment should have the probability of doing less harm than omitting the treatment.

According to some doctors, the second rule of medical care is, "Do something before the patient gets better." This is, of course, meant tongue-in-cheek. But it is true that most conditions cure themselves with no medical intervention, and when the doctor takes some action, the patient will credit the doctor for the cure. Also, there may be a "placebo effect" from preparations with little or no pharmacologic effect.

Placebos are inactive substances with no intrinsic pharmacologic value. Nevertheless, the improvement in symptoms simply from taking the placebo can be very real. About one in three people are susceptible to a placebo effect. In some cultures, such preparations can elicit almost as effective a relief as scientifically proven medications, in which they have little faith.

In fact, simply swallowing a placebo can have a measurable effect before any absorption could possibly occur. The knowledge and act of swallowing, along with the presence of an object in the stomach, causes reflexes and reactions in the nervous system.

Placebos are used in studies establishing the pharmacologic merit of a new drug by comparing the effect of the investigative drug to the placebo. Subjects receiving the placebo and believing they may have taken the new medication, often develop their own set of unwanted side effects such as dizziness, headaches, abdominal symptoms, aches, rashes, and hives.

The placebo effect shows that what the patient expects and thinks the drug should do, is almost as important as what the drug actually does. This also applies to surgery.

Occasionally, in the early years of cardiac-valve surgery, the chest was opened, but the surgery had to be stopped for various reasons. The heart had not been touched. When the patient wasn't told, at the request of his or her family, for example, many showed substantial improvement for as long as six months after the aborted procedure. Nonetheless, another operative attempt would be required.

Treating a specific individual who is sick involves more than performing a procedure or prescribing a pill that is statistically proven to be effective in most people. Effective and safe treatment must also take into account the multiple factors that make each person unique. The limitation of scientific treatment in drug therapy is a perfect illustration of how personal care must be used to supplement impersonal, statistical applications.

CHAPTER 53

The Licit Drug Culture

Prior to the mid-20th century, some of the most effective medications were adopted from folk remedies. This includes digitalis, as previously described, for heart failure; as well as **quinine** for fevers; **salicylic acid**, the precursor of aspirin, for **rheumatism**; and opiates for pain. Exactly how they worked was not understood, despite the growth of the science of pharmacology in the mid-19th century.

Improved understanding of drug mechanisms was based upon progress in the fields of biochemistry and molecular biology. This advancement had slowed during World War II, and then accelerated after that time.

By 1950, the antibiotics penicillin, **chloramphenicol**, and **chlortetracycline,** became available. The effective new derivatives of digitalis were marketed, and cortisone was introduced for rheumatism and other problems. By the end of the 1950s, the anticoagulant Coumadin, derived from dicumarol, was widely released. Ten years later, 30,000 new drug applications had been submitted to the food and drug administration (FDA) for approval.

The FDA was created in 1906, after deliberate adulteration of drugs by manufacturers was proven to be a national problem. The pharmaceutical industry has since come under increasing government supervision. In 1912, rules in regards to labeling and patenting of medicines were established. In 1937, safety became a key regulatory issue, and as of 1962, the efficacy of a new drug had to be established before it could be marketed.

Today, the testing, manufacture, and marketing of all new drugs must be approved by the FDA before they are released. By the time a drug becomes available, it will have required many years of development and evaluation, a process which today costs more than one billion dollars on average for a new drug. And the costs are climbing steadily.

In order for a company to market a new drug, it must conduct studies to demonstrate both its safety and its efficacy for treatment of a specific condition. It can only make claims for a drug if these are backed by a clinical study.

Once the FDA approves a drug for use in one condition, however, doctors are free to use the drug "off- label." This means that the drug may be prescribed as a treatment of a different condition, even though the drug has not been specifically approved for that use by the FDA. In such cases, the drug was studied for use with one condition, but no research was conducted with other conditions, so these latter conditions cannot be listed on the label by the manufacturer. However, different conditions may develop or behave in similar ways, or they may share similar symptoms. For these conditions, a doctor might prescribe a medication "off-label."

Within this system of FDA regulation, drug companies operate in the free marketplace. They may develop any new drug that they choose, subject to market forces. The huge profits available for successful drugs result in too many duplicate, "me too" drugs.

Often a new generation of drugs is only minimally different from prior ones. After a patent expires, companies will release a new and only slightly different version of the drug. Even a small change allows it to be protected under a new patent. Frequently, the older substance is just as effective as the newer one, yet much less expensive, especially when it becomes a generic drug and is no longer protected by a patent.

The attributes of a new drug may benefit only a small proportion of patients, yet the new therapy is frequently hyped and over-promoted. The release of Nexium after the expiration of the patent on Prilosec is a good example of this common practice.

Another unfortunate outcome of the profit-based marketplace is that rare diseases are neglected, since they don't promise great profit potential for the drug companies. When it is clear that there is less profit to be made, drugs developed for these conditions are often abandoned by commercial enterprises. These so-called "orphaned drugs" have received special government support for the development of new therapies that may be helpful to the small population of patients in the general public in need of such treatments.

—∿∿—

In the first half of the 1980s, drug companies were severely criticized for promoting new drugs to doctors by giving gifts of various sorts. As a result, drug companies cut back on this practice and reduced their corps of sales representatives.

Then, of course, drug sales suffered. So, in the latter half of the 1980s, the drug companies adopted strategies for promoting prescription drugs directly to the public. First, they surveyed doctors to determine how they would respond to this approach. Like many surveys, this was intended primarily to instruct those surveyed about the new approach. In this case, it was to prepare doctors for the new era to come in drug marketing.

In the 1990s, the advertisement of prescription drugs to the public came with a fury. Doctors were not happy about this turn of events. Most physicians are not inclined to take the extra time needed to educate their patients on the pros and cons of the newer versus the older medications. While doctors don't like taking the time to explain these differences in medications, they do feel the market pressure when patients mention a new drug. They feel the need to accommodate their patients' interests and respond more rapidly to the availability of the new medication.

As a result of big pharmaceutical companies marketing new drugs directly to the public and the resultant increase in the demand, many excellent and even superior older drugs are ignored in favor of the newer ones. The newer ones are more expensive, but patients who are on prescription plans don't really care. Patients demand the latest medications available, which they feel must be the best, even though this is often not true.

Among other things, our society has become a drug culture. The use of illicit drugs has not increased in our society as much as the demand for and the use of licit drugs. About 80 percent of the US population uses at least one prescription drug or over-the-counter medication on a regular basis.

Many people use numerous drugs. For office visits, I used to ask new patients to bring all of the medications that they had in the house with them to their next appointment. Often, these filled a shopping bag. This not only gave me a chance to review drug interaction problems, but I could also help them discard the old and useless ones. On house calls, I often took the opportunity to inspect patients' medicine cabinets. Many were crammed with outdated medications.

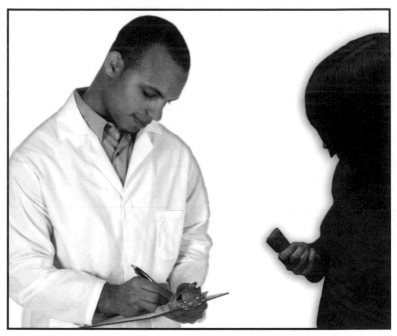

The licit drug culture

—∭—

A patient's level of education, personal theories on health, cultural background, as well as preconceptions from folklore and myths frequently act together to preempt a physician's instructions for use of a drug. Through personal knowledge and understanding of the patient, many physicians can overcome misperceptions about drugs.

Patients frequently don't use the prescribed drugs as instructed. I consistently found that a portion of a course of prescribed antibiotics would remain afterwards, instead of being completely used up as directed. Patients run the risk of not ridding themselves of an infection when they stop the antibiotic too soon—simply because they feel better. That's assuming that they needed the treatment in the first place.

Some patients hold back from using a portion, intending to use it for some future infection, despite the fact that the remaining amount would be insufficient to cure most infections. They run the risk of creating drug-resistant bacteria in their system.

Many patients are prone to the approach, "What the doctor doesn't know won't hurt him." They receive prescriptions from multiple doctors and fail to inform each doctor what the others have prescribed.

This frequently leads to a serious problem, where no one is keeping track of everything that a patient is taking. No one knows whether a patient is getting different drugs for the same purpose, or whether there may be conflicts in actions between the drugs. Pharmacists are aware of these issues only if patients have all of their prescriptions filled at the same pharmacy. Over-the-counter preparations also introduce additional hazards when taken in combination with prescribed medications.

When familiar with all of the drugs a patient is taking, pharmacists may be successful with detecting errors in physicians' prescriptions. Of course, however, pharmacists can make their own errors too, due to misreading prescriptions or filling them with the wrong drugs. One study in 2003 found that the average pharmacy that fills 250 prescriptions a day makes four errors within those 250 medications ordered.

The pharmacist's gratuitous instructions may add yet another layer of confusion and interfere with the physician's treatment. The practice of pharmacists adding their own instructions to the drug labels when filling prescriptions, may help increase the approved use of a drug and reduce adverse reactions. But it also introduces a new type of error. The instructions can modify the physician's intentions and may actually be harmful to patients.

For example, a physician may prescribe a drug for an off-label application, which is within medical standards. The drug label's instructions are only allowed to specify the FDA-approved use of the drug, which is not the use for which the physician has prescribed it. This confuses some patients who actually read the material on the label. Physicians must therefore warn patients about this if they want their instructions followed.

The bottom line is that new drugs can be marvelous and life-saving, but the commercial drug market has driven the development of too many new products. Also, the drug market and the regulatory system attempt to fit all patients into a standard mold, as if they had come off an assembly line. Carefully individualized and personalized use of drugs is essential for safety and effectiveness.

"Take on an empty stomach," for example, is an instruction pharmacists frequently place on medications, especially antibiotics. Some patients may not be able to take a drug this way because it causes stomach upset. They have no way of knowing whether these instructions were added to the container by the pharmacist or were intended by the doctor. They may not bother to contact either the doctor or the pharmacist concerning the instructions and, instead, may decide to simply not take the drug.

Taking a drug other than as directed can indeed change the absorption and effectiveness for an average patient based on studies. The doctor may determine, however, that for a particular patient, taking the drug under nonstandard conditions is better than not taking the drug at all. And learning this may be part of the process of dose adjustment, while determining the optimal level in that particular patient under these altered conditions. The physician knows, or at least should know, the patient better than the pharmacist does.

At times, the instructions on the label required by regulation even have the potential to be fatal. For example, the instructions added for a prescribed diuretic may advise a high intake of foods containing potassium, with the intent to prevent harmful potassium depletion from occurring in the body. I have seen this instruction placed inappropriately on a diuretic that was combined with another medication that already raised the level of potassium. I've checked blood levels for potassium in these patients and found several of them at potentially lethal levels.

Of similar concern is the attempt by pharmacists to broaden the scope of their practice. In the 1950s, I would ask clinic patients, "Who prescribed this medicine for you?"

Some patients would answer, "the doctor on the corner," meaning their local druggist.

In the early 1980s, according to a Commonwealth of Pennsylvania legislator, pharmacists on a sub-committee tried, unsuccessfully, to get legislation introduced which would limit physicians' powers in treating patients. Doctors were to make the diagnosis and pharmacists would manage the treatment.

In the late 1990s, I was treating Tim with the anticoagulant Coumadin and monitoring its effect through the appropriate blood test. He had a sensitivity to Coumadin, so I prescribed another medication that I knew had the potential to modify his sensitivity.

I told him to have his blood checked in several days after the new medication had a chance to change his sensitivity.

The following week, Tim went in to have his prescription for the new drug filled. He mentioned to the pharmacist that he'd been taking samples of the medication, which I had given him.

The pharmacist said, "Go immediately to a hospital emergency room!"

Tim called me, very concerned for obvious reasons.

After reassuring him, I then called the pharmacist and asked why he felt he should disregard my instructions without calling me, and should unnecessarily alarm Tim by sending him to an emergency room.

The pharmacist seemed unaware of the methods that doctors use to monitor the effects of anticoagulants, and had interpreted the potential for a drug interaction as an emergency.

The bottom line is that new drugs can be marvelous and life-saving, but the commercial drug market has driven the development of too many new products. Also, the drug market and the regulatory system attempt to fit all patients into a standard mold, as if they had come off an assembly line. Carefully individualized and personalized use of drugs is essential for safety and effectiveness.

CHAPTER 54

A Treatment for Every Human Flaw

As progress in genetics, medical technology, and drug therapies continue to advance the frontiers of healthcare, the expectations of the American public become almost unlimited. Increasingly today, even physiological variations among individuals are now being proposed as diseases. This shifts the primary burden of personal health improvement from the individual to the healthcare industry.

Where a condition does not have a clear-cut cause, those individuals falling well outside of the statistical norm are now regarded as abnormal. Thus, by the normal distribution curve, four percent of a group—those more than two standard deviations from the mean—may be regarded as abnormal for a measurement of any individual characteristic. And the criteria for measurement of a particular characteristic shifts over time. Thus, eventually, everyone could be deemed abnormal with respect to some characteristic or another.

People today expect to be treated for not only every condition, but almost every discomfort, symptom, unusual personal characteristic, or anxiety, with some drug or other. And it can't be just any drug. It must be the latest, which automatically is believed to be the best. As noted in the preceding chapter, the most recent is the most expensive, but not always better than an older brand. Advertising of the newest drugs directly to consumers feeds the frenzy.

For example, a generation ago, kids and their parents by and large ignored scratches and bruises, not requiring any treatment. Today, however, many do seek treatment for these trivial injuries.

I recently saw a doting mother who was watching the club's tennis pro run her talented 12-year-old son from one back corner of the tennis court to the other.

"I'll have to give him an Advil tonight," she said.

This was for the normal muscular aches that kids in the past accepted as an ordinary part of growing up, requiring no special treatment.

The sense of entitlement to physical perfection and total comfort is an expensive predisposition in American society today. Individual variations and minor conditions are not diseases that need to be treated.

New examples of abnormal anxiety categories are proposed nearly monthly. Some diagnosed with **post-traumatic stress disorder,** PTSD, have detectable neurophysiologic abnormalities. One anxiety that has been around for awhile is SAD, the wintertime **seasonal affective disorder**. It used to be called "cabin fever." However, it was eventually proven to be caused largely by physiologic abnormalities from reduced sunlight exposure and earned its designation as a disease.

One of the newer syndromes relatively rampant among young adults has been commonly termed "SEA sickness," for self-esteem asthenia. Another is genealogical bewilderment stress, or "GBS," which may be found in those who are anxious because they do not know their ancestral history.

Eventually, the claim will be made that every type of human anxiety, major or minor, has a basis in disturbed brain function. Drugs will be found for treating these real or imagined conditions. In addition, herbal and natural treatments will be promoted as cures.

—⁘—

In the 1990s, about 85 percent of proposed legislation in Pennsylvania had some health aspect. We are reaching the point at which almost every aspect of private or public activity is considered fair game for inclusion in the medical domain. Only one federal judge has been declared legally sane. Should we expect certifications of sanity from every public servant, particularly presidential candidates?

—〰—

Most aspects of lifestyle are by choice, yet many consider their lifestyle forced upon them by circumstances or factors outside of their control. Health treatments for preventing and moderating chronic conditions such as hypertension and arteriosclerosis must involve the participation of the individual patient. Changes in lifestyle are important in preventing and treating disease.

In the last decade of the 20th century, 70 percent of the increase in drug expenditure in the us was for comfort care. The same was true for the increase in surgical expenditures.

The sense of entitlement to physical perfection and total comfort is an expensive predisposition in American society today. Individual variations and minor conditions are not diseases that need to be treated.

CHAPTER 55

Straying from the Herd

Contrary to what many people believe, science is susceptible to fads, fashion, and serendipity, just like other human endeavors. Deliberate progress through planning has been effective in only a few areas of science. What usually happens is that a new technique, procedure, or gadget is developed, and this is then applied to every situation that seems suitable. The means becomes the end.

Purists seek a solution to a specific problem. They develop a new or special piece of equipment to achieve that end. The resultant device is not an end in itself.

Most of those who consider themselves researchers, believe they should be able to work in an area of their interest and expertise as the inclination moves them. This is disputed by those who believe that research should be goal-oriented—that is, directed to solving a specific problem for the social good, or more specifically, for the purpose of the group that is paying for the research.

Hence, much research by drug companies may be directed to the need, but it is the need as they see it. The company's primary need in free-market medicine, is to satisfy its stockholders by pursuing the path to the higher monetary return on the investment.

Another approach used when true innovation is difficult, is to simply change the existing nomenclature used within a system or specialty, to give the impression of progress. One of the consequences of this approach, intended or not, is to discourage the more senior workers in the given field. Often, the changes are based on only a few new facts. These then become the basis for attempts to extensively reorganize the known methodology.

The classic example of giving an old approach a new name,

has been the introduction in recent decades of "holistic care" as a supposedly new concept. It promotes the treatment of the individual as a whole person. Hippocrates is regarded as the father of medicine, and he introduced this concept in the 5th century B.C. It's simply called "personal care."

The creation of the "Metabolic Syndrome," discussed earlier, is another example of an attempt at a major conceptual shift through nothing more than a reorganization of existing information. This term refers to a group of metabolic risk factors, including abnormal blood fats and cholesterol, diabetes mellitus, and hypertension, which are aggravated by the secondary risk factors of excessive body weight and poor diet. This cluster of risk factors were known long before the name was coined.

Another example occurred in the early 1970s, when L. L. Weed proposed that a defined database be collected on each patient. This has come to be known by the acronym "SOAP," which stands for Subjective (history), Objective (physical), Assessment (diagnoses), and Plan. These are simply new names for taking a patient's history, conducting a physical examination, coming up with a diagnosis, and creating a treatment plan…the long-established approach to patient care.

The new approach did help to standardize the care methods and record keeping, but it also attempted to standardize physicians' thinking. Through such standardization, third parties found it easier to track, organize, systematize, and evaluate physician's medical practices more precisely. The standardized approach provided better understanding for third parties and helped in managing a complex system.

A similar introduction of a "new" approach was suggested in the early 1990s, with the term "evidence-based medicine." This implied that prior practice had not been based on inductive reasoning and was little more than the reading of entrails and tea leaves.

In my experience, evidentiary medical practices, which are based on clinical trials among large sample populations, actually only help with less than 5 percent of the work performed by a practicing physician. Study results provide nothing more than a starting place for what will become the doctor's truly individualized and personalized care for a specific patient.

—⟋⟍—

The first-hand knowledge of the various pathologic aspects of diseases, and their complex interactions in a particular patient, are as important for successful patient care as the information from the related standardized studies. Many physicians misuse the evidentiary approach by treating patients as if they were average subjects based on the statistics from the studies. Individualization and personal care are neglected.

The first clinical studies were undertaken in the mid-1700s with scurvy treatment and smallpox inoculation. The statistical tools for study design and evaluation, however, were not developed until the 1920s. One of the first large, multi-center trials took place at the end of the 1940s. The study was with anticoagulants for acute myocardial infarction, but this was crude and without contemporary controls. As of today, the cumulative number of published trials has grown to more than 40,000.

Many trials concern therapy, especially drug therapy, and are not only multi-centered but international in scope, some with tens of thousands of subjects. Many are more useful in application to the needs of large populations rather than those of individuals.

Trials are conducted for several reasons. One is to evaluate a drug or product for effectiveness and safety, so that it can be marketed. These studies are designed so that a determination can be made as to whether the new drug is superior to a placebo or is at least equal to, if not superior, to another available drug.

The criteria for selecting candidates that qualify for inclusion in the trial are broad and may be representative of only a small subset of patients treated by practicing physicians. The hope is that the information derived from the group can be extrapolated to individual patients. But no study has been done that can't be faulted in its extrapolation to the individual.

These large studies provide no more than guidelines to a physician caring for an individual patient, whom the doctor also evaluates according to patho-physiologic principals. Many of the studies, given the bias in the selection of ill subjects, simply prove that sick people are sicker than their well counterparts.

Most studies generate as many questions as they answer. From some of the studies with an extremely large number of participants, such as the studies on the use of hormone-replacement therapies in women, conflicting conclusions have been drawn.

Some subgroup responses are unexpected and differ from the majority of the study participants. This difference often requires a confirmation study using patients with these special characteristics.

Very few particular patients in a physician's practice have all of the same characteristics of those in a large study. Clinicians need to know how a treatment is going to work on their specific patients, each a unique being.

One suggestion has been that all of the data from these large studies should be made available to practicing physicians through a website on the internet. A physician can then enter the individual characteristics of a patient. The applicability of the study conclusions to this specific individual would be analyzed based on the results from that specific subgroup in the study. This analysis would be immediately available online to the physician.

The parties most interested in the promotion of evidence-based medicine are drug companies. They need to conduct the studies, pay for them, and then use the results to promote particular new drugs. Other interested parties include "herd" managers, such as group insurers, and social engineers who are involved in the management of large populations and have little experience with individual patients in the clinic.

I suspect that some of these very large studies in time will be regarded as dogma, much as the evidentiary medicine promoters now regard the small studies of the past. The assumption is that physicians relying on personal experience have been on the wrong track and their practices need to be changed. In reality, the opposite is true.

Doctors who are deeply involved in the personal care of patients frequently adopt individualized treatments that are far from those promoted for the herd. Fortunately, this usually provides a higher quality care for the specific patient.

CHAPTER 56

Am I Sick?

The objective of all medical care might be summed up best by the recognized goal of rehabilitation medicine: "After prevention fails and a diagnosis is made, the aim of care is to restore the patient to maximum physical, mental, emotional, psychiatric, vocational, and social well-being."

How is well-being defined? Is it simply the absence of disease? If so, how is disease defined, and who determines whether an individual does or does not have a disease? Finally, are we talking about the individual alone or the population as a whole, i.e., the herd?

According to a World Health Organization conference in 1970, the standard for good health should be self-determined by each individual. In the US, however, it is generally assumed to be the absence of disease as determined by others.

Medical care usually begins when the individual and often his or her immediate confidantes—spouse, family, or friends—decide that he or she is ill and that self-help has failed. Only then does the individual seek professional medical care.

Most people today have a pretty good idea about what is wrong with them when they go to a doctor. They are seeking reassurance as to the nature of their illness, as well as help toward a speedier recovery.

The higher the individual's level of education, the more apt he or she is to be among the "worried-well." These people seek reassurance and treatment earlier than most patients. Many worried-well people tend to expect extensive testing to determine if they may harbor an incipient disease or are at risk for certain illnesses.

At the opposite extreme are those who are unaware of or dismiss health issues because of ignorance or culture. Often, their specific symptoms or complaints are ignored or are difficult for them to recognize and describe.

I have cared for those who know they are ill only when they can't get out of bed in the morning because of extreme weakness. I've seen others who keep falling down when walking, not recognizing some obvious symptom such as tremendously swollen legs and very significant weight gain from retained fluid. Still others I've seen realize they are not well when they can't finish their usual day's work because of extreme fatigue.

Some simply ignore the potential of illness because they can't afford medical care. With the decline in the number of free clinics, impoverished people today use hospital emergency departments for initial care. By the time they do so, a condition that may have been easily treatable earlier may now require hospitalization.

Physicians' styles of addressing different types of patients vary, depending upon training and specialty area. Physicians all have a tacit contract to attend to the patient's medical welfare within the sphere of their own expertise and limitations, but they may have very different perceptions of their responsibilities resulting from this contract. Merely meeting the standards of care recommended by a medical organization does not fulfill all of the physicians' obligations to the patient.

As I've noted before, people do not come off assembly lines like cars. Physicians must modify and tailor standard treatments, depending upon their general knowledge of how a specific patient's body systems work and how these functions respond to or are modified by specific disease processes. Doctors must also understand how each patient is affected by specific treatments. Physicians must understand not only how this individual is different, but also how personal factors, other than those listed in the standards, affect the management of the patient and the illness.

These factors may be determined only through an understanding of the detailed personal variations of the individual patient. And the resulting care must be applied on a personal basis.

In recent decades, technology-based treatment has led to less personal attention, along with increasing costs and other major changes in the care of patients. These trends have converged, leading to a powerful interference with the important process of focusing medical care on the personal factors of the individuals.

PART V

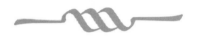

Paying the Price

CHAPTER 57

Servants of Two Masters

When a patient pays a doctor directly and is responsible for the full fee, a mutual accountability is created that promotes a healthy relationship between the two parties. Not only are doctors ethically required to place the patient's health interests first, but the fee paid directly by the patient alone provides an economic incentive for the doctor to satisfy the patient. This, in turn, helps the doctor to build a following, a practice.

This traditional system of direct payment by patients was in place until the 1950s. Since then, it has gradually been modified and distorted in a number of ways, so as to obscure the traditional, two-party, mutual accountability.

In essence, the physician today has two masters—the patient and the healthcare organization that employs the physician. Medicine has become a job rather than an independent profession.

In 1939, the Roosevelt Administration prepared a plan to nationalize healthcare. In view of our impending involvement in World War II, however, the plan was temporarily shelved. During the war, employer-based health insurance was encouraged and became more widespread.

Immediately after the War, the plan for the nationalization of healthcare was introduced once again. Congress rejected this idea when insurers and others insisted that it should not be a government-run program, but instead should be administered by the commercial insurance industry. Employer-based health coverage grew.

Finally, with the advent of Medicare and **Medicaid** in the 1960s, partially nationalized healthcare was established. Soon, employers, along with government agencies and insurers, felt that dealing with a loose system of independent physicians was like herding cats. Such a system was too difficult to manage. Personal medical care delivered from community doctors' offices was disparagingly referred to as a primitive "cottage industry" by many third parties.

By the 1980s, insurers, employers, and hospitals had created large healthcare systems that collected potential patients into groups or herds. Patients were soon regarded as clients or customers.

Today, few patients pay the doctor directly for all of their medical bills. They tacitly allow the employers to turn their medical purse over to the third-party system that manages them as part of the herd.

The group costs are controlled through several mechanisms that ration care. One is the insurance underwriting system that distributes the cost of care through the pool of insured. Another mechanism is the health maintenance organization or other similar system that contracts with doctors to deliver care for fees that are less than the doctors' usual fees.

Various incentives are offered in order to keep the costs of services low. One of the rationing mechanisms limits patient procedures by agreement. Administrators establish the rules and make decisions about patient care that are based upon the welfare of the organization's purse rather than the welfare of the patient. These decisions not only work to the disadvantage of the patient, but also penalize the doctor.

Whether an employee or independent practitioner, the physician today—who is primarily paid by the healthcare organization—has a supervisor in medical decisions regarding the patient. The ethical standards of care of course remain, but the contemporary physician does not have the same economic incentives to satisfy the patient, as compared to the traditional, fully self-employed physician, who is paid directly and in-full by the patient.

In essence, the physician today has two masters—the patient and the healthcare organization that employs the physician. Medicine has become a job rather than an independent profession.

For several reasons, neither the patient nor the physician is likely to be satisfied with this type of far-less personal relationship. Patients today can no longer rely upon a continuity of care provided by the same physician. Also, since the doctor is not adequately reimbursed for time spent with the patient, the office visit has become a brief interaction, and is much less personal and reliable.

Patients expect more testing as a substitute for personal care. Many physicians are happy to provide tests, which take little time to order in their overcrowded schedules. And they are happy to refer patients to specialists.

Many referrals today are for problems that were ordinarily handled by primary physicians in the past. Specialists can sort these out, but in so doing, also feel obligated to conduct more specialized testing than indicated. The decrease in the level of personal care is one reason for the rise in malpractice litigation. This type of defensive medicine is also more expensive.

The development of innovative medical technology has become a double-edged sword. It is life-saving, but it has also driven the cost of care higher and higher, to astronomical proportions compared to 50 years ago.

The attempt to control the dramatic rise in costs has resulted in a shift in medical economics. Funding for the time required for relatively inexpensive personal care, as well as the relationship between doctor and patient, have declined. This reduction in cost for personal care has been more than offset by the unnecessary increase in the use of more expensive technology. The entire progression has been counterproductive.

The problem is propagated by our culture and the medical

education system. Many patients as well as physicians value technology above personal care. They regard extensive testing as higher quality care. Also, physicians seem less aware of controlling costs today than in earlier decades.

This system of inverted values, replacing the personal doctor-patient relationship with impersonal technology, is endemic to the medical research and educational system, which are the institutions that train our doctors today.

CHAPTER 58

Don't Worry About Money

People choose to become physicians for many reasons. Most freshman medical students' interest in medicine is altruistic to a large degree. Unfortunately, many lose this as a priority by senior year. Faculties of many medical schools have a primary interest in research and super-specialization. The glamour of these role models and the promise of technology gradually supersede the altruism.

Students in the 1940s had been raised during the Great Depression, and many of them wanted to pursue medicine for purely economic reasons. College tuitions in 1942 were astoundingly low. The undergraduate tuition at the University of Wisconsin, a state university, was $50 per year, and the medical school tuition was $150 annually.

Doctors appeared to make an easy living, even during the Great Depression. In 1942, the dean told my incoming freshman class that first-year, pre-medical students had the lowest grade-point average of any major. It attracted many of the more academically challenged for economic reasons.

The career wasn't as easy as it may have appeared, however, and the living was not necessarily as good. In that era, it wasn't until physicians were in their mid-40s that they had earned as much cumulatively as their high-school classmates who had become apprenticed in a trade right out of high school.

The only time that income or medical economics were mentioned in medical school was as an aside in a third-year lecture by Ovid Meyer, M.D., Professor of medicine. He simply told us, "Don't worry about money. It'll take care of itself."

—⁂—

In 1947, the stipend for my internship at Research Hospital was $50 a month in addition to free room, board, and laundry. This was twice the $25 stipend paid to interns in the previous year. In 1948, I earned $100 per month during my residency.

Many highly regarded internship positions paid nothing more than room and board. Pennsylvania Hospital, the nation's first hospital, was the last in the country to pay interns. That was in 1960. When it did, however, the Hospital then charged for room, board, parking, and laundry. It was mostly a wash. Interns with families at some Philadelphia hospitals qualified for food stamps.

Most doctors at the time went on to become general practitioners. Ed Jones, my fellow resident at Research Hospital, started a general practice in a small town near Kansas City. Throughout the Midwest and especially in the Great Plains states, the general practitioner was not just the only doctor in town. He was the only one for miles around. After about five years, he would be burned out, but by then he had saved enough money to take on a residency for specialty training.

Some doctors found subspecialties more inviting in that they permit better organization of one's time. Specialists also tended to practice in larger communities where other specialists were practicing. This gave them coverage for weekends off-call and for vacations. This is one of the attractions of group practices.

Occasionally, a doctor who had been in solo general practice wanted and badly needed some relief, so he would bring in another doctor. Often, these were specialists such as obstetricians, surgeons, orthopedists, or urologists. Many of the large clinics of today were started and built by solo general practitioners.

When I was looking for a place to settle down and practice, I visited cardiologists in Fort Wayne, Philadelphia, Burlington, Kansas City, Milwaukee, and other areas. I was impressed with how the Great Depression had left its mark. Most of these specialists hedged their practices in some way so that they could shift quickly into general medicine. A cardiologist in Fort Wayne, for example, admitted that he was doing 15-percent general medicine for that reason.

State legislatures expected the state-supported medical schools to provide general practitioners for the state. Prior to the 1940s, this was not difficult as specialization and the specialty boards were just becoming established. After World War II, however, the increasing influence of the specialty boards was felt at the local level. The battle for positions and certifications between generalists and specialists was heating up in the late 1940s and early 1950s across the country, and Kansas City was no exception.

Prior to World War II, most members of hospital staffs were generalists. There was little specialty training. In Kansas City, many had been in the same intern class at Kansas City General Hospital. Some of those going into surgery took an additional year of pathology or surgery. One would go out as a general practitioner and do surgery. His classmate would go out as a surgeon and do general practice.

After World War II, however, the generalists got their wings clipped. Those physicians who were certified by the increasingly influential specialty boards gradually became more dominant on the hospital staffs. The self-designated surgeons had been grand-fathered into the specialty boards, that is, they were certified without testing. And the general practitioners who did surgery but were uncertified had their range of surgical procedures progressively restricted by their colleagues—who didn't necessarily have any more surgical training or capability.

Many of these surgeons were doing general practice as well. This provided a patient referral base that was much more dependable than relying on other doctors for referrals. This was also one of the persisting effects of the Great Depression.

Doctors starting out in practice at the same time often trained together. They know each other's capabilities and have confidence in one another. Each helps the other's practice grow through mutual referrals.

This interdependency could cause difficulties when a young associate was brought in by an established senior. Often, the distribution of the income was based on the number of new patients referred to the practice. When the young doctor was told by a referring doctor that he was preferred because he was more up to date, the established doctor in the practice might claim the referral because, "Smith always refers to me." This type of disagreement was responsible for the dissolution of many partnerships.

Other group practices threatened to break up over more mundane matters. One internist in a group of four, said that a day didn't go by that the group wasn't threatened by a breakup over very inconsequential issues—such as what quality of typing paper or even toilet paper that should be used in their office.

During early post-World War II in Kansas City, many of the generalists did not refer patients to non-surgical specialists such as neurologists or cardiologists. They felt that a more precise diagnosis was of little help, as nothing more could be done than what they were already doing. Patients were sent directly to the surgeon who could do more. In those instances where surgery was not indicated, some specialty surgeons would refer the patient to a medical specialist.

Soon, of course, the subspecialists took the lead in the training centers. These technology experts imbued the next generation of medical students with the sense that clinical care of the patient was of less importance than conducting the latest tests and procedures. With the rapid rise in the cost of technology and other aspects of care, funding issues began to have an increasing impact on medicine.

CHAPTER 59

Worries About Money

In 1939, as a teenager in Milwaukee, I had surgery for scrotal swelling from fluid that had collected around the testicles. Based on theory rather than fact, the surgeon performed bilateral **hernia** surgery. This surgery was entirely unnecessary. I had no hernias and there was a simpler, standard procedure for correcting the swelling.

I stayed in a private hospital for 16 days and wasn't allowed out of bed for 14 days. I had no complications. I was simply a subject of training for a few doctors and nurses. Student nurses insisted that I take deep breaths to prevent pneumonia.

I couldn't stand straight for a week. It cost my dad $9 out-of-pocket. His company insurance paid the rest.

The economics of healthcare in day-to-day medical practice was much more apparent at that time. Patients' care was self-rationed based on their ability to pay. Employer-paid health insurance like my father's was unusual.

In the 1940s, the cost for a hospital bed was about $5 per day. Businessmen on hospital boards at the time wondered how hospitals could charge so little with their expensive 24-hour-a-day employees, when hotels couldn't afford to rent rooms for less than $10 per day. Contributions to hospitals from their communities made up the difference.

In the 1930s and 1940s, Blue Cross organizations spread across the country. Some were started by radiologists, surgeons, and pathologists to pay for in-hospital care. In Kansas City, the cost of radiology procedures, such as upper gastro-intestinal series and barium enemas, were covered only for patients admitted to the hospital. So doctors would admit them to the hospital for one day.

Blue Cross changed the minimum requirement for coverage

to two days in the hospital, and then to three days. All this accomplished was to lengthen patient stays approved by doctors just to cover the test charges. Finally, Blue Cross gave up and paid the outpatient procedure charges. The flood gates were ajar.

—m—

Until the 1960s, Blue Shield covered surgical procedures as well as doctors' charges for inpatient care. It did not cover specialty consultants. Most private insurance coverage of nonsurgical hospital treatment was disease-specific. The more affordable policies paid a fixed amount for diagnoses such as infantile paralysis, cancer, stroke, or myocardial infarction. The coverage of nonsurgical admissions broadened after 1966 when Medicare was introduced.

By the 1970s, a large difference existed between the hospital's full charges, which were based on expenses and the mix of patients, and the much lower reimbursements permitted by Medicare, Medicaid, and Blue Cross. Private payers and insurance companies were expected to make up this difference by paying the fully billed rate. This still accounts for the outrageously high hospital bills that uninsured people receive today.

Hospital costs rose spectacularly after World War II, when the bare-bones operations required during the Depression and the war came to an end. With the ensuing prosperity, the hospital boards followed the lead of corporate America. The décor, departments, and salaries ballooned.

In the 1940s and 1950s, most doctors were careful about costs to the patient, and some were too careful. At times, the limitations placed on testing were penny-wise and pound-foolish. Patients often needed to return prematurely because of the doctor's failure to test for adequate control of the admitting disease, such as diabetes, or for preventable complications that would have been detectable prior to discharge.

—m—

A recession in 1957-58 hit just after I'd set up a private practice in Independence, Missouri. I found that this did not have as devastating an effect on medical care as the Depression of the 1930s. This was attributable in part to unemployment insurance. Men would come in during a lay-off, unconcerned.

"What are you doing with your free time?" I asked one man.

"I'm painting the house."

Wives went to work part-time until their husbands were recalled.

A number of established doctors noted the cyclic nature of their practices. When they were very busy, the flow of net income would be low. When the demand eased up, the cash flow suddenly increased due to the lag-time in billing and payment.

A urologist I knew in Independence used to take his vacations during these ebbs in demand. Most doctors could have relied on this security, but few actually trusted it enough to take the opportunity to enjoy the respite.

CHAPTER 60

Paid in Lobsters

During the era in which patients paid all of their medical fees directly, physicians charged whatever the traffic would bear. Full payments compensated for the free treatment of the poor who were unable to pay. As of the 1950s, this free-market approach was particularly relevant for those who were attempting to build a practice of the middle-class and well-to-do patients.

People often judge the competence of doctors by how much they charge. Nobody wants bargain-basement brain surgery.

In 1958, I gave a talk at a medical conference and had dinner with another presenter. He was a hematologist with a practice on Park Avenue in New York City, who happened to have a unique billing method. He said he'd never billed a patient for a specific amount. His patients were asked to pay whatever they thought his services were worth. Overall, the doctor claimed he received more money than if he had billed at a set rate. One might conclude that he had no patients with average incomes in his practice.

In the mid-1960s, the laissez faire medical billing system was destined to change. Medicare and Medicaid established approved fee schedules for those physicians wishing to care for these patients. They were soon followed by Blue Shield and other insurance companies, with their preferred provider networks.

US legislators had no idea just how much free medical service was given to the elderly and indigent before the introduction of Medicare and Medicaid, which paid for the elderly and the impoverished, respectively. Lawmakers didn't seem to appreciate the potential financial impact of this voluntary welfare system that was already in place, and they made no attempt to understand it.

For several years, both patients and doctors were suspicious of Medicare. When the distrust was overcome, and most of the prior welfare services were transferred into the Medicare and Medicaid systems, the costs of the new programs grew much faster than expected nationwide.

An ophthalmologist friend of mine had been doing three to five free cataract operations per week for indigent patients at Wills Eye Hospital in Philadelphia. After Medicare was introduced, the surgery which he had been performing without charge was then being reimbursed at $300 per procedure. He didn't say how much, if any, of his Medicare windfall he had to turn over to the Hospital.

Of course, this free service that he had been giving had been factored into his other medical care charges, which made up the difference. After starting to receive Medicare reimbursement, I'm sure that he, like all other doctors at the time, did not reduce his fees. Thus, the new government programs were inflationary.

Many physicians starting a practice in urban areas were able to support themselves within a short time, largely as a result of the income from these new programs. Others in larger urban centers would work part-time as company physicians, in addition to their private practices. This stifled the ability for some to build their practice. The new doctors were either too comfortable or too afraid to rid themselves of this income security. Today, most physicians start out as employees of a medical group.

People often judge the competence of doctors by how much they charge. Nobody wants bargain-basement brain surgery. In the 1960s, I read about one doctor in his early 60s who wanted to cut back his practice and did not want to hire an associate. He increased his fees in order to discourage new patients. His practice grew. He increased the fees again. His practice continued to grow. He continued increasing the fees, and he remained busier than he'd ever been.

In depressed times, many doctors were paid in kind. In rural areas, this would be farm produce. Most doctors still receive gifts at holidays, including fruit baskets, baked goods, candy, and the like. One patient would give me home-grown figs; another, goodies from the family bakery.

Roger was my patient for many years. He couldn't work. I never charged him or Medicaid. But he was a very resourceful individual. He saw to it that I was made a "Kentucky Colonel," an "Arkansas Traveler," an "admiral in the Nebraska Navy," and received a "Key to the City of New Orleans."

But that wasn't all.

One of his most tasteful payments was a fresh, 15-by-20-inch, two-tiered strawberry shortcake, given to him by a friend of his who was a pastry chef at the Old Bookbinders Restaurant in Philadelphia. This cake was topped only by the crate of 26 live lobsters, which he had delivered to my office from an acquaintance of his in Maine.

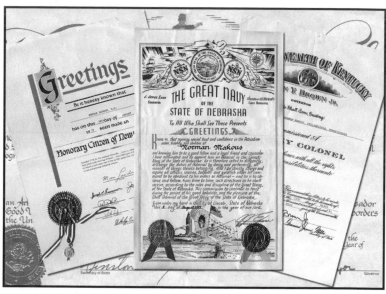

In-kind payments to Dr. Makous for services rendered

—∿—

Whenever a friend became a patient, it provided a challenge. I found that when they were not charged at all, they were reluctant to call for advice or come in for a visit. They felt it was an imposition, since they were receiving free services. This reduced the level of care they received compared to regular paying patients. They felt trapped by the friendship and didn't want to insult me by changing doctors.

I found that imposing a small nominal charge for services eliminated their reluctance to seek advice. They appreciated the care as well as the reduction in fee.

When I started practice, professional courtesy was the norm. Physicians didn't charge for the care of fellow physicians or their families. Some extended this courtesy to dentists and the clergy. In Philadelphia, however, this was not the practice among all physicians, particularly psychiatrists.

Later, as more and more physicians had medical insurance, the practice was to accept the insurance payment as full payment. Today, professional courtesy is a thing of the past. All physicians carry medical insurance and are usually billed for the copayment like any other patient, although it can be waived at times.

Fee-splitting in the legal profession, for example, is regarded as a finder's fee and is generally appropriate. In medicine, it's always considered unethical. The concern is that the referring doctor may be influenced more by the size of the monetary kickback than by the welfare of the patient. The patient deserves the best consultant or surgeon. Monetary concerns shouldn't enter into the consideration.

Of course, factors other than the exchange of money influence referral patterns. Physicians who train together tend to refer patients to each other and help build each others' practices. They know each others' strengths and limitations, which can benefit the patient.

Patients may, however, require specialty care beyond that provided by specialists in the same group, yet they may not receive the appropriate referral. This is a particular problem in multi-specialty group practices that have a policy of not referring patients outside of the group. If they do so, they may be subject to disapproval within the group, including a financial penalty.

One of the original justifications for fee-splitting was the disproportionate compensation collected by the surgeon as compared to the referring physician. The family physician got up in the middle of the night and made the house call. He made the diagnosis of **acute appendicitis,** arranged for an immediate operation, and admitted the patient to the hospital. He then went to the hospital to await completion of the surgery with the family. In these early days, this whole ordeal might incur a charge of $10.

The surgeon, on the other hand, would spent an hour overall and charge $150. The surgeon could not turn part of his fee over to the family physician. This is considered unethical fee-splitting. One solution considered ethical by many was to use the family physician as an assistant at surgery, even though the surgeon may not have needed this additional help. This justified the charge of an assistant's fee by the referring physician. However, the surgeon didn't necessarily reduce his own fee.

Generally, doctors do make a comfortable living, but for most, it is well-earned. Many of the internists I knew in the Kansas City area were working 70 to 80 hours per week, as I was. Several were putting in more than 90 hours per week. In recent decades in the Philadelphia area, the average was around 60 hours per week. Many physicians who are also employees expect shorter work weeks and more time off in trade for their lower-income levels.

Like many other employees in our society, physicians' incomes have remained flat over the past 15 years. Nonetheless, it remains a financially rewarding profession.

CHAPTER 61

A Pot of Molasses

Overall, the cost of care in hospitals is substantially greater than the cost of care by physicians. In the latter part of the 20th century, hospital costs rose significantly, due to changes resulting from the new technologies. The methods of funding the costs of patient care, particularly with the involvement of government oversight, changed dramatically during that period.

My experiences on the staff at Pennsylvania Hospital for nearly 50 years gave me an inside view of these changes and their impact on patient care. Pennsylvania Hospital, established in 1751, was the first institution in the nation designed and built as a hospital. The original building's cornerstone is still displayed about four feet below the current street level. Benjamin Franklin was one of its founders.

The Hospital grounds occupy an entire city block between Eighth and Ninth streets and between Spruce and Pine streets, a mile from the center of the city. It was built on pastureland with a stream. The original red brick wall separates the grounds from the sidewalk and streets. The southern third of the premises still has the original lawn. The herb garden was restored in recent years.

In the 1960s, Pennsylvania Hospital was regarded as a sleepy, bucolic institution by many in the medical profession, particularly those at the hospital of the University of Pennsylvania, a thriving research center at 34th Street. To many people in nearby south Philadelphia, the Hospital was cold, aloof, or foreboding, in part because of its wall. In view of its inconspicuous staff turmoil, I came to regard it as a simmering pot of molasses.

When I first arrived at Pennsylvania Hospital in 1953, the handful of private rooms was out of the 19th century. Few had toilets and some didn't even have a sink and running water. The Hospital had emerged from the tradition of volunteer hospitals, employing staff who would work for little or no pay. Some of the employees had been recent patients, and a number of those were disabled. They were generally untrained.

—ҡ—

The medical practice at the hospital provided an interesting contrast to the reactionary practices in Kansas City and the Midwest. Organized medicine in the US still held the fear of the socialization of medicine, which was introduced in Great Britain right after World War II. There, the government had taken on the responsibility of providing everyone with medical care. In Kansas City, any doctor who had an office within a mile of a hospital was thought to be in danger of being "taken over" and made an employee of the hospital.

In sharp contrast to the Midwest, most of the doctors' offices at Pennsylvania Hospital were in buildings owned by the Hospital, in a perfect position to be taken over, yet there was no concern about this eventuality. In the larger urban areas like Philadelphia, physicians and patients had many more options than those in communities with only one or two hospitals. In these urban areas, hospitals were much less likely to acquire medical practices.

The Pennsylvania School of Medicine was founded in the 1780s at Pennsylvania Hospital. Jacob Ehrenzeller was the first house-staff member. As a trainee, he basically was an indentured slave for four years in the early 1780s. Interns in modern times serve there for two years.

In the 1950s, Pennsylvania Hospital had an association with both the University of Pennsylvania and Thomas Jefferson medical schools, but was independent with its own board and endowment. The large, house staff basically ran the Hospital, which was devoted primarily to care for the poor. In 1997, the University of Pennsylvania made Pennsylvania Hospital part of its health system.

The hospital board at the time was involved in hands-on, day-to-day management. The Board's House Committee didn't get out of the linen closets, monitoring supplies and other operational minutia until sometime after H. Robert Cathcart was appointed chief executive officer in 1952.

By the late 1940s, the Hospital began to experience a deficit. The usual community support from corporate grants and other donations was inadequate to prevent erosion of the endowment. The Hospital Board's proposed solution to the deficit was to merge with Graduate Hospital. After committing to this marriage in 1954, the Board had second thoughts. They retained the chief consultant for the New York City hospitals, who was a physician, lawyer, and accountant. His charge was to evaluate the merger and make recommendations.

After nine months of study by his team, his conclusions were announced at a heavily attended, general medical staff meeting. It was held in the main auditorium, located off of the foyer opposite the main entrance, just behind Benjamin West's large painting of "Christ Healing the Sick."

The consultant's conclusions were as follows: first, a merger with Graduate Hospital would not solve the problems of either hospital, as neither could provide the other with what they each needed; and second, the problems were the fault of the physicians on the medical staff.

This last conclusion was ridiculous. Only a handful of doctors had any financial stake in the institution. Most admitted no patients and few patients were referred from one's private practice. Only a few of the doctors on the staff were full-time. Garfield Duncan, M.D., chief of medicine, was the only one who was able to make a living in private practice there. Dr. Joseph Vander Veer was head of cardiology at two hospitals, the other being Bryn Mawr Hospital, where he also had an office.

Many young physicians started at Pennsylvania Hospital but couldn't make a living. They ended up practicing in the suburbs, where the more affluent people lived. Most of the 400 doctors who were active on the staff contributed their time to teach. Before World War II, Dr. Duncan said he had spent seven years in the outpatient clinics before gaining the privilege to teach on the wards as an attending physician.

The merger with Graduate Hospital was annulled. Six years later, a long-range building development program began to replace some of the antiquated structures.

Hospital administrators at many institutions felt that the influence of doctors in hospital management was excessive, so they were involved in a constant campaign to reduce physician influence. At Pennsylvania Hospital in 1960, the doctors' dining room was eliminated. The doctors' coat room was moved from the entrance to a less accessible location in the building. After considerable staff protest, an area for staff dining was created in the general dining room, which allowed for medical conversation out of earshot of patient's families, and the coat room was moved to a more convenient place.

Hospital administrators had three different internal groups to manage, in addition to patients and the public. It was like a three-mast sailing ship without a captain. The medical staff was in charge of one mast, the nursing staff had another, and the administrative department controlled the third. Each group of staff members had its own ideas about where the ship should be going, and the president was at the helm trying to keep the befuddled vessel from capsizing.

In order for the hospital to qualify for significant government funding, it had to have a major affiliation with a University. The Pennsylvania Hospital had always been part of the University of Pennsylvania, but the association with it, and later with Jefferson, was considered a minor one. In 1958, the Hospital staff elected to go with the University as a major affiliation. This meant, among other things, that the entire staff had to be appointed to the University's faculty.

Most of the department and section heads had primary appointments as full professors. Later, this became a battle over academic-track designations. Those not in the research track were given a "clinical" designation, frequently over their objections. Whenever the hospital contract was renegotiated with the University, great turmoil would occur as a result of this provision. Hospital management and staff attempted to negotiate from a position as an institution that was equal to the University, not accepting the fact that—from the University's financial point of view—the hospital was just another component, like an animal laboratory or a library.

By the early 1960s, 15 percent of the Hospital's income was derived from research grants. In 1963, the Hospital's Board adopted a resolution affirming that Pennsylvania Hospital was primarily an institution devoted to patient care, not primarily a research institution. President Johnson's blueprint for "The Great Society" was on the horizon. Soon, patient care would eclipse research as the key beneficiary of the government's cornucopia.

When Medicare was launched in 1965, the impact on hospital care nationwide was monumental. Medicare regulations allowed a hospital to calculate its expenses on which reimbursement was based by one of three methods. The formula selected by most hospitals was based on the percentage of the hospital area devoted to in-patient care.

At Pennsylvania Hospital, 15 percent of the total hospital area was used for outpatient services. This meant that 15 percent of the president's salary and other overhead was disallowed as an eligible Medicare expense. As a result of the reimbursement formulas, the services traditionally provided by the hospital changed. Space not devoted to in-patient care had to go.

Outpatient clinics were the first to go. Initially, the clinics were moved to doctors' offices, but in time, other non-hospital areas on the expanding hospital campus were devoted to clinic services. For hospitals retaining a clinic, the floor area was reduced so that it comprised a much smaller percentage of the total hospital area.

For those hospitals that had an affiliated nursing school, all related expenses had been included in most hospital budgets. This line item, too, was not covered by the Medicare reimbursement formula. The solution was to eliminate the nursing school. The nursing faculty remained on the hospital payroll but they were now devoted to in-hospital, in-service training.

Part of the justification for the increased in-service nurse trainers was the claim that many of the nurses with University degrees had less practical experience than those nurses trained at hospital nursing schools. The new University graduates therefore were required to have additional training in hospitals. By the early 1970s, Medicare reimbursed 108 percent of nursing wages, based on the rationale that Medicare patients required more nursing care than younger patients.

The introduction of Medicare also significantly changed the training of physicians. To qualify for reimbursement, surgeons had to be present in the operating room while supervising trainee residents. It made the usual policy of supervising several residents operating on patients in different rooms unacceptable for reimbursement. Likewise, with the medical services, the residents and interns were to be more closely supervised by a staff physician than they had been in the past.

Since this period in the 1960s, hospitals always seemed to be building, creating new beds and other patient-care facilities. For hospitals accepting Medicare patients, any new rooms that were built could be used as single rooms only. Double rooms, multi-bed rooms, and large wards were not allowed.

Hospitals, even nonprofit hospitals, profited through borrowing money for the new construction. Not only could they receive reimbursements based on the portion of the loan principal paid annually, but also based on the sizable interest for the debt service. Thus, they were able to deduct from their income more than 100 percent of the actual cost of construction as an expense over five or six years. Congress finally eliminated this anomaly in order to reduce the addition of unnecessary beds.

Many communities reduced their costs for medical care of the indigent by eliminating city and county General Hospitals. Extra beds in private hospitals were supposed to be devoted to the indigent. This was a big change, as the city and county community hospitals had been excellent training facilities for physicians.

CHAPTER 62

You'll Just Have to Take Us to Court

With the influx of the new government funding, the 1960s and 1970s was a time of great expansion in hospital facilities, personnel, activities, and costs, which caused a great deal of turmoil in a hospital's internal politics.

More than two-thirds of hospital costs are in salaries. Up until the 1960s, the administrative employees were generally untrained and unskilled. Then, as of the mid-1960s, the heads of administrative departments were college-trained. Their departments received name changes and grew in responsibilities as well as size of staff.

Pennsylvania Hospital had always been sparkling clean. This tradition continued after the housekeeping department was renamed "environmental services," and the staff doubled from 60 to 120 members within four months. By the late 1960s, most hospitals needed new, around-the-clock security departments. Government regulations required more record keeping, which required more clerical support.

The fact that Pennsylvania Hospital had no tree of authority was an administrative flaw that soon became apparent. Hospital President Robert Cathcart kept his fingers on the detailed workings of every department, until he became too busy attending to external matters. It appeared that his administrative staff could say "No" to staff requests, but couldn't say "Yes."

The President's office door, which I called the "kitchen door" due to its frequency of use, was open every Saturday morning and anybody was welcome to walk in and talk with him. He headed off a great deal of staff discontent in this way.

By 1970, medical staff affairs were dismal. Many new beds had been added and the Hospital was having trouble adapting to the increased number of physicians who were in private practice with offices on the campus. However, of the 400-plus doctors on the staff, less than 100 were actively admitting patients.

Prior to the mid-1960s, many local physicians had been ignored, as they were not eligible for a University appointment. Then, with the need to fill beds, they were recruited to the staff anyway, with admitting privileges, in order to increase the patient census. As soon as the beds got tight and admitting patients became difficult, the staff appointments for many of these local physicians were not renewed, and they were summarily dumped. As a result, many of these disgruntled physicians discontinued referring patients to specialists at the Hospital.

Department directors weren't treated much better. They were recruited as if the Hospital was a University, and these directors were initially given what was promised. After they arrived, however, the hospital administration would not invest further in their efforts to improve their respective departments.

The chiefs used various techniques to circumvent the lack of administrative cooperation. One chief of surgery simply ignored his administrative functions. Another section head ordered equipment without notifying the administration or seeking authorization. The administrators knew how to effectively deal with that behavior. It was right up their alley. They just said, "No."

Several highly regarded academic heads were recruited but backed out at the last moment, sensing potential problems. A new chief of medicine arrived in the mid-1960s, but he only lasted two years. He couldn't have self-destructed faster if he'd tried. Frustrated by the Hospital and by other department heads, he started setting up a private clinic separate from the Hospital's clinics. His mistake was that his clinic was to include laboratory and radiology sections, which would compete with the Hospital's. That's all it took for his ousting.

One new chief of surgery left after two years, taking an offer that he couldn't refuse. It was for the same position at a University hospital. He'd been told by his mentor, the retiring chief at this university hospital, that he'd never be named chief of surgery. Although he was named as chief of surgery, he resigned from this position in two years as well over the administrative load, just as he had done at Pennsylvania Hospital.

—⁓—

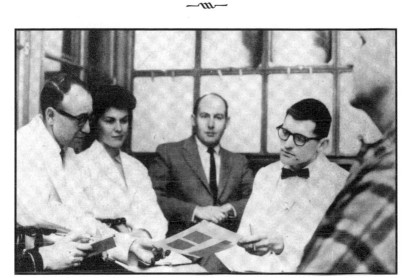

Dr. Makous (second from right) chairs a Pennsylvania Hospital committee meeting

The department heads at Pennsylvania Hospital were salaried and therefore distrusted by most of their department members, who supported themselves in private practice. In an attempt to have a voice in Hospital administration, three of us in the Department of Medicine started the "Thomas Bond Association." It was composed of physicians who, like us, were in private practice at the Hospital but were not employed by the Hospital. It lasted about 10 years.

I was named president of the Bond Association in its second year. Under the new State Sunshine Law, I started to attend the meetings of the hospital's medical staff Executive Committee, a group composed primarily of department heads and a few elected medical staff members. The Hospital president or his representative attended ex-officio.

These meetings were held in the president's office at a long table that could seat about 20 people. One end was used by the president as his desk. As time went on, I moved from the adjacent, sitting-room portion of the office, to a seat at the Committee table whenever one was open. Soon, I was taking part in the deliberations.

After several years, during a vote, the Executive Committee chairman turned to me and said, "Norm, you didn't vote."

"I know. I'm not a member of the Committee," I reminded him.

The medical staff bylaws were not only unusual, but were also apparently designed to obfuscate. The starting dates of officers were unstated, although their duration in office was made known. There was a nominating committee, but its duties were described in another section of the bylaws. These duties were to nominate members to a committee of an obscure rehabilitation fund that was used for undisclosed purposes, and may have had no funds in it. The committee did not nominate medical staff officers.

I rewrote a large section of the bylaws, correcting a number of confusing discrepancies. The Hospital president approved of my revisions when I showed them to him, before I presented them to the Executive Committee. The Executive Committee referred them to the Bylaws Committee for review. The Bylaws Committee returned with their recommendations in a month—namely that they didn't see any reason for the changes. Nobody disagreed. No vote was taken.

I spoke up. "We all know what is intended by the bylaws, but down the road, in years to come, others may not."

Nobody disagreed.

Turning to the chairman, I said, "Is there any reason the minutes can't reflect our interpretation of the bylaws?"

"Why no!" He said. "I don't see why not."

Again, nobody disagreed.

At the next meeting, the minutes of that previous meeting stat-

ed that the Executive Committee had accepted the bylaw changes I had recommended in their entirety. There never was a vote. These minutes were accepted without dissent or comment.

The Executive Committee meeting minutes were written by the Hospital's administration, which was interested in their historical value. Minutes back as far as the 1780s were in its archives. They generally were rather bland and said little to reflect the issues or debates. One of the Executive Committee members insisted on writing his version of the minutes. All he got was grief. They usually had to be rewritten several times.

After the general medical staff began electing officers, the Executive Committee meetings were no longer elitist. So, the department heads created a Planning Committee, through which they conducted their business and debate outside of the general medical staff's purview.

On one other occasion, the Executive Committee actions were especially notorious. A new section head within a medical staff department was being selected in mid-spring. The contract with the University of Pennsylvania required Pennsylvania Hospital to submit, for the University's approval, the names of not only department heads but also of department section heads. The hospital's medical staff bylaws reflected this requirement.

On July 1st, however, several months in the future, a new agreement was to go into effect by which section heads no longer needed University approval. Therefore, the Executive Committee decided it would not submit the name of the new head. The committee didn't merely ignore the current contract or postpone approval for several months until after July 1st. No, the Executive Committee just voted to "lay aside the staff bylaws."

I couldn't believe it. "You can't disregard the bylaws any time you want," I protested.

The Executive Committee Chairman said, "Norm, you'll just have to take us to court."

This exchange never appeared in the carefully manicured

minutes, but the Hospital administration did take note. An administrative trainee called me four months later to discuss the outrageous action. There were no ramifications and nothing ever came of this misstep, as far as I knew.

These are just a few examples of the territorial conflicts between medical staffs and hospital administration, and the shifting currents of medical practice, during the period of strong growth of the hospital in the 1960s and 1970s. It was a microcosm of trends and concerns at all hospitals nationwide.

CHAPTER 63

War! Total War!

The frequency of malpractice litigation has risen steadily since the 1950s. Since then, it has contributed its share to the burgeoning overall costs of medical care.

The only professor to mention legal matters during my training in medical school was an orthopedic surgeon. He told of being subpoenaed by a plaintiff's attorney in Northern Wisconsin. The professor had to travel more than 300 hundred miles to testify. He had never been involved in the care of the plaintiff, and the lawyer had never even talked to the doctor at any time concerning the matter.

As soon as he had been sworn in at the trial, the plaintiff's lawyer put up an x-ray and started asking the surgeon technical questions about it.

The surgeon responded casually, saying, "well, it looks like an x-ray alright. I guess that's the backbone there and maybe the ribs."

Over the years, it has become apparent that many of those claiming injury earn their settlement the hard way. The injured person's recovery is delayed, often deliberately, until the matter is resolved, which can take years. By that time, their health is often destroyed by the delayed recovery they deem necessary to support their suit until settlement.

The point he was making to us was that a witness cannot be forced to testify as an expert unless he has factual knowledge concerning the specific case in question. He can be forced to testify only at the level of knowledge and understanding of an informed layman. The surgeon may well have been willing to testify as an expert had the lawyer consulted him in advance. But then it would have cost the lawyer and his client more than the $20 that the surgeon was actually paid. The medical malpractice industry was still in its infancy at that time.

The physician couple for whom I substituted for two months in Northern Wisconsin in 1952, had acquired their well-established practice from a bachelor physician who had fled to Alaska, where it was less crowded and where the hunting and fishing were better. He was reputed to be very critical of the care given by the seven other doctors in town. The rate of malpractice suits in the area was four-times the state average.

My annual malpractice premium there was $100, much higher than the $15 annual premium required earlier when I was called to active duty with the Navy in 1950. In recent years, the premium for a non-procedural cardiologist in the Philadelphia area has been running at about $15,000 a year. In some surgical specialties, the malpractice premium is as high as $150,000.

Over the course of more than 40 years, I have been deposed well over 100 times and testified in court more than 50 times. In addition, I wrote opinions on more than 300 cases for both defense and plaintiff attorneys. I started out as a defense expert 85 percent of the time. By the time I retired, that ratio had reversed.

About half of the cases involved workers' compensation matters concerning city employees—mostly firemen and some policemen. The other half of the matters involved doctors and hospitals.

Over the years, it has become apparent that many of those claiming injury earn their settlement the hard way. The injured person's recovery is delayed, often deliberately, until the matter is resolved, which can take years. By that time, their health is often destroyed by the delayed recovery they deem necessary to support their suit until settlement.

Initially, I was annoyed at lawyers' general lack of understanding of medical issues. I thought that the doctors' ignorance of the law was exceeded only by the lawyers' ignorance of medicine. I wanted to educate them. Many lawyers felt that with their cases, the medical matters were less important than their knowledge of the law. The successful ones, however, knew it was both. I was the one who received the education.

The attitude of winning at all costs is intrinsic to the practice of law and prevalent on both sides of every case. This has helped escalate the cost of medical litigation to astronomical proportions. As of 2008, some estimates are that the proportion of medical costs attributed to malpractice insurance and litigation has reached 10 to 15 percent. This has grown from less than 1 percent when I entered medicine.

Over time, I learned that competence and ineptness were equally split among defense and plaintiff attorneys. By and large, however, plaintiff attorneys were better prepared. They were usually more experienced than the younger defense attorneys retained by the insurance companies. The younger ones were paid less and were less motivated, as well as less experienced.

After a medical liability insurance system crisis in the 1970s drove many insurers from the state, the Pennsylvania Medical Society established its own medical liability insurance company. This not only helped reduce insurance fees, but also allowed doctors to challenge more suits. The general belief was that insurance companies settled many defensible suits simply because it cost them less money than going to court.

Disputes concerning suit litigation or settlement between the doctors and the insurance companies were to be resolved by a committee of doctors from the Medical Society. I sat on this committee for six years, two as chairman. This gave me a fair insight into malpractice litigation statewide.

Judges demonstrated attitudes ranging from strict impartiality to overt bias. I found bias to be more evident outside of the larger metropolitan areas. Testifying in several cases in small towns in Central Pennsylvania, I found that no matter how atrocious a physician's actions had been, the judge and the jury preferred to overlook them, rather than risk losing one of their doctors who might leave to practice elsewhere.

In one instance, I was called in as a cardiology expert for the US Postal Service. The 300-pound defense counsel briefed me concerning the impending trial before the US District Court in Philadelphia. He wanted me to understand litigation from his viewpoint.

"A trial has nothing to do with justice," he told me. "A trial is war! Total war! Justice is up to the legislators."

He won this war.

The attitude of winning at all costs is intrinsic to the practice of law and prevalent on both sides of every case. This has helped escalate the cost of medical litigation to astronomical proportions. As of 2008, some estimates are that the proportion of medical costs attributed to malpractice insurance and litigation has reached 10 to 15 percent. This has grown from less than 1 percent when I entered medicine.

The cost of malpractice litigation and insurance is coming under control in some states as a result of legislation setting limits on awards for pain and suffering. As the rationing of medical care by third parties continues to grow, so will litigation. Many people feel that capping these awards is the only way to control litigation costs. In any event, the overall proportion of medical expenses caused by litigation continues to increase.

CHAPTER 64

Nose in the Tent

The rising cost of medical care has been a major concern since World War II. As a board member of a number of medical societies and government agencies, I closely followed the issues relating to these rising costs for several decades.

With the introduction of Medicare and Medicaid in 1965, the federal government became deeply involved in medical-care delivery. It created the Regional Medical Programs, requiring medical facilities that expected to treat Medicare patients to obtain a Certificate of Need for all new capital expenditures. This included hospital additions, catheterization laboratories, and x-ray facilities. This was intended to reduce duplication and the expensive competition between hospitals.

In the 1970s, Congress replaced the Regional Medical Programs with Health System Agencies. I had been on the board of the Philadelphia Regional Medical Program, and I was then appointed to the Philadelphia Health System Agency interim board. I became president of its west Philadelphia Advisory Council.

One of the Council's major functions was to review and make recommendations on any project involving US government grants or funding requested by institutions within the Council's area. This included all projects that required a Certificate of Need. In reviewing the applications for these certificates, I found the spread of technology to be intriguing.

The concept that highly technical, expensive, and low-volume medical procedures should be limited to the large medical centers, started with the introduction of more advanced technical procedures for neurosurgery in the 1920s. This concept grew over the decades with new thoracic surgery procedures in the 1930s, and cardiac procedures in the 1960s. Mandating Certificates of Need in the mid-1960s was the first attempt by the government to control the costly spread of technology.

Despite rationing of new facilities through the use of these regulatory methods, cardiology catheterization laboratories rapidly spread in the 1960s, from the large medical research centers to suburban and smaller community hospitals. This was followed by the spread of cardiac surgery capabilities by the 1980s.

Computerized axial tomography, more commonly known as the CT scan, was introduced in the 1970s. When the CT radiological scan equipment became available, the government attempted to limit these very expensive new units to only a few hospitals in each region. The intention was to enforce a rationing of expensive services, which would have resulted in "queuing," or lining-up for treatment, as happens in England and other countries with rationed care.

Favoring certain hospitals, however, upset the dynamics of hospital usage by specialists. It created a disparity in care services. Unless these CT centers were equally inaccessible to all hospitals, the hospitals with the scanners would be in a position of providing a higher level of technical service than other hospitals. As a result, these hospitals would have ended-up with a disproportionate number of specialists on their medical staffs.

The creation of these CT centers as a means of limiting the use of expensive treatments to certain hospitals, was actually one of the intentions of the legislation. It was a rationing mechanism.

The approval of the units and their Certificates of Need was often obtained through the political process. As a result of this disparity as well as the lobbying on behalf of community hospitals, many of the CT units became free standing. They may have been located on a community hospital campus, but they were administratively separate from the hospital. If the CT units were part of the hospital, Medicare and Medicaid payment for patient care would be denied unless the hospital itself had been given a Certificate of Need.

Eventually, it became evident that many people with non-urgent health problems who lived outside of a metropolitan area, far from any medical research center, would delay their evaluation, or even avoid having one altogether, if it meant that they had to go to a hospital in a metropolitan center. They were only comfortable going to their familiar local hospital.

This issue first became evident in the 1960s, in the region between New York City and Baltimore, when catheterization laboratories had spread widely and began opening in the suburbs. Their utilization increased dramatically. People wondered why they hadn't had access to these services earlier. Local usage was based on familiarity, ease of access, and comfort with the local hospital, as well as dislike by many of the "big city" experience. If the need wasn't urgent, they postponed the procedure.

Intense community loyalty to the local hospital was evident when a suburban Philadelphia hospital chain tried to close one hospital's maternity service, which would have forced women to go to another of the chain's hospitals nearby. Community rebellion forced them to abandon the plan.

Because it was circumvented through politics, the government's attempt to control the spread of expensive procedures through the Certificate of Need process had little impact in the long run in limiting these special services. Today, CT scan capabilities and other expensive technologies are widely available in community hospitals.

Another attempt at government rationing of care was made through monitoring of Medicare claims. Upon its introduction, Medicare's fiscal intermediary was Pennsylvania Blue Shield, for which I was serving on a doctor advisory board. Initially, Pennsylvania blue shield attempted to deprive the advisory board of comment on the Medicare program, but was quickly forced to admit it to our purview.

Eventually, the Medicare physician advisory committee was

separated and run by the US Health Care Finance Administration and supervised by its related regional office. I remained on both advisory committees for several years.

One of Blue Shield's activities as Medicare intermediary was to monitor the coding of office visits. This was done to determine reimbursement for services received by Medicare patients, just as they did for their private business programs. They had statistical parameters for overuse, but none for underuse. Their claim was that monitoring over-utilization was in the interest of quality of care.

Actually, overuse was monitored by Blue Shield because cost control, not quality of medical care, was their concern. If quality had been their primary goal, they would have addressed under-utilization as well. When I raised this issue at an advisory board meeting, it was summarily dismissed.

Medicare established three levels of care for an office visit. The duration of the visit was the key component in determining the care level.

I learned about how zealously they enforced these codes when my office assistant miscoded their services for a period of time. This resulted in a number of overpayments to me that raised a statistical red flag, and they investigated based on over-utilization. There were no consequences after we returned the overpayments. As a result, I had a much better understanding of their monitoring system.

—ɯ—

Another type of reimbursement closely monitored by Blue Shield—in an attempt to control Medicare costs—was in situations of concurrent care, which is defined as in-hospital care by more than one physician. At one point, Blue Shield refused to pay me for a significant amount of care provided concurrently with another physician. I knew that under certain circumstances, reimbursement for concurrent care was allowed for Medicare patients by the Health Care Finance Administration. I went through various appeal procedures, to no avail. I finally asked for a physician review, which was my last step before going to an arbitration court. Actually, I could have done this initially. The verdict was in my favor.

Because of my negative experience with respect to concurrent care, I wrote a paper on the serious problems created by the policy of intermediaries like Blue Shield that fail to follow Medicare regulations. It was reviewed at the American Society of Internal Medicine. Its president and its executive vice president, who had been a top executive at the American Medical Association, visited Pennsylvania and leaned on the leadership of the Blue Shield Medicare program. This resulted in a change in blue shield's method of evaluating concurrent care, allowing payment in appropriate cases.

When a system can be faulted, it is vulnerable to change. Whenever I've had a problem, instead of running to the leadership for a solution through personal intervention, I would go through the recommended method of resolution in order to test its effectiveness. This approach provides insights into the operation of the system, and allows discussion of the problems, which on occasion, leads to changes.

—〰—

Government first got its "nose in the tent" in the medical arena by increasing research funding after World War II. Once Medicare was established in the 1960s, government presence in medicine continued to grow by leaps and bounds. While government attempts to control costs are worthy, the methods often have had unintended effects in the American system of free-market medicine.

Diminished quality of care or perceived disparities in care resulting from rationing is not tolerated by the American public. While the upward spiral in the costs of care continues, effective methods of cost control that are fair to all, have not been found.

CHAPTER 65

Splintering and Bundling

The cost of medical care is driven by the growth of technology, which in turn, is driven by our culture. As a result, medical costs are out of control.

Many of the costs are met by the government through Medicaid and Medicare. Private insurers account for most of the balance, except for the expenses of the 17 percent of the population who has no coverage.

Employers select the insurers and pay for the cost of insurance as an employee benefits expense. The insurance company managers provide coverage under careful rationing, with an eye on the group purse.

Individuals with coverage, who are thus relieved of the financial responsibility for their own care, feel entitled to the most advanced care. Attempts to control costs are unpopular if they limit access to all of the fruits of technological progress. As a result, the attempts to limit the costs are directed toward those who deliver the care—the doctors and hospitals.

Personal care, which is the face-to-face time between doctor and patient, can help to rein-in the costs of a care system driven by technology. Yet, as discussed throughout this book, the personal aspect of medical care has declined in recent decades.

When the insurance companies and government programs began attempts to control medical costs, it was easier for them to focus on systematizing hospital costs rather than systematizing the costs for individual physicians. The hospital is the place where more expensive care is concentrated. The justifiable response of hospital management toward many of the new regulatory requirements was to add an additional layer of administration on that which had already existed. This further inflated the cost of care.

In 1984, hospital reimbursement for Medicare patients was brought under some control with the introduction of payment by Diagnosis Related Groups. Blue Cross and the health management organizations, referred to as "HMOs," also controlled reimbursements to hospitals. By the 1990s, after HMOs began to have a significant impact on medical costs, hospitals no longer were regarded as cash cows, but became cost centers. If the hospital was owned by the system, then the most successful hospital manager was one who could save the most money by closing a so-called "unnecessary" hospital.

At first, physicians were lured into accepting Medicare patients by a fee schedule that often exceeded the physician's usual charge. Also, they were initially reimbursed for indigent care at the rate of 35 percent of their usual charges, and later at a rate approaching 50 percent.

Then, the ratcheting reduction of Medicare reimbursements began. Initially, reimbursement for regular care was at about 70 percent of the physician's usual charge. Gradually, this has been reduced to less than 60 percent, and it will eventually approach the rate for indigent care, I suspect.

Physicians' responses have been predictable. Non-procedural physicians—those who do no surgery—are not reimbursed equitably for the time they devote to patients for their non-procedural "cognitive care." In other words, time for personal care is not covered. Physicians have lobbied so that reimbursement can be based on the overhead it takes to provide care.

General practitioners are reimbursed at lower rates than specialists. Part of the basis for the inequity in fees was based on the difference in overhead. This has accounted for some of the variation in reimbursements found between different areas of the same state, as well as differences in reimbursements between regions of the country.

Medicare addressed this in the 1980s. Medicare reimbursements were based upon the training of the specialist and upon the practice's overhead determined through several local economic factors. This was assisted through establishing Medicare's Resource-Based Relative Value Scale.

In addition, reimbursement by Medicare is not the same throughout the country. Services are not treated equally. Because of this inequity, in some areas and states, many physician specialists have left to practice elsewhere.

Most people who have group insurance as employees are not aware that the primary financial obligation of their physicians is to the insurer who pays them. And the insurers continually negotiate reductions in fees and services from the physicians. This mechanism rations the available medical resources to the insured public. While public awareness of this careful allocation of resources has grown somewhat, the rationing of care for the insured is ultimately a hidden process.

In addition to Medicare and Medicaid, other third parties attempting to control medical care costs through the reduction of physicians' reimbursements were the Blue Shield agencies and the HMOs. Surgeons began charging for separate parts of a procedure. Medicare referred to this as "splintering," and combined the charges at a lower reimbursement rate. Physicians referred to this as "bundling."

By the mid-1980s, few internal medicine residents finished their training without mastery of some invasive diagnostic procedure for which they could receive an additional reimbursement. In fact, many internists already in practice took additional training in procedures new to them, such as proctoscopic examinations for rectal disease.

Reimbursement for these procedures was expected to help make up for the reduced payments they were receiving for the cognitive care provided through office visits. Ultimately, this hasn't helped very much.

Another demand on the medical dollar results from the splintering of medical care into numerous subspecialties and areas of non-physician-administered technical expertise. By the 1990s, Medicare recognized 130 of more than 200 subspecialty groups demanding their share. These demands will increase as more subspecialty areas are created and recognized. For example, a fast-growing group of subspecialties has been created in genetics.

Most people who have group insurance as employees are not aware that the primary financial obligation of their physicians is to the insurer who pays them. And the insurers continually negotiate reductions in fees and services from the physicians. This mechanism rations the available medical resources to the insured public. While public awareness of this careful allocation of resources has grown somewhat, the rationing of care for the insured is ultimately a hidden process.

The time required for physicians to counsel patients is a very important part of personal care, but reimbursement for this type of care is inadequate. Third parties doubt that counseling patients is cost-effective. They seem to regard physicians as basically over-trained for counseling, like using a SWAT team to maintain domestic harmony in the household. This economic pressure is turning physicians into technicians.

Much of what many primary-care physicians are expected to do for patients today relates to preventive care. This takes time, but they are not being reimbursed for it. Health Maintenance Organizations, belying their name, by and large did not start encouraging much in the way of preventive care until the 1990s. The cost-effectiveness of the approach is assumed today, but the only scientific evidence that supports this applies to immunizations and specific procedures such as colonoscopy and **mammography**.

Since physicians are not reimbursed for counseling, many do so only by handing out written material and leaving the questions and discussions to assistants. Providing advice on obesity and smoking are examples of this. Since this is a public health service, perhaps it is better addressed in that domain of our culture.

The gradual reduction in physician reimbursement also has had other effects on the practice of medicine and the delivery of care. In some parts of the country, the physician loses money accepting new Medicare patients. Since physicians are not required to accept everyone as a patient, some of the elderly have had difficulty finding a primary-care physician.

Many institutions have discontinued their geriatric services. What the elderly need is more compassionate care. This requires less technological care and more physician time. Medicare regards this as low-level personal care. Its reimbursement for this time is inadequate. As a consequence, Medicare will continue to pay more for testing and referrals to high-fee consultants.

As part of the consequence of the low-reimbursement policy, medical care is becoming a multi-tiered system. The patient is still the hub, but is regarded less as an individual and more as a member of a group. The patient's advocate, the primary-care doctor, is becoming harder to find.

The low reimbursement levels for the personal physician and the financial incentives of free-market medicine are driving new doctors into the specialties and super-specialties. Family doctors are forced to act less as personal physicians and more as leaders of impersonal teams. Doctors' direct contact with their patients is thereby greatly diluted.

CHAPTER 66

Rearranging the Deck Chairs

Today, patient care often starts with triage by a mechanized phone system. The phone extension choices are different for emergencies, appointments, changing appointments, prescription refills, test results, general questions, talking to a coordinator, talking to a patient-care technician, billing questions, or the office manager, to name a few. No number will connect you directly to your doctor, but that's not new.

Office visits, at least in the larger practices in urban areas, consist of running the gamut of assistants before seeing the physician, and that often is a brief contact. In some practices where the next open appointment is weeks away—if your problem is urgent—you can still be seen immediately. You may, however, be seen by everyone but the doctor.

Hopefully, the doctor is kept informed and is making some of the decisions in the direction of your care. This military-service model of care triage may be fine for young and vigorous patients, but generally this is not a good model for a practice with elderly or chronically ill patients.

In some large practice situations, the doctors are not on the premises. Care is presumably guided by a physician who is at a different site miles away. One version of this type of care is the "Nurse in a Box" at shopping malls, similar to the storefront, "Doc in a Box," of a few years ago.

Rural and homecare by nurses has also increased in recent years. In some areas, nurse practitioners have been caring for many people as the only immediate caregiver available. They practice under the aegis of a physician who may be at a distant location. Whether these non-physicians can fill the void and deliver quality care more cost-effectively and satisfactorily has yet to be determined. State legislators are gradually expanding the scope of practice for nurse practitioners.

People who are ill, as well as the worried-well, have varying degrees of anxiety. They expect and need reassurance. As the physician no longer is paid for the time required, more people have gone to alternative-care practitioners in the past 20 years, than those who have sought traditional medical care. In some instances, this can delay early disease detection and more effective treatment.

Increasingly, hospital care is delivered by hospitalists. These are doctors who are full-time in the hospital and have no office practice of their own. There have always been doctors who do not care for their patients who are in need of hospital care. They refer them to doctors on the hospital staff. This is increasing as hospital stays are reduced to a minimum. More patients now require the more intense and expert care that the well-trained hospitalists provide. The quality of care is generally better. The downside is that the continuity of care by the personal physician is interrupted.

Phone contact among the physicians is greatly reduced today compared to past eras. Communication, if any, from one physician to another, is restricted to a briefly written report that is delayed in its transmittal. It is only a fair substitute for a conversation. This poor communication reduces the quality of care and increases the risk to the patient for medical errors.

Most people today expect more from medical care, which has heightened the level of health anxiety. As most have insurance, people generally seek medical attention earlier than they would if personally responsible for payment. Even if they have an incipient illness, due to the earliness of the visit to the doctor, their complaints are non-specific and physical findings on examination are less helpful.

These patients generally find that the personal contact with the doctor, who takes a history and performs a physical examination, is reassuring. Doctors, however, find that the personal contact and examination is less rewarding in early disease, as well as in the absence of disease. This reinforces the prevalent belief that these personal contacts have little to offer and that testing is superior to examination. Consequently, much of the history and even the physical examination itself is delegated to assistants.

The doctor orders more tests and performs more procedures as a substitute for time with the patient. Much of this testing is unnecessary and costly. As a result, patients remain anxious and, in turn, expect more testing.

As another consequence, patients seek unnecessary and costly second opinions. They often bypass the personal physician and go directly to a specialist based on their self-diagnosis, which of course may be erroneous.

Specialists, in turn, feel obligated to use the diagnostic procedures of their specialty area—whether indicated or not. The tests or procedures can be justified. They rationalize that the medical legal liability is reduced.

Today, in our culture of individualism, personal rights, and high expectations from technology, the end result of this spiral of frustration is that patients have become more litigious. This, in turn, unnecessarily inflates the cost of care.

Many consultant specialists have turned themselves into technicians. They do not attempt to determine for themselves whether a procedure is indicated. Often, it's easier and less time-consuming to perform a procedure for which they are reimbursed, than to take the time—for which they may not be reimbursed—to fully evaluate the appropriateness of a test. Many specialists no longer bother to consult with the referring physician in order to decide upon the best course of management.

If a physician does refer a patient for a procedure, even one that is not needed, the consultant specialist can defend doing it much more readily than not doing it. While the liability risk is usually low, the cost to the system of numerous unnecessary tests and procedures is high.

The missions of the third-party insurers and the physicians are in conflict. What the third-party payers regard as unnecessary testing and procedures in their management of the herd's purse strings, is often contrary to the needs of the patient and the physician whose primary obligation is to the patient. The physician orders tests that are based on individual need. Third-party insurers may determine that these are unnecessary based on group statistics.

A disease missed or mistreated by the physician through lack of testing or failure to perform a procedure is a 100-percent failure that may prove fatal in a given patient. For the third parties managing the purse of the herd, these 99 of 100 tests represent an excellent rate of successful rationing and fulfillment of their financial responsibility.

The significant increase in litigation over the years arises from patients' dissatisfaction based upon many of the factors mentioned above. This reflects a feeling that they are powerless, and are not always treated with respect. Many of these suits have no significant merit, but some people feel it is the only manner in which they can obtain satisfaction from such a system.

The cost of malpractice insurance has outstripped the inflation factor during the past 50 years. The expense of these premiums has made a significant contribution to the increase in the cost of medical care. Physicians in some specialties have moved to another state where malpractice insurance rates are lower. This has deprived some communities of essential medical care.

A number of approaches are suggested and are presently under evaluation to control medical costs. One example is the proposal that the physician reimbursement be based on the quality of care that is given. This reduces costs in part because testing and referral to specialists is reduced. This also results in some instances of "gaming the system" by doctors, who do not accept older patients or those with chronic illnesses.

Many proposals have been made to improve medical care in order to reduce the cost of care. Among them is the interest in reducing medical errors and integrating the medical information technology. Most of these proposals only tweak care in the hope of controlling costs. The real issue is avoided. Technology is the costly culprit in the decline of personal care. In the absence of overt and clear rationing policies, these measures amount to painting bulkheads, swabbing the decks, and rearranging the deck chairs on a sinking ship.

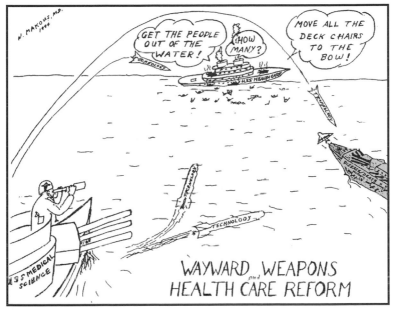

Collateral damage, by Norman Makous, Philadelphia Medicine, Volume 91, Number 2, Feb. 1995

PART VI

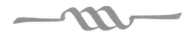

Conclusion: Personal Care is Key

CHAPTER 67

The One-Hoss Shay Syndrome

As we have seen, medical care today is driven by technology and our cultural values. These in turn have driven the cost of care steadily upward.

During the last century, many diseases and medical conditions have fallen victim to science as a result of technological advances. These are in the provinces of immunizations, diagnostic methods, surgical procedures, and drug therapy.

Prevention has improved with advances in immunizations. More infectious diseases have succumbed to new and better vaccines. Improved treatment has prevented and reduced complications of many chronic diseases.

Technology has contributed much to the improvement in diagnostic techniques. Computerized axial tomography, the CT scan, has improved x-ray diagnosis. **Magnetic resonance imaging,** MRI, uses magnetic waves to complement x-ray diagnosis. Ultra-sound probes the body to produce images of organs and abnormalities. Many new, more accurate, and very rapid blood tests aid in diagnosis.

Even more impressive results are seen with advances in surgery and anesthesia. Healing assistance techniques have shortened post-surgery recovery times. Many procedures that previously required hospital admission in the past, can now be performed safely on outpatients.

Abdominal **keyhole surgery** with laparoscopic instruments reduces damage, which speeds healing and convalescence. Severely damaged heart valves and blood vessels can be replaced with artificial as well as natural ones, when other techniques fail to correct the damage.

Many joints in the body can be replaced with **prostheses**. Brain-controlled artificial limbs are being developed. Implanted electronic pacemakers and defibrillators for normal and abnormal heart rhythms are available. Management of organs such as the bladder affected by nervous system dysfunction is electronically possible. Organ transplants of the kidney, heart, lungs, and liver are long-lasting. Also spectacular is the success of surgery to correct potentially fatal heart defects in the fetus while still in the womb.

The determination of an individual's genetic makeup helps to identify and treat not only inherited disorders, but also susceptibility to infections, cancer, and other diseases. There are those who believe that genetic testing and medicine is the future of medical care. This certainly will be part of the future, but the complexity of the environment within the cell is almost as great as that outside of the cell. Genetic testing is no diagnostic magic bullet and must be treated like any test.

Genetic susceptibility to a disease is a risk factor and not a certainty that the disease will develop. As with any risk factor, the importance of these findings must be considered carefully and compassionately as part of an individual's total personalized care. Otherwise, even with counseling, genetic issues may induce more anxiety than they will relieve in many people.

In the US today, we worship at the altar of technology. During this period of marvelous advances in medical science, our culture of equality and individualism has created a sense of entitlement to medical care. Everyone wants his or her share of the latest miraculous developments. Compensation for the cost of medical care for all individuals, using the best medical methods available, is expected.

—ɯ—

Ideally, from a community's point of view, individuals are expected to contribute more to the general social well-being than they take away from it. They should be able to care for themselves. As far as the general health of the community is concerned, the investment to provide for this through immunizations, preventing the spread of contagious diseases, ensuring pure water, clean air, safe foods, refuse disposal, and general safety, would bring more bang for the buck than investment in individual healthcare.

In the US today, we worship at the altar of technology. During this period of marvelous advances in medical science, our culture of equality and individualism has created a sense of entitlement to medical care. Everyone wants his or her share of the latest miraculous developments. Compensation for the cost of medical care for all individuals, using the best medical methods available, is expected.

While technology saves lives and its benefit to individuals with less common diseases has often been spectacular, increasingly, much of the cost of care is devoted to optional comfort care through drugs and surgery. This is in addition to the less spectacular alleviation of the effects of common diseases and the overall prolongation of life.

As a result of medical interventions, life expectancy has increased from 46 years in 1900 to more than 78 years today. One specter raised by the lengthening of life is that the pool of adults who are susceptible to diseases, both degenerative and infectious, is growing.

When the pool of unimmunized and susceptible individuals for a specific contagious disease reaches 30 percent or more, the risk of an epidemic rises. It is therefore possible that a pool of adults susceptible to infectious diseases will develop from those now surviving non-infectious childhood diseases, through the wonderful successes of technology. If so, the size of this pool will swell and increase the susceptibility of the entire population to epidemics.

Today, a longer, more comfortable life of a higher quality is all but a promise. Many diseases can be cured and death can be thwarted. But some look upon all death as just another disease, not as an inevitable outcome of living, and preventable only in the short run. To some, death is a consequence of aging, and aging is a primary disease waiting to be conquered.

The ultimate goal of medical science is therefore viewed as the conquest of aging and, by extension, of death. Accepting death as inevitable is deemed a failure of science, and science does not accept failure as an option.

Since, in this view, we are all born with the incipient disease of death, then, as with any disease, the prolongation of a life of acceptable quality becomes another healthcare challenge. The ultimate goal of medical science is therefore viewed as the conquest of aging and, by extension, of death. Accepting death as inevitable is deemed a failure of science, and science does not accept failure as an option.

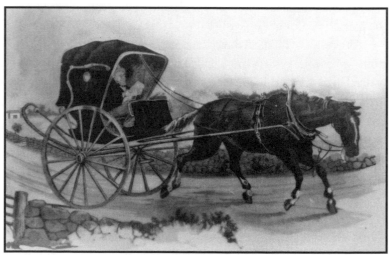

"The Wonderful One-Hoss Shay"
Image provided by Special Collections at University of Southern California

To some of us, this attitude makes about as much sense as conducting research to find a disease that will cause the "one-horse shay syndrome." In Oliver Wendell Holmes' poem "The Wonderful One-Hoss Shay," the vehicle is built of very durable materials with a predetermined useful life. Suddenly, on its 100th birthday, the carriage instantly becomes a heap of dust, the remains easily swept up. As it is now, we die in pieces, in an incremental manner that is very costly, especially during the last four months of life.

The sense of entitlement among Americans to a longer, higher-quality life with a painless death, has resulted in some significant challenges. If we are not going to break the bank, meeting the needs of our aging population compassionately will become increasingly difficult.

The opposite extreme, **euthanasia** in the name of compassionate care, is a slippery slope that must be avoided. For some proponents, the hidden motive of cost control is that of economy, saving our society the cost of old age. It represents a social value that will never be acceptable in our society.

Most individuals today meet the inevitability of death in the near future with some equanimity as long as they feel that their pain and suffering are addressed, and that they are not being abandoned. Those, however, who will never accept death, are willing to endure the sufferings that result from pursuing every last option to the bitter end, "cost be damned."

This attitude leads to never-ending treatment, drug course after drug course, procedure after procedure, transplant after transplant, and the endurance of every possible experiment. During this process, large debts may be incurred and the financial resources of individuals and families, not to mention those of our society, can be completely consumed.

Given the underlying sense of entitlement to medical care, many individuals today expect the public purse to pay for such extreme measures.

CHAPTER 68

Medicine's Dirty Little Secret

Extending the life of an individual generally does not save society money in the long run. Coronary artery angioplasty or bypass surgery may save the life of a 40-year-old man and return him to work, but it doesn't eliminate the coronary artery atherosclerosis that is the basic cause of the blockage in need of relief.

Bypass surgery gives the individual a second chance to reverse the atherosclerosis, but permanent improvement requires the continuous use of medications, plus changes in lifestyle so severe that few are able to effect them. Over time, younger individuals will need additional procedures, possibly even a heart transplant.

In general, every new diagnostic procedure costs more than the one it is replacing. More information may be generated by new tests than by older ones, but in many situations, the additional information is more than what was needed in a specific case. The diagnostic procedure should fit the need.

When elaborate tests such as CT scans are used as screening tools on healthy individuals, "case finding," which is identifying a disease at a very early stage, frequently doesn't justify the diagnostic cost. And if it does, the procedural treatment may be overused long before it may be a necessity. Diagnostic case finding is unnecessarily expensive and doesn't necessarily extend life.

With many forms of surgical treatment, success results in ever broadening indications that include more and more people. This has been the case with joint replacement, as one example. As the prostheses improve and the risk from the surgery decreases, an increasing number of older people are having knees or hips replaced with artificial joints. And they are doing it at such an early stage of the disease that it is too soon to tell if the joint condition will be chronically disabling. The replacement may be unnecessary. This trend would also apply to organ transplants, except that the supply of organs imposes a limitation.

The prospective introduction of a practical artificial heart would be another example. Unlike heart transplants, the supply of devices will be virtually unlimited. Besides requiring additional surgical staff, this innovation will introduce the new expense of a cadre of therapists and repair persons of various expertise. Eventually, the next replacement becomes more effective and less costly.

As the technology of the mechanical replacement improves, individuals will qualify for it earlier and earlier in the course of their heart disease, especially where the risk of sudden death is greater. To reduce this example to an absurdity, if the artificial device eventually becomes better than nature's heart, the replacement will be indicated in infants. The cost per procedure may fall, but so many more procedures would be done that the overall costs would rise rapidly.

Eventually, healthcare will reach the maximum acceptable proportion of our economy. After this point, we will have to make some tough decisions about who receives certain aspects of care, and what care they receive. The questions we will then have to ask are, "How will these decisions be made? And, who will make them?"

Who will bear the rising costs? Illness no longer is accepted as solely an individual's financial responsibility. Our society is increasingly adopting the concept that someone else must pay if an individual cannot afford it.

Insurance is a form of lottery that is an acceptable way of inconspicuously spreading the cost of illness. Today, people look upon it as a prepayment for all medical care, not just for major illnesses.

When there is personal assumption of some cost, the utilization of care decreases, as does the overall cost of care, and there are no negative health consequences.

Medical care now consumes 17 percent of the gross domestic product (GDP), and this proportion is rising steadily with no end in sight. The introduction of new and expensive technologies available to the general population increases this cost.

Eventually, healthcare will reach the maximum acceptable proportion of our economy. After this point, we will have to make some tough decisions about who receives certain aspects of care, and what care they receive. The questions we will then have to ask are, "How will these decisions be made? And, who will make them?"

Recently, when I mentioned cost control to a young colleague of mine, he said, "You mean medicine's dirty little secret?" When healthcare cost control is thought of by the negative term of "rationing," it seems appalling to Americans.

Medical care has always been rationed. When individuals are fully responsible for the cost of their own care, the care is self-rationed. If rationing applies to everybody and is overt, it has been accepted, just as food and gas rationing were during World War II. But, when rationing is covert, as it is with medical underwriting today, it is poorly understood and not accepted, especially when it is applied to one's own health.

Given America's core concept of equality, we are particularly intolerant of the concept of rationing. It is perceived as discriminatory toward some groups, and therefore unacceptable.

Fair, non-discriminatory rationing calls upon the difficult ethics of distributive justice. It must not only be overt and unbiased, but it must also be perceived as completely fair or it will be met with great resistance.

Chapter 69

The Value of Personal Care

A lament heard with each generation of middle-aged doctors is, "I'm sure glad I'm not starting in practice today."

When I heard that in 1948, it meant that the biochemical paradigm that was replacing anatomy in medicine was too much for them. Or else, that the increased income tax put in place during the War and then never reduced, was a huge burden. The same comment in the 1980s meant that the third-party involvement in medical care was intrusive and unnecessarily demanding.

That which you have never experienced, you are less apt to miss. In the late 1980s, a psychiatrist friend reported that when he complained during a lecture to his residents about the intrusion of various third parties into the practice of psychiatry, one of the residents interrupted him.

"But doctor, we don't understand what you're talking about. We don't know anything else," the resident said.

Many senior doctors who do remember times in which they were more independent have quit practice early because of what is referred to as "the hassle factor." This refers to the increased paperwork on behalf of third parties, and the resultant intrusion into the care of their patients.

If the present course of medical care continues, physicians may adapt, but their numbers will decrease as a proportion of the general population. Ultimately, initial care will be delivered by those with less training and by alternative care practitioners.

American medicine is among the most technically advanced of any country in the world. The 17 percent of our GDP that we spend on medical care is more than half again as much as the average country.

The percent of the GDP spent on medical care will continue to rise steadily. An end does not seem to be in sight. Despite this increasing expenditure, however, life expectancy, maternal and infant mortality, and medical care coverage of the US population falls short of nearly 20 other countries in the world—and some of these do not even have first-world economies. Medicaid and Medicare have helped to broaden medical insurance coverage for many years now, but about 17 percent of our population still is not covered by medical insurance.

The proportion of the GDP that we spend today on medical care is just a fraction of what will be required in the future. Consumer demand and the continuing advances in technology will exert unrelenting pressure on the GDP.

Within this context, our social humanitarian and egalitarian bent is giving rise to an increasing demand for health coverage of all citizens. We are the only country worldwide that is applying the capitalistic, free-market approach to the delivery of healthcare.

If all US citizens are to receive some degree of healthcare coverage, key questions include, "Who will pay for it? Who will manage it? And, how much care will be guaranteed?"

Many in the US today insist that if universal healthcare is to be approved, it must be delivered by the private sector with government oversight only. This requirement is what killed universal care in the US when it was initially proposed in 1946. Even if the private sector approach to universal care were to be adopted, the cost will continue to rise dramatically. Without rationing, we are likely to reach the point of bankruptcy of our economy sooner.

Universal care is not a panacea, but it may be better for more individuals than what we offer today. Whether it is delivered by the government or by the private sector, it will be subject to political manipulation as well as exploitation by commercial enterprises. One example of the political effect is that Medicare's Health Care Regions around the country have different reimbursement criteria for the same services. Much of this is the result of variations in lobbying success among regions.

The British health system is held up as a model of universal care. Its apparent success in controlling costs since its introduction in 1948 is attributable to three major factors. For 40 years, no new hospitals were built. These capital expenditures were postponed. Also, physician reimbursement rates were progressively reduced. Many of the physicians employed in the system are immigrants from second-world countries willing to accept these reduced payments. Lastly, the British temperament and culture is much more tolerant of rationing than we are in the US.

Rationing will be essential in the US. However, as we devote more and more of our GDP to healthcare, it will have to accommodate the American sense of fairness.

Also in the US, the prevalence of individualism will result in a medical system with its own special characteristics. Compassionate and personalized care can help to accommodate the American need for individualism. Perhaps this should be termed, "universal personal care."

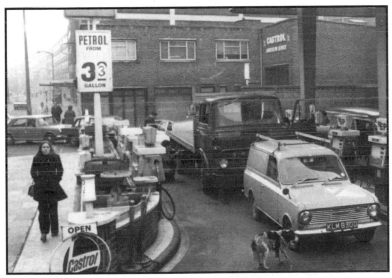

Rationing a la 1974
Evening Standard/ Hulton Archive/ Getty Images, Inc.

CHAPTER 70

The Future of the US Healthcare System

The cost of medical care in the US is widely discussed, but the product is undefined! What is the actual intended goal of medical care? Is it merely to relieve pain and suffering and prevent immediate death? Or is it also to prolong meaningful life as long as possible by all available means? These are very different goals.

Prevention includes the treatment of risk factors, both genetic and lifestyle factors, which place a person at risk for developing a disease. Prevention also involves immunizations to prevent infectious diseases. "All available means" involves treatment with drugs and surgery, including body-part replacement and transplantation.

How much of this health and medical care can the country afford? If everyone in this country receives all of the healthcare to which they believe they are entitled, it could eventually consume the US economy. As in George R. Fisher's book, *The Hospital That Ate Chicago*, we would have "The Health System that Consumed the US."

To be perceived as fair and compassionate, society's goals for medical care of the individual must be the same for everyone in the community. Given the central value of equality in the US, we must differentiate between what an individual needs from what the individual wants.

The differences in the medical-care goals between those of the individual versus those of our society must be recognized. In the US, we have not agreed upon a definition of good individual health. We tend to define disease as a variation from normal on a statistical basis, and good health as the absence of any variation.

As mentioned earlier, the World Health Organization defines good individual health using personal standards. It consists of complete physical, mental, and social well-being as each individual defines it, not as others define it. It is not simply freedom from disease.

For the individual, the goals of healthcare should be: the prevention of death when it's not inevitable, relief of pain and suffering, the treatment of disease, and the restoration of health. These are obvious needs. The inclusion of all comfort care, which is not a need but a want, is debatable. And correction of all individual variations from the norm, another want, is certainly an unnecessary luxury.

From the perspective of society, the goals should include: the prevention and control of contagion; hygienic management of food, water, sewage, air, and other environmental matters; and promoting workforce health, independence, safety, and security. Preventive healthcare may be more important to the community as a whole, than is the medical care of a single individual.

To be perceived as fair and compassionate, society's goals for medical care of the individual must be the same for everyone in the community. Given the central value of equality in the US, we must differentiate between what an individual needs from what the individual wants.

Life is one of the inalienable rights set forth in the declaration of independence. Is the right to good health part of that right to life? Is health an entitlement, like our other Constitutional rights? If so, then it is an entitlement for everyone.

This raises other questions. How long is the life to which one is entitled? And how high must the quality of that life be?

When or how do we define a threat to health as a threat to life? Is such a threat only applicable to those conditions that require immediate, life-saving intervention? How many minutes, hours, days, weeks, or years must the person be able to survive without treatment in order for such a health threat to qualify as a threat to life?

If everyone has the right to medical care, who should pay for it, and how will it be funded? Which rights should be available only to those who are able to pay?

On the other hand, perhaps society's health goals should be based only upon the public needs of society, such as safety from epidemics or workforce requirements, and individual wants and needs should be considered private concerns. If so, which needs are public and which are private?

All of these issues must be considered in coming up with a consensus regarding the goals of the US healthcare system. Prolonging life for everybody as long as possible, by all available means possible, and at all costs is not realistic. Our society cannot afford everything that is and will be possible.

If medical care is an entitlement, our society shall have to determine how much medical care it can afford. This involves rationing, by definition. In countries in which equality is less valued than in the us, and cultural diversity is lower, rationing of healthcare is accepted more readily.

One common method is rationing by queue, which results from the calculated limitation of resources. Another method, long in use but perhaps little known, has been rationing of care through age discrimination. For example, organ transplants frequently are not available to those above a certain age.

In the US, rationing of medical care has always been with us. It is less overt, and the term "rationing" is avoided. We refuse to acknowledge it. Rationing is turned over to a third-party group-management system, where an individual's healthcare needs are limited by the group's financial resource criteria and profit-making goals. The criteria and decision-making process are hidden from the general public.

Individuals have little input as to how their care is rationed. Distinctions must be drawn between the care of the individual alone, the care of the individual as a member of a group, and the care of the individual as a member of society as a whole.

Personal care delivered by experienced general practitioners can be much more cost-effective than that provided through large systems. Large groups minimize the primary physician's role, which encourages the use of high-grade technology from specialists, much of which is not needed. In the latter system, patient anxiety is much higher, which further feeds the overuse of technology.

In any case, if everyone is entitled to healthcare, rationing is a necessity. To achieve a consensus on methodology, both the goals and the limitations of healthcare in such a US health system should be recognized and thoroughly discussed. These should be debated whether the system is called socialized medicine, national healthcare, or universal healthcare. It should be discussed whether the system becomes a single-payer system delivered by the government or delivered by private intermediaries, or if it remains a version of the for-profit, free-market system we now have.

The elements that should be included in basic medical care should be openly recognized and debated. While Medicare and Medicaid have paved the way for acceptance of comprehensive healthcare—which contains key elements of rationing—the lion's share of the debate lies ahead. Again, to be effective, the system must be equitable, and it must be perceived as equitable.

The concepts of social security and universal medical care were both first introduced in Germany in the late 19th century. It took many decades and the crisis of the Great Depression before the US Social Security program was finally created. Universal healthcare has now been debated for more than a century. It will be unfortunate if a national health crisis of a proportion similar to the Great Depression is required in order to establish a healthcare system that provides coverage to all.

CHAPTER 71

Happier and Healthier

I hope this narrative about my experiences has illustrated how, historically, the personal relationship between doctor and patient greatly helped the doctor in understanding the health conditions of the patient. It also provided patients with the reassurances they needed.

The most important component of this vision for the future, however, is providing more personal care of higher quality. Understanding the importance of restoring the doctor-patient relationship to its central role will add to the quality of our healthcare, helping to solve a multitude of problems.

I have attempted to show too, how the use of technology has increased in healthcare today and what both its intended and unintended effects have been. It has been lifesaving and greatly contributed to the many improvements in treatment, but it has also intruded upon the personal relationship between doctor and patient, one that is essential to providing the insight, understanding, and compassion that people need in their medical care. Yet, impersonal technical care has largely replaced the personal care once given by the physician.

Furthermore, the high cost of technology has been a key economic factor in encouraging this trend. The importance of controlling costs will become more critical as we adopt a universal healthcare system, paid at least in part through the public purse.

Providing equitable distribution of care will require a public consensus on how the limited resources will be rationed. The methods and values incorporated in the rationing process must be openly discussed and debated.

The most important component of this vision for the future, however, is providing more personal care of higher quality. Understanding the importance of restoring the doctor-patient relationship to its central role will add to the quality of our healthcare, helping to solve a multitude of problems.

Personal medical care will not only supplement the positive impacts of technical tests and procedures, it will also provide central direction and help to eliminate unnecessary procedures and costs. Greater patient satisfaction will provide increased fulfillment among medical professionals. This will result in a generally happier and healthier society.

Norman Makous, M.D.
June 30, 2009

APPENDICES

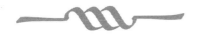

Appendix I

Index

Bolded words also appear in the Glossary, Appendix 2.

APPENDIX 2

Glossary*

ablation (ab-la´shən) [L. ablatus carried away] removal or destruction of a part, especially by cutting.

abscess (ab´ses) [L. abscessus, from ab away +cedere to go] a localized collection of pus buried in tissues, organs, or confined spaces.

acute appendicitis, the sudden development of symptoms from inflammation of the appendix which is a fingerlike attachment at the beginning of the large bowel (colon).

acute coronary syndrome, clinical presentation ranging from unstable angina through acute myocardial infarction; also called ACS.

acute myocardial infarction, one occurring during the period when circulation to a region of the heart is obstructed and tissue necrosis is occurring; it is usually characterized by severe pain, pallor, perspiration, nausea, and dizziness.

Addison's disease, a chronic type of adrenocortical insufficiency, characterized by hypotension, weight loss, weakness, and a bronze-like hyperpigmentation of the skin. It is due to tuberculosis- or autoimmune-induced destruction of the adrenal cortex, which results in deficiency of aldosterone and cortisol and is fatal in the absence of replacement therapy.

adhesion (ad-he´zhən) [L. adhaesio, from adhaerere to stick to] 1. the stable joining of parts to each other, as in wound healing or some pathological process; sometimes done artificially such as in bonding materials to a tooth. 2. a fibrous band or structure by which parts abnormally adhere.

adrenaline (ə-dren´ə-lin) see **epinephrine**.

advanced directive, a legal document through which an individual indicates medical choices regarding accepting or refusing life-sustaining procedures in the case of mental incompetence or maintaining an unconscious state; also known as an **advanced healthcare directive** or a **living will**.

Portions from Dorlands Medical Dictionary. Reprinted by permission.

aldosterone (al-dos'tər-ōn) the major mineralocorticoid secreted by the adrenal cortex; it promotes retention of sodium and bicarbonate, excretion of potassium and hydrogen ions, and secondary retention of water.

Alzheimer's disease, a progressive central neurodegenerative disorder; it may be inherited or sporadic. The first signs of the disease are slight memory disturbance or changes in personality; deterioration progresses to profound dementia over 5 to 10 years on average. Women are affected twice as often as men, and onset may occur at any age; the disorder is currently divided into early-onset and late-onset forms, with the dividing age being approximately 65 years, but there is no clinical distinction between the two forms.

amyloidosis (am"ə-loi-do'sis) [amyloid-+-osis] a group of conditions characterized by the accumulation of insoluble amyloid in various organs and tissues of the body. The associated disease states may be inflammatory, hereditary, or neoplastic.

anasarca (an"ə-sahr'kə) [ana-+sarco] generalized massive **edema**.

anatomy (a-nat'-me) [ana-+-tomy] the science of the structure of the body and the relationship of its parts.

anemia (ə-ne'me-ə) [an-[1]+-emia] a reduction below normal in the concentration of red blood cells or hemoglobin in the blood, measured by volume of packed red cells; it occurs when the equilibrium is disturbed between blood loss (through bleeding or destruction) and blood production.

anemic (ə-ne'mik) pertaining to or characterized by **anemia**.

anesthesia (an"es-the'zhə) [an-[1]+esthesia] 1. loss of sensation, usually by damage to a nerve or receptor; also called numbness. 2. loss of the ability to feel pain, caused by administration of a drug or by other medical interventions.

aneurysm (an'u-riz"əm) [Gr. aneurysma a widening] a sac formed by the dilatation of the wall of an artery, a vein, or the heart; it is filled with fluid or clotted blood, often forming a pulsating tumor.

angina (an-ji'nə) (an'jĭ-nə) [L.] 1. **a. pectoris**. 2. any spasmodic, choking, or suffocative pain.

angina pectoris, a paroxysmal thoracic pain or discomfort, often radiating to the arms, particularly the left, sometimes accompanied by a feeling of suffocation and impending death; subdivided into stable and unstable angina pectoris; **nocturnal angina** occurs in bed at night.

angiocardiogram (an"je-o-kahr´de-o-gram) the film produced by **angiocardiography**.

angiocardiography (an"je-o-kahr"de-og´rə-fe) [angio-+cardiography] x-ray imaging of the heart and great vessels after contrast material is injected into a blood vessel or one of the cardiac chambers; images obtained can be analyzed to measure various heart functions.

angioplasty (an´je-o-plas"te) [angio-+-plasty] a procedure which reduces areas of narrowing in the blood vessels of the heart; **angioplastic surgery**.

anticoagulant therapy, the use of anticoagulants such as heparin, warfarin, or dicumarol, popularly referred to as "blood thinners," to discourage thrombosis or clotting.

anticoagulation (an"te-) (an"ti-ko-ag"u-la´shən) the prevention of clotting of the blood.

aorta (a-or´tə) [l., from Gr. aortē] the main artery in the chest and abdomen from which the arterial system branches. It arises from the left ventricle of the heart. (see "Appendix 3, Diagram of the Heart.")

aortic coarctation (ko"ahrk-ta´shən) [L. coarctatio, from cum together +arctare to make tight] see **coarctation of aorta**.

aortogram (a-or´to-gram) the radiographic record resulting from aortography.

aortography (aor-tog´r-fe) [aorta+-graphy] radiography of the aorta after the intravascular injection of a liquid visible by x-ray.

apex cardiogram (a"peks-kahr´de-o-gram) a tracing of a simple displacement curve from the heart as detected on the surface of the body; abbreviated ACG.

appestat (ap´ə-stat) [appetite +stat] the brain center concerned with controlling the amount of food intake.

arrhythmia (ə-rith´me-ə) [a-¹+rhythm+-ia] any irregular rhythm of the heartbeat.

arsenic (ahr′sə-nik) [L. arsenicum, arsenium, or arsenum; from Gr. arsēn strong] a nonmetallic element, it is toxic by inhalation and ingestion and can cause cancer. Now rarely used in medicine, it is important only in the treatment of certain tropical parasitic diseases.

arsphenamine (ahrs-fen′ə-mēn) the first medicine specific for the treatment of syphilis, yaws, and similar infections, later replaced by oxophenarsine and then by penicillin.

arteriosclerosis (ahr-tēr″e-o-sklə-ro′sis) [arterio-+sclerosis] any of a group of diseases characterized by thickening and loss of elasticity of arterial walls; there are several common forms, including **atherosclerosis**. Also called arterial sclerosis and vascular sclerosis.

arthralgia (ahr-thral′jə) [arthr-+-algia] pain in a joint.

arthritis (ahr-thri′tis) [arthr-+-itis] inflammation of a joint; see also **rheumatism**.

aspirate (as′pĭ-rāt) 1. to draw a foreign substance, such as the gastric contents, into the respiratory tract during inhalation. 2. to treat by aspiration. 3. the substance or material obtained by aspiration.

assay (as′a) determination of the amount of a particular constituent of a mixture, or determination of the biological or pharmacological potency of a drug.

atherosclerosis (ath″ər-o-sklə-ro′sis) [athero-+sclerosis] a common form of arteriosclerosis with formation of deposits of yellowish plaques containing cholesterol, lipoid material (fats), and lipophages (fat ingesting cells) in the large and medium-sized arteries.

atria (a′tre-ə) [L.] plural of **atrium**.

atrial fibrillation, an arrhythmia in which the atria, instead of contracting intermittently, quiver continuously in a chaotic pattern, causing a totally irregular, often rapid ventricular rate.

atrial septal defects, **atrioseptal defects**, congenital cardiac anomalies in which there is an opening in the wall between the right and left atria.

atrium (a′tre-əm) [l., from Gr. atrion hall] one of two chambers of the heart, **right atrium** and **left atrium**, that afford entrance to the ventricles of the heart. (see "Appendix 3, Diagram of the Heart.")

aureomycin, brand name of an antibiotic in the tetracycline family.

autoclave (aw´to-klāv) [auto-+ l. clavis key] an apparatus for sterilization by steam under pressure.

bacterial endocarditis, infective **endocarditis** caused by any of various bacteria most commonly involving the heart valves.

ballistocardiogram (bə-lis″to-kahr´de-o-gram″) the tracing made by a **ballistocardiograph**.

ballistocardiograph (bə-lis″to-kahr´de-o-graf″) an apparatus for recording the movements of the body caused by cardiac contractions and associated blood flow; it has been used to determine cardiac output and other aspects of cardiac function.

balloon angioplasty, angioplasty using a balloon catheter that is inflated to open an artery from the inside.

barbiturate (bahr-bic h´ r- t) any of a class of sedative-hypnotic agents derived from barbituric acid or thiobarbituric acid. Many barbiturates were widely used as sedatives or hypnotics, but benzodiazepines have replaced them in most uses.

barium enema, a suspension of barium injected into the intestine and visible to x-ray examination.

bends (bendz) pain from bubbles of nitrogen in the limbs and abdomen occurring as a result of rapid reduction of high air pressure.

beriberi (ber″e-ber´e) [singhalese, "I cannot," signifying that the person is too ill to do anything] a disease caused by a deficiency of thiamine (vitamin B1) and characterized by nerve inflammation, heart malfunction, and edema. The epidemic form is found primarily in areas in which white (polished) rice is the staple food.

beriberi heart disease is heart disease caused by **beriberi**.

beta blocker, **beta-adrenergic blocking agent**, a drug that induces blockage of adrenaline on the nerve receptors.

biochemistry (bi″o-kem´is-tre) [bio-+chemistry] the chemistry of living organisms and of vital processes; physiological chemistry.

biopsy (bi´op-se) [bio-+ Gr. opsis vision] the removal and microscopic examination of tissue from the living body, performed to establish precise diagnosis.

blood pressure, the pressure of the blood on the walls of the arteries, dependent on the energy of the heart action, the elasticity of the walls of the arteries, and the volume and viscosity of the blood. The maximum or **systolic blood pressure** occurs near the end of contraction of the left ventricle of the heart. The minimum or **diastolic blood pressure** occurs between heart beats.

boric acid (bor'ik) a mild acid used as a weak topical antiseptic on intact skin and in ophthalmic solutions. Also used as a pesticide to kill ants and cockroaches.

breech delivery, delivery of a baby when the buttocks are presented first.

brucellosis (broo"sə-lo'sis) infection caused by species of brucella. in animals such as cattle, sheep, goats, pigs, deer, and rabbits, it may cause infertility or abortion. In humans coming in contact with such animals or their infected food products or tissue, it is a generalized infection characterized by fever, sweating, weakness, malaise, and weight loss. Also called malta fever and undulant fever.

bubonic plague, the most common form of plague, the Black Death of fourteenth century Europe, prevalent in rodents, transmitted by fleas, typically characterized by abrupt onset of fever, chills, weakness, and headache, followed by pain, and tenderness in the lymph nodes.

Buerger's disease, an inflammatory and obliterative disease of the blood vessels primarily of the lower extremities, occurring chiefly in young men and leading to gangrene.

bypass (bi'pas) 1. an auxiliary channel, such as around a blocked segment in the circulatory system or alimentary tract. 2. surgical creation of such a channel, e.g., **coronary bypass.**

C-reactive protein, a globulin that reacts with the somatic C-polysaccharide of the pneumococcus in vitro.

cachectic (kə-kek'tik) pertaining to or characterized by **cachexia.**

cachexia (kə-kek'se-ə) [cac-+ Gr. hexis habit +-ia] a profound constitutional disorder, of general ill health, malnutrition, and physical wasting.

calcium gluconate, a calcium salt of gluconic acid, administered intravenously or orally in the treatment of hypercalcemia and as a nutritional supplement.

cardiac catheterization, passage of a thin tube through a vein in an arm or leg or the neck and into the heart, permitting the securing of blood samples, determination of intracardiac pressure, detection of cardiac anomalies, planning of operative approaches, and determination, implementation, or evaluation of appropriate therapy.

cardiac tamponade, acute compression of the heart caused by the collection of blood or fluid in the pericardium from rupture of the heart, penetrating trauma, or progressive effusion.

cardiopulmonary resuscitation, the artificial substitution of heart and lung action in cardiac arrest or apparent sudden death from any cause. The two major components of CPR are artificial respiration and compression or **closed chest manual cardiac massage.**

cardioverter (kahr´de-o-vur″tər) an energy discharge type of condenser that delivers a direct-current shock to the heart to restore a normal rhythm.

catheterization (kath″ə-tur″-ĭ-za´shən) 1. the insertion of a catheter or thin tube. 2. the use of a catheter.

catarrh (kə-tahr´) inflammation of a mucous membrane, particularly of the head and throat; also called **catarrhal fever.**

catecholamine (kat″ə-kol´ə-mēn) one of a group of biogenic amines mimicking the effect of adrenaline; examples are dopamine, norepinephrine, and epinephrine.

Caesarean section, incision through the abdominal and uterine walls for delivery of a baby. Also called abdominal delivery.

chelation (ke-la´shən) combination with a metal in complexes in which the metal is part of a chemical ring.

chelation therapy, the use of a chelating agent to remove toxic metals from the body, used in the treatment of heavy metal poisoning. In complementary medicine, also used for the treatment of atherosclerosis and other disorders.

chloramphenicol (klor″əm-fen´ĭ-kol) a broad-spectrum antibiotic effective against bacteria and certain spirochetes, and in the treatment of typhus; administered orally or applied topically.

chloroform (klor´ə-form) a colorless, volatile liquid with a strong ether-like odor and a sweetish, burning taste; it is toxic when ingested. Once widely used as an inhalation anesthetic and analgesic, and as an antitussive, and counterirritant.

Chloromycetin (klor″o-mi-se′tin) trademark for preparations of chloramphenicol.

chlortetracycline (klor″tet-rə-si′klēn) a broad-spectrum antibiotic, the first of the tetracycline group to be discovered.

Chlorthiazide, a diuretic that causes elimination of urine by altering electrolyte absorption; used to treat edema, hypertension, and diabetes.

cholesterol (k-les′tr-ol) [chole-+sterol] a key constituent of cell membranes in higher animals, mediating their fluidity and permeability. Most cholesterol is synthesized naturally by the liver and other tissues, but some is absorbed from dietary sources, with each kind transported in plasma by specific lipoproteins. Cholesterol can accumulate or deposit abnormally, and is strongly associated with progression of atherosclerosis. Two main types of cholesterol have been identified: low-density-lipoprotein (LDL) cholesterol, which can create harmful atherosclerotic deposits, and high-density-lipoprotein (HDL) cholesterol, which is helpful in metabolism.

closed chest manual cardiac massage see **cardiopulmonary resuscitation.**

coagulation (ko-ag″u-la′shən) [L. coagulatio] formation of a blood clot.

coarctation (ko″ahrk-ta′shən) [L. coarctatio, from cum together +arct- are to make tight] **stenosis.**

coarctation of aorta, a narrowing, usually severe, of the aorta.

collagen disease, any of a group of diseases that, although clinically distinct and not necessarily related, have in common widespread pathologic changes in the connective tissue; they include lupus erythematosus, scleroderma, rheumatic fever, and rheumatoid arthritis.

colonoscope (ko-lon′o-skōp) [colon+-scope] an elongated flexible endoscope for visual examination of the entire colon.

colonoscopy (ko″lən-os′kə-pe) examination by means of the **colonoscope.** also called **coloscopy.**

computerized axial tomography, a scan in which the emergent x-ray beam is measured by a scintillation counter; the electronic impulses are recorded on a magnetic disk and then are processed by a computer for reconstruction display of the body in cross-section on a computer screen. Also called computed tomography, CAT scan or **CT scan.**

congestive heart failure, a clinical syndrome due to heart disease, characterized by breathlessness and abnormal sodium and water retention, often resulting in edema. The congestion may occur in the lungs, abdomen, and lower extremities.

control (kǝn-trōl′) 1. a standard against which experimental observations may be evaluated. 2. a patient or group differing from that under study (the treated or case group) by lacking the disease or by having a different or absent treatment or regimen; the controls and case or treated subjects usually otherwise have certain similarities to allow or enhance comparison between them.

conversion disorder, a mental disorder characterized by loss of voluntary motor or sensory functioning suggesting physical illness, such as seizures, paralysis, dyskinesia, anesthesia, or blindness, with no physiological basis. A psychological basis is suggested by exacerbation of symptoms at times of psychological stress, avoidance of unpleasant responsibilities, or attention provided by the symptoms. Many patients exhibit a lack of concern about the impairment caused by the symptoms; histrionic personality traits are also common. Symptoms are neither intentionally produced nor feigned, and are not limited to pain or sexual dysfunction.

conversion hysteria, former name for a subtype of hysterical neurosis; currently classified as **conversion disorder.**

cor pulmonale, acute, acute overload of the right ventricle due to pulmonary hypertension, usually resulting from acute pulmonary embolism; **cor pulmonale, chronic,** heart disease characterized by hypertrophy and sometimes dilation of the right ventricle secondary to disease affecting the structure or function of the lungs, but excluding those pulmonary disorders resulting from congenital heart disease or from diseases primarily affecting the left side of the heart.

coronary (kor′ǝ-nar″e) [corona] a term applied primarily to the arteries in the heart muscle.

coronary artery disease, atherosclerosis of the coronary arteries, which may cause angina pectoris, myocardial infarction, and sudden death.

coronary bypass, coronary artery bypass, a section of vein or other conduit grafted between the aorta and a coronary artery to circumvent an obstructive lesion in the coronary artery.

cortisone (kor′tĭ-sōn) a natural steroid produced in the adrenal cortex. The synthetic hormone exerts its pharmaceutical effects through its metabolic conversion to cortisol, which affects the metabolism of glucose, protein, and fats, and also regulates the immune system and affects many other functions.

Coumadin (koo′mə-din) trademark for preparations of warfarin sodium. See also **warfarin.**

coumarin (koo′mə-rin) 1. an agent derived from tonka bean, sweet clover, and other plants, and also prepared synthetically. It contains a factor, dicumarol, that inhibits coagulation of the blood. Its derivatives are used widely as anticoagulants in the treatment of disorders in which there is excessive or undesirable clotting, such as thrombophlebitis and pulmonary embolism. 2. any derivative of coumarin or any synthetic compound with coumarin-like actions.

creatinine (kre-at′ĭ-nin) the product of creatine excreted in the urine; measurements of excretion rates are used as diagnostic indicators of kidney function and muscle mass.

CT scan, see **computerized axial tomography**.

cyclopropane (si″klo-pro′pān) a colorless, flammable gas with a characteristic odor and pungent taste that was once used as an inhalational anesthetic; now little used because of its flammability.

defibrillator (de-fib″rĭ-la′tər) an electronic apparatus used to counteract atrial or ventricular fibrillation by the application of brief electroshock to the heart, either directly or through electrodes placed on the chest wall. When placed in the body, called an **implantable cardioverter-defibrillator, or automatic implantable cardioverter-defibrillator.** See also **cardioverter.**

dementia (də-men′shə) [de-+ 1. mens mind] a general loss of cognitive abilities, including impairment of memory as well as one or more of the following: aphasia, or disturbed planning, organizing, or abstract thinking abilities.

diabetes (di″ə-be′tēz) [Gr. diabētēs a syphon, from dia through +bainein to go] any of various disorders characterized by passage of a large volume of urine.

diabetes mellitus, a chronic syndrome of impaired carbohydrate, protein, and fat metabolism owing to insufficient secretion of insulin or to target tissue insulin resistance. It occurs in two major forms: type 1 or juvenile diabetes and type 2 or adult onset diabetes. They differ in etiology, pathology, genetics, and treatment.

dialysis (di-al′ə-sis) [Gr. "dissolution"] 1. the process of separating colloids (macromolecules) from crystalloids (ions and low-molecular-weight compounds) in solution by the difference in their rates of passage through a semipermeable membrane, through which crystalloids can pass readily but colloids pass very slowly or not at all. 2. **hemodialysis.**

diastolic pressure, diastolic blood pressure, the minimum blood pressure which occurs between heartbeats. See **blood pressure.**

dicumarol (di-koo′m-rol) 1. a coumarin anticoagulant found in spoiled sweet clover; animals eating the clover may develop the hemorrhagic condition known as sweet clover disease. 2. a synthetic preparation of the same substance, used as an oral anticoagulant.

digitalis (dij″ĭ-tal′is) [L. "fingerlike"] 1. the dried leaf of Digitalis purpurea, the purple foxglove, used to treat congestive heart failure and most supraventricular tachycardias; digitalis and the other digitalis glycosides act by increasing the force of myocardial contraction and by decreasing the heart rate. 2. collectively, the digitalis compounds.

digitoxin (dij″ĭ-tok′sin) a cardiac glycoside obtained from Digitalis purpurea, D. lanata, and other Digitalis species; it has the same actions and uses as **digitalis;** administered orally, intramuscularly, or intravenously.

digoxin (dĭ-jok′sin) a cardiac glycoside obtained from the leaves of Digitalis lanata, having the same actions and uses as **digitalis;** administered orally, intramuscularly, or intravenously.

diphosphate, any compound in which a base molecule is attached to two phosphoric acid molecules.

diphtheria (dif-thēr´e-ə) [Gr. diphthera leather +-ia] an acute infectious disease caused by strains of Corynebacterium diphtheriae, acquired by contact with an infected person or carrier; usually confined to the upper respiratory tract. It may obstruct breathing and cause death by suffocation.

dissecting aneurysm, longitudinal splitting of the arterial wall resulting from hemorrhage; it usually affects the **aorta** (aortic dissection) but may also affect other large arteries.

diuresis (di"u-re´sis) [Gr. diourein to urinate, to pass in urine] increased excretion of urine.

diuretic (di"u-ret´ik) [Gr. diourētikos promoting urine] 1. pertaining to or causing diuresis. 2. an agent that promotes diuresis. e.g., a **mercurial d.**

diverticulitis (di"vər-tik"u-li´tis) inflammation of colonic diverticula, the hollows or pouches in the intestinal wall, which may undergo perforation with abscess formation. Sometimes called left-sided appendicitis.

dropsy (drop´se) [L. hydrops, from Gr. hydōr water] archaic term for **edema.**

ductus (duk´təs) [L.] a duct: anatomic nomenclature for a passage with well-defined walls, especially such a channel for the passage of excretions or secretions.

ductus arteriosus, a fetal blood vessel connecting the left pulmonary artery directly to the descending aorta; in normal development, it closes at birth.

duodenum (doo"o-de´nəm) (doo-od´ə-nəm) [L. duodeni twelve at a time] the first or proximal portion of the small intestine, much shorter than the following portions, extending from the pylorus to the jejunum; so called because its length is about 12 finger breadths.

dye-dilution curves, an indicator dilution curve in which the indicator is a dye, usually indocyanine green; it is used in studies of cardiac output and other aspects of cardiovascular function.

dynamics (di-nam´iks) that phase of mechanics which deals with the motions of material bodies taking place under different specific conditions.

Ebstein's anomaly, a malformation of the tricuspid valve (see "Appendix 3, Diagram of the Heart"), in which the valve leaflets adhere to the wall of the right ventricle; usually associated with an atrial septal defect. Also called Ebstein disease.

ECG, see **electrocardiogram.**

echocardiogram (ek″o-kahr′de-o-gram″) the record produced by **echocardiography.**

echocardiography (ek″o-kahr″de-og′rə-fe) a method of graphically recording the position and motion of the heart walls or the internal structures of the heart and neighboring tissue by the echo obtained from beams of ultrasonic waves directed through the chest wall. Also called ultrasonic cardiography. See also **ultrasonography.**

ectopic beat, an abnormal heart beat originating at some point other than the sinus node.

edema (-de′m) [Gr. oidma swelling] the presence of abnormally large amounts of fluid in the tissues. It may be local, such as from venous obstruction, or systemic, such as from heart failure.

effusion (ə-fu′zhən) [L. effusio a pouring out] the escape of fluid into a body part or tissue.

electrocardiogram (e-lek″tro-kahr′de-o-gram″) [electro-+cardiogram] a graphic tracing of the variations in electrical activity of the heart muscle and detected at the body surface. The first wave form in the tracing, the p wave, is due to excitation of the atria; the next part, the qrs wave complex, is due to excitation of the ventricles; and the t wave shows recovery of the ventricles. Abbreviated **ECG** or EKG.

electrocardiographic recorder, the device that produces the graphic tracing for an **electrocardiogram** by detection of variations in electrical potential between two points on the body caused by the electrical impulses of the heart muscle.

electrocardiographic tracing, the graphic tracing produced in an electrocardiogram.

electro-cardioversion (kahr′de-o-vur″zhən) the restoration of normal rhythm of the heart by electrical shock.

embolectomy (em″bə-lek′tə-me) [embolus+-ectomy] surgical removal of an **embolus**.

embolic (em-bol′ik) pertaining to an **embolus** or to **embolism**.

embolism (em′bə-liz-əm) [L. embolus, q.v.] the sudden blocking of an artery by a clot or foreign material which has been brought to the site of lodgment by the blood current from another part of the circulatory system.

embolus (em′bo-ləs) [Gr. embolos plug, from en in +ballein to throw] a mass, which may be a blood clot or some other material, that is brought by the bloodstream through the vasculature, lodging in a vessel too small to allow it to pass, obstructing the circulation.

emphysema (em″fə-se′mə) [Gr. "an inflation"] 1. a pathological accumulation of air in tissues or organs. 2. **pulmonary e.**

endocarditis (en″do-kahr-di′tis) [endocardium+ -itis] inflammatory alterations of the **endocardium**, usually characterized by infection on the surface of the endocardium or in the endocardium itself, and most commonly involving a heart valve. It may occur as a primary disorder or as a complication of or in association with another disease.

endocardium (endo-kahr′de-um) [endo+ Gr. kardia heart] the membrane lining the cavities of the heart.

enema (en′ə-mə) [Gr.] a liquid injected or to be injected into the rectum.

epinephrine (ep″ĭ-nef′rin) 1. a catecholamine hormone secreted by the adrenal gland and active in the nervous system. It is released in response to hypoglycemia, stress, and other stimuli and is a potent stimulator of the adrenalin receptors of the sympathetic nervous system and the heart rate. 2. a synthetic preparation of epinephrine, used topically as a local anesthesia, and intravenously as a cardiac stimulant. Also called adrenaline (Great Britain).

erythema (er″ə-the′mə) [Gr. erythēma flush upon the skin] redness of the skin produced by congestion of the capillaries.

erythrocyte, one of the blood cells found in human blood; a yellowish, biconcave disk, adapted by its hemoglobin content to the transport of oxygen; it turns red when carrying oxygen; also called a **red blood cell** or a corpuscle.

ethacrynic acid (eth″ə-krin´ik) a diuretic used in the treatment of edema associated with congestive heart failure, or of hypertension, often in combination with other drugs; administered orally.

ether (e´thər) [L. aether, from Gr. aithēr "the upper and purer air"] 1. a colorless, volatile, flammable liquid with a characteristic odor; the first inhalational anesthetic used for surgical anesthesia (1846), now little used because of its flammability. Also called diethyl e. and ethyl e.

ethylene (eth´ə-lēn) a colorless, flammable gas with a sweet taste and odor, formerly used as an inhalational anesthetic.

euthanasia (u″thə-na´zhə) [eu-+ Gr. thanatos death] 1. an easy or painless death. 2. the deliberate ending of the life of a person suffering from an incurable and painful disease.

extubate (eks-too´bāt) [ex-+ 1. tuba tube] to remove a tube from. For example, to remove a tube from the trachea that assists in breathing.

femoral artery, the artery that supplies blood to the legs and lower extremities.

flicker fusion, the threshold at which an intermittent light stimulus appears to be completely steady to the observer.

florida phthisis, see **phthisis.**

fluoroscope (floor´o-skōp) a device used for examining deep structures by means of x-rays; it consists of a screen covered with crystals of calcium tungstate on which are projected the shadows of x-rays passing through the body placed between the screen and the source of irradiation.

fluoroscopic (floor″o-skop´ik) pertaining to fluoroscopy.

fluoroscopy (flu-ros´kə-pe) examination by means of the fluoroscope.

flutter (flut´ər) a rapid vibration or pulsation.

furosemide (fu-ro´sə-mīd) a diuretic used in the treatment of edema associated with congestive heart failure, as an adjunct in the treatment of acute pulmonary edema, and in the treatment of hypertension, usually in combination with other drugs; administered orally, intramuscularly, or intravenously.

gangrene (gang´grēn) [L. gangraena; Gr. gangraina an eating sore, which ends in mortification] death of tissue, usually in considerable mass, associated with loss of blood supply and followed by bacterial invasion and putrefaction.

gastroenterologist (gas″tro-en″tər-ol´ə-jist) a specialist in **gastroenterology.**

gastroenterology (gas″tro-en″tər-ol´ə-je) [gastro-+entero-+-logy] the study of the stomach and intestines and the nature and treatment of their diseases.

glaucoma (glaw-) (glou-ko´mə) [Gr. glaukōma opacity of the crystalline lens (from the dull gray gleam of the affected eye)] a group of eye diseases characterized by an increase in intraocular pressure that causes pathologic changes in the optic disk and typical defects in the field of vision.

glioblastoma (gli″o-blas-to´mə) [glio-+blastoma] a general term for malignant forms of brain tumors; **glioblastoma multiforme,** the most malignant type of brain tumor, grows rapidly and is usually found in the brain hemispheres.

glycyrrhizin, the main sweet tasting compound from liquorice root. Chemically, glycyrrhizin is a glycoside of glycyrrhizic acid.

gonorrhea (gon″o-re´ə) [gono-[1]+-rrhea] usually a sexually transmitted disease. In males, it is marked by urethritis with pain and pussy discharge; in females, it is commonly asymptomatic, although it may extend to produce abscesses.

hardening of the arteries, popular term for **arteriosclerosis.**

heart block, impairment of conduction of the electric impulse in heart excitation, either permanent or transient, and due to anatomical or functional impairment. It is subclassified as first, second, or third degree **(high heart block)** and is frequently used specifically to denote atrioventricular block.

hemodialysis (he″mo-di-al´ə-sis) the removal of impurities from the blood by virtue of the difference in the rates of their diffusion through a semipermeable membrane. Also called dialysis, kidney dialysis, and renal dialysis.

hemoptysis (he-mop´tĭ-sis) [hemo-+ Gr. ptyein to spit] the expectoration of blood or of blood-stained sputum.

hemorrhage (hem´ə-rəj) [hemo-+-rrhage] the escape of blood from the vessels; bleeding.

hemostat (he´mo-stat) a surgical clamp for constricting a blood vessel.

heparin (hep´ə-rin) [Gr. hēpar liver] a potent natural anticoagulant released by blood cells and present in many tissues, especially the liver and lungs; also produced synthetically.

hepatitis (hep″ə-ti´tis) [hepat-+-itis] inflammation of the liver.

hernia (hur´ne-ə) [L.] the protrusion of part of an organ or tissue through an abnormal opening.

histoplasmosis (his″to-plaz-mo´sis) infection resulting from inhalation, or sometimes ingestion, of spores of Histoplasma capsulatum, found in droppings from chickens, pigeons, starlings, blackbirds, and bats. It is usually asymptomatic, but in a few cases it may cause acute pneumonia, anemia, or a flu-like illness with joint swelling.

hydrochlorothiazide (hi″dro-klor″o-thi´ə-zīd) a thiazide diuretic used for treatment of hypertension and edema; administered orally.

hypertension (hi″pər-ten´shən) [hyper-+tension] high arterial blood pressure.

hyperventilation (hi″pər-ven″tĭ-la´shən) overbreathing, a state in which there is an increased amount of air entering and leaving the lungs; results in excess carbon dioxide loss from the body, which eventually leads to a chemical imbalance in the blood.

hypochondriac (hi″po-kon´dre-ak) a person affected with **hypochondriasis**.

hypochondriasis (hi″po-kon-dri´ə-sis) [so called because it was supposed by the ancients to be due to disturbed function of the organs of the upper abdomen] a psychological disorder characterized by a preoccupation with bodily functions and the interpretation of normal sensations (such as heart beats, sweating, peristaltic action, and bowel movements) or minor abnormalities (such as a runny nose, minor aches and pains, or slightly swollen lymph nodes) as indications of serious problems needing medical attention.

hypodermaclysis, the delivery of fluids under the skin.

hypoxia (hi-pok´se-ə) reduction of oxygen supply to tissue below physiological levels despite adequate supply of blood.

hysterectomy (his″tər-ek´tə-me) [hystero-+-ectomy] the operation of excising the entire uterus.

implantable pacemaker, see **pacemaker.**

implanted cardiac defibrillator, see **defibrillator.**

infectious mononucleosis, a common, infectious disease caused by the Epstein-Barr virus, characterized by fever, membranous pharyngitis, lymph node and splenic enlargement, lymphocyte proliferation, and atypical lymphocytes. It affects primarily adolescents and young adults and is spread by saliva transfer and possibly other modes; in children the infection is largely subclinical. Also called glandular fever and kissing disease.

inhalation pneumonia, see **pneumonia.**

intra-arterial blood pressure, see **blood pressure.**

intravascular dynamics, dynamics within a blood vessel; see **dynamics.**

intravenous (in″trə-ve´nəs) within a vein or veins.

intravenous injection, an injection made into a vein.

intubation (in″too-ba´shən) [L. in into +tuba tube] the insertion of a tube into a body canal or cavity; frequently refers to insertion of a tube into the trachea to assist with breathing.

iron lung, a popular name for the Drinker respirator, a type of ventilator consisting of a metal tank enclosing the body of the patient with the head outside. It was formerly in wide use, but its use has now decreased in favour of less cumbersome ventilators.

jaundice (jawn´dis) [fr. jaunisse, from jaune yellow] a condition characterized by elevated bilirubin and deposition of bile pigments in the skin, mucous membranes, and sclera, with resulting yellow appearance of the patient; also called icterus.

keyhole surgery, see **laparoscopic surgery.**

lactate (lak´tat) a salt of lactic acid; **one-molar l. solution,** a dilute solution of lactic acid salt.

laparoscope (lap´ə-ro-skōp″) a thin, telescope-like instrument with a light and a lens that is inserted into the abdomen to inspect it. Also called celioscope and peritoneoscope.

laparoscopic (lap″ə-ro-skop´ik) performed using a **laparoscope.**

laparoscopic surgery, surgery performed using a **laparoscope.**

leukocyte, a cell of the immune system defending the body against both infectious disease and foreign materials; also called a **white blood cell.**

lidocaine, a local anesthetic delivered by infiltration injection or by topical application; also administered intravenously for use as a cardiac antiarrhythmic.

lidocaine hydrochloride, the salt product of **lidocaine.**

locum te´nens, locum te´nent, a practitioner who temporarily takes the place of another.

lupus (loo´pəs) [L. "wolf" or "pike"] 1. name formerly given to numerous types of localized destruction or degeneration of the skin caused by cutaneous diseases. 2. **lupus erythematosus.**

lupus erythematosus, see **lupus** and **systemic lupus erythematosus.**

lymph node, tissue varying from 1 to 25 mm in diameter, situated along the course of lymphatic vessels. The lymph nodes are the main source of lymphocytes of the peripheral blood and serve as a defense mechanism by removing noxious agents, such as bacteria and toxins; probably play a role in antibody production.

magnetic resonance imaging, a method of visualizing soft tissues of the body by applying an external magnetic field that makes it possible to distinguish between hydrogen atoms in different environments; also called **MRI.**

malaria (mə-lar´e-ə) [it. "bad air"] an infectious disease endemic in many warm regions of the world, caused by **protozoa** of the genus Plasmodium, usually transmitted by the bites of infected mosquitoes. It is characterized by prostration with high fever, shaking chills, sweating, and anemia; death may result from its complications. It may follow a chronic or relapsing course.

mammography (mə-mog′rə-fe) radiography of the mammary gland. **digital mammography,** a method for breast radiography that converts x-rays into electric signals producing digital images that can be seen on a computer screen and stored; the radiation dose is lower than that of traditional mammography.

mapharsen, brand name for oxophenarsine, a drug developed in 1937 from the product of liver metabolism of **arsphenamine.** Found to be less toxic than arsphenamine, the standard for treatment of syphilis since 1909.

Medicaid, a US government program, financed by federal, state, and local funds, providing hospitalization and medical insurance for persons of all ages within certain income limits.

medical thyroidectomy, pharmacologic suppression of **thyroid** function. see **thyroidectomy.**

Medicare, a US government program providing hospitalization insurance and voluntary medical insurance for persons aged 65 and over and for certain disabled persons under age 65.

mercurial (mər-kūr′e-əl) [L. mercurialis] pertaining to mercury.

mercurial diuretic, see **diuretic.**

mercury (mur′kūr-e) a metallic element, liquid at ordinary temperatures. Mercury and its salts have been used medicinally, but because of the risk of mercury poisoning, their use has diminished.

metabolic syndrome, metabolic syndrome X, a syndrome including at least three of the following: abdominal obesity, hypertriglyceridemia, low level of high-density lipoproteins, hypertension, and high fasting plasma glucose level. It is associated with an increased risk for development of diabetes mellitus and cardiovascular disease. Also called syndrome X.

mitral stenosis, a narrowing of the left atrioventricular valvular orifice (mitral orifice) of the heart; see **stenosis.**

mitral valve prolapse, hooding of mitral valve leaflets so that they are thrust backward into the left atrium, often causing mitral regurgitation or leakage; also called floppy mitral valve.

Mohs Method, Mohs surgery, a technique of microscopically controlled serial excision of high-risk, nonmelanoma skin cancers. Early on, the tissue was removed after being fixed with zinc chloride paste (Mohs chemosurgery); later this was modified to a more tissue-sparing technique in which serial excisions of fresh tissue would be done with microscopic analysis. Also called Mohs technique.

mononucleosis (mon″o-noo″kle-o´sis) see **infectious m.**

morphine (mor´fēn) [L. morphina, morphinum] the principal narcotic derived from opium having powerful analgesic action. It is used for relief of severe pain, antitussive, adjunct to anesthesia, and in treatment of pulmonary edema. Abuse of morphine leads to dependence.

MRI, see **magnetic resonance imaging.**

Munchausen syndrome, a condition characterized by habitual presentation for hospital treatment of an apparent acute physical illness, the patient giving a plausible and dramatic history, all of which is false.

myocardial infarction, gross death of an area of heart muscle as a result of interruption of the blood supply.

myocarditis (mi″o-kahr-di´tis) [myo-+carditis] inflammation of the heart muscle.

myocardium, the involuntary, striated muscle found in the walls of the heart.

myxosarcoma (mik″so-sahr-ko´mə) [myxo-+sarcoma] a malignant tumor composed of primitive connective tissue cells and stroma; also called mucous tumor.

narcotic (nahr-kot´ik) [Gr. narkōtikos benumbing, deadening] 1. pertaining to or producing narcosis. 2. an agent that produces insensibility or stupor, applied especially to the opioids, i.e., to any natural or synthetic drug that has actions like those of morphine.

neoplasm (ne´o-plaz-əm) [neo-+-plasm] any new and abnormal growth or tumor; specifically a new growth of tissue in which the growth is uncontrolled and progressive. May be benign or malignant, which has the properties of invasion and metastasis.

nitroglycerin (ni″tro-glis´ər-in) 1. a colorless to yellow liquid formed by the action of nitric and sulfuric acids on glycerin. It explodes on concussion, but is safe if diluted with inert material. Exposure to excessive amounts causes headache, blurred vision, vomiting, hypotension, and syncope, and possibly cyanosis and methemoglobinemia. Prolonged exposure causes tolerance, and abrupt discontinuation can cause withdrawal symptoms. 2. a pharmaceutical preparation of nitroglycerin, diluted with lactose, dextrose, alcohol, propylene glycol, or other excipient for safety and officially called diluted nitroglycerin; it has antianginal, antihypertensive, and vasodilator properties and is used in medicine for the prevention and treatment of angina pectoris, the treatment of congestive heart failure, as an adjunct in the treatment of myocardial infarction, and for blood pressure control or controlled hypotension during surgery. Administered by absorption through the oral mucous membranes, orally, intravenously, topically, or with a transdermal patch.

nocturnal angina see **angina pectoris.**

occlude (ə-klood´) 1. to fit close together. 2. to close tight, as to bring the mandibular teeth into contact with the teeth in the maxilla. 3. obstruct.

one-molar lactate solution, see **lactate.**

opiate (o´pe-ət) 1. a remedy containing or derived from **opium.** 2. hypnotic (def. 2).

opium (o´pe-əm) [l., from Gr. opion] the air-dried milky extract obtained from the unripe capsules of papaver somniferum or P. Album, commonly known as the poppy flower. Various derivatives of opium, including morphine and codeine, are used for their narcotic and analgesic effects.

osteoarthritis (os″te-o-ahr-thri′tis) [osteo-+arthr-+-itis] a degenerative joint disease seen mainly in older persons. It is accompanied by pain, usually after prolonged activity, and stiffness, particularly in the morning or with inactivity.

pacemaker (pās´ma-kər) the artificial cardiac pacemaker is a medical device which uses electrical impulses delivered by electrodes contacting the heart muscles, to regulate the beating of the heart; required when the heart's natural mechanism is absent or defective; **implanted pacemaker, internal pacemaker,** an artificial cardiac pacemaker completely inserted into the subcutaneous tissue.

palpation (pal-pa´shən) [L. palpatio] a physical diagnostic technique of applying the fingers with light pressure to the surface of the body to determine the consistency of the parts beneath.

Pantopon, trade name for a preparation of opiates made up of all of the alkaloids present in opium in their natural proportions as hydrochloride salts; it can sometimes be tolerated by persons who are allergic to morphine.

patent ductus arteriosus, abnormal persistence of an open passage in the **ductus arteriosus** after birth, the direction of flow being from the aorta to the pulmonary artery, resulting in recirculation of arterial blood through the lungs.

pathognomonic (path″og-no-mon´ik) [patho-+ Gr. gnōmonikos fit to give judgment] specifically distinctive or characteristic of a disease or pathologic condition; a sign or symptom on which a diagnosis can be made.

pathologic (path″o-loj´ik) indicative of or caused by an illness.

pathology (pə-thol´ə-je) [patho-+-logy] 1. the branch of medicine that deals with the essential nature of disease, especially of the structural and functional changes in tissues and organs of the body that cause or are caused by disease. 2. the structural and functional manifestations of disease.

Pel-Ebstein fever, a cyclic fever occasionally seen in Hodgkin disease or certain other diseases, characterized by irregular episodes of fever of several days' duration, with intervening afebrile periods lasting for days or weeks.

penicillin (pen″ĭ-sil´in) any of a large group of antibacterial antibiotics derived from strains of fungi of the genus Penicillium. The penicillins, despite their relatively low toxicity for the host, are active against many bacteria, especially gram-positive pathogens (streptococci, staphylococci, pneumococci); clostridia; some gram-negative forms (gonococci, meningococci); some spirochetes (treponema pallidum and T. pertenue); and some fungi. Certain strains of some target species, e.g., staphylococci, secrete an enzyme that inactivates penicillin and confers resistance to the antibiotic.

Pentothol, trade name of a drug used to cause drowsiness or sleep before surgery or certain medical procedures; also used to stop seizures and for other medical conditions.

peptic ulcer, an ulcer of the mucous membrane of the alimentary tract caused by action of acidic gastric juice.

pericardial effusion, the accumulation of an abnormally large amount of fluid in the **pericardium.**

pericarditis (per″e-kahr-di′tis) [pericardium+-itis] inflammation of the **pericardium.**

pericardium (per″ĭ-kahr′de-əm) [l.; peri-+ Gr. kardia heart] 1. the fibrous sac that surrounds the heart and the roots of the great vessels. The base of the pericardium is attached to the central tendon of the diaphragm.

peripheral vascular disease, disease of the blood vessels outside the heart and brain; often a narrowing of the vessels that carry blood to the legs, arms, stomach or kidneys; two types: **functional peripheral vascular diseases** which don't involve defects in blood vessel structure; can be short-term effects triggered by conditions such as temperature, stress, machinery or smoking; **organic peripheral vascular diseases** which are caused by structural changes in the blood vessels, such as inflammation and tissue damage that block normal blood flow.

peritoneal dialysis, hemodialysis through the abdominal cavity; the dialyzing solution is introduced into and removed from the abdominal cavity. Unwanted solutes leave the blood because of a concentration gradient across the peritoneal membrane.

phlebitis (flə-bi′tis) [phleb-+-itis] inflammation of a vein; when accompanied by a **thrombus** (clot) formation it is called **thrombophlebitis.**

phonocardiography(fo″no kahr″do og′rə fe)[phono ı cardiography] the graphic representation of heart sounds, murmurs, or any acoustic phenomena emanating from the heart; in clinical use, the term usually includes recording of the pulse tracings, and is often combined with other noninvasive methods such as echocardiography. **Intracardiac phonocardiography,** the graphic registration of sounds produced by action of the heart by means of a recording device passed into one of the heart chambers through a tube.

phthisis (thi′sis; ti′sis) [Gr. phthisis, from phthiein to decay] a wasting away or degeneration of the body or a part of the body usually from tuberculosis; **Florida phthisis,** pneumonia that involves the degeneration of most of both lungs.

Pitressin (pĭ-tres´in) trademark name for vasopressin, a pituitary gland hormone that stimulates contraction of muscles of capillaries and arterioles, raising the blood pressure; it also promotes contraction of the intestines and the uterus.

placebo (plə-se´bo) [L. "I will please"] any dummy medical treatment; originally, a medicinal preparation having no specific pharmacological activity against the patient's illness, given solely for the **psychophysiological** effects of the treatment; more recently, a dummy treatment administered to the control group in a clinical trial so that the effects of the experimental treatment can be compared to a base level; the experimental treatment must produce better results than the placebo in order to be considered effective.

placebo effect, 1. the sum total of psychological and physiological effects associated with the physician-patient relationship, the patient's expectations and apprehensions concerning the treatment and the effects of taking a medication or treatment. 2. the measured effects on a patient in a controlled study who is receiving the **placebo.**

placenta previa, a complication of pregnancy in which the placenta develops in the lower uterus so that it covers the cervical opening.

pneumonia (noo-mo´ne-ə) [Gr. pneumōnia] inflammation of the lungs; often categorized according to causative organism or location; **inhalation pneumonia,** pneumonia due to the inhalation of irritating substances.

polio, see **poliomyelitis**

poliomyelitis (po″le-o-mi″ə-li´tis) [polio-+myel-+-itis] an acute infectious disease occurring sporadically or in epidemics and usually caused by a poliovirus. It is characterized clinically by fever, sore throat, headache, and vomiting, often with stiffness of the neck and back. In the minor illness these may be the only symptoms. The major illness is characterized by involvement of the central nervous system, with stiff neck, localized muscle pain, and sometimes paralysis. There may be subsequent atrophy of groups of muscles, ending in contraction and permanent deformity. Also called **polio.** The major illness is also called infantile paralysis and acute anterior polio.

polypharmacy (pol″e-fahr´mə-se) [poly-+ Gr. pharmakon drug] 1. the administration of many drugs together. 2. the administration of excessive medication.

popliteal artery, continuation of **femoral artery** into the knee and calf.

posttraumatic stress disorder, an anxiety disorder caused by exposure to an intensely traumatic event; characterized by re-experiencing the traumatic event in recurrent intrusive recollections, nightmares, or flash-backs, by avoidance of trauma-associated stimuli, by generalized numbing of emotional responsiveness, and by hyperalertness and difficulty in sleeping, remembering, or concentrating. The onset of symptoms may be delayed for months to years after the event. Terms formerly used for disorders of this type include gross stress reaction, shell shock, and combat or battle exhaustion or fatigue. Also known as PTSD.

preceptor, a skilled medical practitioner or faculty member who supervises students in a clinical setting to allow practical experience with patients.

preeclampsia (pre″e-klamp′se-ə) a complication of pregnancy characterized by hypertension, edema, or protein in the urine; when convulsions and coma are associated, it is called eclampsia.

procainamide (pro-kān′ə-mīd) a cardiac depressant used in the treatment of cardiac arrhythmias, administered orally, intramuscularly, or intravenously. Also called **procainamide hydrochloride.**

proctoscope (prok′to-skōp) [procto-+-scope] a speculum or tubular instrument with appropriate illumination for inspecting the rectum. Also called a rectoscope.

proctoscopic examination, an examination of the rectum using a **proctoscope.**

prostatitis (pros″tə-ti′tis) inflammation of the prostate.

prostheses (pros-the′sēz) [Gr.] plural of **prosthesis.**

prosthesis (pros-the′sis) [Gr. "a putting to"] an artificial substitute for a missing body part, such as a limb, eye, or tooth, used for functional or cosmetic reasons, or both.

prothrombin time, the rate at which blood will coagulate; used to monitor administration of anticoagulants.

protozoa (pro″to-zo′ah) a single-celled organism of the animal kingdom.

pseudocyesis (soo″do-si-e´sis) [pseudo-+-cyesis] false pregnancy; the presence of signs of pregnancy without occurrence of conception and development of an embryo; it may be due to psychogenic factors, to a tumor, or to endocrine disorders.

psychophysiologic (siko-fize-o-loj´ik) [psycho-+physiologic] having a relationship between physiological and psychological processes; **psychophysiological.**

psychosomatic (si″ko-so-mat´ik) [psycho-+somat-+-ic] pertaining to the mind-body relationship; having bodily symptoms of psychic, emotional, or mental origin; also called **psychophysiologic.**

pulmonary artery, the vessel that carries blood from the heart to the lungs. (see "Appendix 3, Diagram of The Heart.")

pulmonary edema, abnormal accumulation of fluid in the lungs characterized by intense difficulty breathing, and if severe, by expectoration of frothy pink fluid and bluish skin color due to insufficient oxygen levels. Also called wet lung.

pulmonary embolism, the closure of the pulmonary artery or one of its branches by an **embolus** or blood clot, sometimes associated with **pulmonary infarction.**

pulmonary embolus see **pulmonary embolism**

pulmonary emphysema, a condition of the lung characterized by an abnormal increase in the size of air spaces in the terminal bronchioles.

pulmonary infarction, localized necrosis of lung tissue caused by obstruction of the arterial blood supply, most often due to pulmonary embolism.

pulmonary neoplasm, new or abnormal growth of tissue in the lungs; see **neoplasm.**

pulmonary valve stenosis, pulmonary stenosis, narrowing of the opening between the **pulmonary artery** and the **right ventricle,** usually located in the valve leaflets.

pulsus paradoxus, an exaggeration of the normal variation in the pulse during the inspiratory phase of respiration, in which the pulse becomes weaker as one inhales and stronger as one exhales. Also called paradoxic pulse.

quinidine (kwin´ĭ-dēn) the extract of **quinine** obtained from various species of plants or prepared from quinine. It has cardiac depressant activity, and is as potent an antimalarial as quinine.

quinine (kwin´in) (kwin-ēn´) (kwi´nīn) [L. quinina] an extract of the cinchona plant which suppresses malarial parasites. Once widely used to prevent and control malaria, it has been largely replaced by less toxic and more effective synthetic antimalarials, and is now used chiefly in the treatment of malaria that is resistant to other antimalarials. Quinine also has analgesic, fever-reducing, and cardiac depressant properties.

rales (rahls) a series of short nonmusical noises, heard primarily during inhalation; also called crackles.

red blood cell, see **erythrocyte.**

red blood cell sedimentation rate, the rate at which red blood cells precipitate out from a well-mixed specimen of venous blood, measured by the distance the top of the column of cells falls in a given time interval under specified conditions.

renal dialysis, see **hemodialysis.**

rheumatic fever, a feverous disease resulting from infection with beta hemolytic streptococci, characterized by inflammation of connective tissue, especially the heart (rheumatic heart disease), blood vessels, and joints (rheumatic arthritis).

rheumatism (roo´mə-tiz-əm) [L. rheumatismus; Gr. rheumatismos] popular name for any of a variety of disorders marked by inflammation, degeneration, or derangement of connective tissue, especially the joints; symptoms include pain, stiffness, or limitation of motion; rheumatism confined to the joints is more precisely called **arthritis.**

Rocky Mountain spotted fever, an acute, infectious, sometimes fatal disease caused by a rickettsia infection, usually transmitted by the bite of an infected tick; it occurs only in north and south america. It is characterized by sudden onset; chills; fever lasting 2 to 3 weeks; a rash; muscle pain; severe headache; and prostration.

salicylic acid (sal´ĭ-sil´ik) a derivative obtained from white willow bark and wintergreen leaves, and also prepared synthetically; used as a topical treatment for a variety of skin disorders including acne, dermatitis, plantar warts, and corns. Its sodium salt is an analgesic.

sarcoma (sahr-ko´m) [sarc-+-oma] any of a group of tumors usually arising from connective tissue; most are malignant.

scarlet fever, a streptococci infection characterized by pharyngitis, tonsillitis, and a rash progressing from the trunk and neck to the limbs and face. Other symptoms include a red or white strawberry tongue. Also called scarlatina.

schizophrenia (skit″so-fre´ne-ə) [schizo-+phren+-ia] a group of mental disorders characterized by disturbances in thought, mood, sense of self, relationship to the external world, and behavior.

seasonal affective disorder, a cyclically recurring mood disorder characterized by depression, extreme lethargy, increased need for sleep, overeating, and carbohydrate craving; it intensifies in one or more specific seasons, most commonly the winter months, and is hypothesized to be related to melatonin levels. Also called SAD.

secondary hypertension, high blood pressure associated with a variety of primary diseases, such as renal disorders, disorders of the central nervous system, endocrine diseases, and vascular diseases. See **hypertension.**

sigmoid colon, the s-shaped part of the colon that lies in the pelvis, extending from the pelvic brim to the third segment of the sacrum; it is continuous above with the descending colon and below with the rectum. Also called pelvic c. and sigmoid flexure.

sigmoidoscope (sig-moi´do-skōp) a rigid or flexible scope with appropriate illumination for examining the sigmoid colon.

sigmoidoscopy (sig″moi-dos´kə-pe) inspection of the sigmoid colon through a **sigmoidoscope.**

sinoatrial node, see **sinus node.**

sinus beat, a natural pulsation of the heart, originating in the **sinus node**; see **sinus rhythm.**

sinus node, the collection of nerves and tissue positioned on the wall of the right atrium which receives impulses through the autonomic nervous system to initiate the heartbeat; a normal sinus node activates the muscles of the atria and ventricles in a coordinated fashion to create an effective heartbeat; also called the **sinoatrial node.**

sinus rhythm, normal heart rhythm originating in the **sinoatrial node.**

sodium fluoride, a dental hygiene and disease preventive agent used in the fluoridation of water and applied topically to the teeth.

sputum (spu'təm) [L.] matter ejected from the respiratory tract through the mouth.

stenosis (stə-no'sis) [Gr. stenōsis] an abnormal narrowing of a duct or canal.

stenotic, pertaining to **stenosis.**

stenotic valves, abnormally narrowed valves.

subcutaneous (sub″ku-ta'ne-əs) beneath the skin; also called hypodermis.

subspecialist, in internal medicine or surgery, a doctor who has chosen to receive additional, more in-depth training and board certification in the diagnosis and management of a specific type of disease such as infectious diseases or cancer, or diseases affecting a single organ system, such as heart and circulation.

sympathectomy (sim″pə-thek'tə-me) [sympathetic+-ectomy] the transection of any part of the sympathetic nervous pathways. Operations may be named according to the location of the nerve operated on, as cervical, dorsal, or lumbar.

sympathetic nerve, one of the nerves of the **sympathetic nervous system.**

sympathetic nervous system, the portion of the autonomic nervous system that regulates functions such as heart rate, pupil diameter, intestinal motility, and urinary output; always active at a basal level (called sympathetic tone) and becomes more active during times of stress.

syndrome (sin'drōm) [Gr. syndrome concurrence] a set of symptoms and signs that occur together and may have more than one cause.

syphilis (sif'ĭ-lis) [Syphilus, a shepherd infected with the disease in a poem by Fracastorius (Girolamo Fracastorio, Italian physician and poet, 1483–1553); the poet may have derived the name from Gr. syn together +philein to love, or from Gr. siphlos crippled, maimed] an infectious disease caused by the spirochete treponema pallidum, usually transmitted by sexual contact or acquired in utero. Untreated, syphilis usually progresses through three clinical stages (primary, secondary, and tertiary), with a latent period (latent syphilis) intervening between the first two and the last. The time of duration of each stage varies.

systemic lupus erythematosus, a chronic, inflammatory, often feverous disorder of connective tissue that proceeds through remissions and relapses; it may be either acute or insidious in onset and is characterized by involvement of the skin, joints, kidneys, and serosal membranes. The etiology is unknown, but it may be due to a failure of regulatory mechanisms of the autoimmune system.

systolic pressure, systolic blood pressure, the maximum pressure that occurs near the end of contraction of the left ventricle of the heart. See **blood pressure.**

tachycardia (tak″ĭ-kahr′de-ə) [tachy-+cardia] excessively rapid heart beat; the term is usually applied to a heart rate above 100 beats per minute in an adult at rest.

tetanus (tet′ə-nəs) [Gr. tetanos, from teinein to stretch] an acute, often fatal infectious disease caused by the bacillus Clostridium tetani; it usually enters the body through a contaminated puncture wound such as from a nail, splinter, or insect bite.

tetracycline (tet″rə-si′klēn) 1. any of a group of related broad-spectrum antibiotics; some are isolated from certain species of streptomyces and others are produced semisynthetically. The group includes chlortetracycline, doxycycline, methacycline, minocycline, oxytetracycline, rolitetracycline, and tetracycline (def. 2). Tetracyclines are effective against a wide range of bacteria; they are also effective against certain **protozoa.** 2. a semisynthetic antibiotic produced from chlortetracycline, having the same wide spectrum of antimicrobial activity as other members of the tetracycline group; administered orally.

Tetralogy of Fallot, a congenital heart defect that changes the normal flow of blood through the heart.

theophylline (the-of′ə-lin) a compound occurring in tea leaves and prepared synthetically; acts as a smooth muscle relaxant, central nervous system and cardiac muscle stimulant, and bronchodilator. Used as a bronchodilator in the prevention and treatment of symptoms of asthma, chronic bronchitis, emphysema, or other chronic obstructive pulmonary disease; administered orally or intravenously.

thiamine (thi′ə-min) vitamin B1, a water-soluble compound found particularly in pork, organ meats, legumes, nuts, and whole grain or enriched cereals and breads. Deficiency of the vitamin can result in beriberi and is a factor in alcoholic neuritis.

thiazide (thi′ə-zīd) any of a group of diuretics that act by inhibiting the reabsorption of sodium and stimulating chloride excretion, with resultant increase in excretion of water. They also increase the excretion of potassium, which can cause hypokalemia (low potassium) requiring potassium supplementation. Thiazides are used for the treatment of edema due to congestive heart failure or chronic hepatic or renal disease and, alone or in combination with other drugs, in the treatment of hypertension.

thiocyanates (thi″o-si′ə-nāt) compound derived from hydrogen cyanide; found in tobacco smoke, with higher levels in those who use tobacco.

Thiomerin, a mercurial diuretic introduced in 1950, which could be delivered subcutaneously, under the skin.

thrombo-embolus, a clot (thrombus) that breaks loose and is carried by the blood stream to plug another vessel.

thrombophlebitis (throm″bo-flə-bi′tis) [thrombo-+phlebitis] vein inflammation (phlebitis) associated with formation of blood clots (thrombosis).

thrombosis (throm-bo′sis) [Gr. thrombōsis] the formation, development, or presence of a blood clot.

thrombus (throm′bəs) [Gr. thrombos clot] a stationary blood clot along the wall of a blood vessel, frequently causing vascular obstruction.

thyroid (thi′roid) [Gr. thyreoeidēs, from thyreos oblong shield +eidos form] pertaining to the **thyroid gland** (glandula thyroidea); an **overactive** thyroid gland or an underactive thyroid gland can lead to certain medical complications.

thyroidectomy (thi″roid-ek′tə-me) [thyroid+-ectomy] 1. surgical removal of the **thyroid** gland. 2. **medical** elimination of thyroid function.

timoptic (ti-mop′tik) trade name for a preparation of timolol maleate, a beta blocker, used topically in **eye-drops** to lower pressure inside the eye in the treatment of glaucoma and ocular hypertension; also used orally in the treatment of hypertension, recurrent myocardial infarction, and the prevention of migraine.

tincture of belladonna, an alcoholic preparation containing extracts of belladonna leaf; it has been used as an antispasmodic for disorders of the gastrointestinal tract.

trachea (tra´ke-ə) [l., from Gr. tracheia artēria] 1. the cartilage tube descending from the larynx and branching into the right and left main bronchi in the lungs. Also called the windpipe.

tracing (trās´ing) see **electrocardiographic tracing.**

trans-fat, the common name for a type of unsaturated fat molecule containing one or more double bonds between the carbon atoms, leaving fewer bonds available for hydrogen. The consumption of trans fats increases one's risk of coronary heart disease by raising levels of bad LDL cholesterol and lowering levels of good HDL cholesterol. Health authorities worldwide recommend that consumption of trans fat be reduced to trace amounts.

Trichomonas (trik″o-mo´nəs) [tricho-+ Gr. monas unit, from monas single] a genus of parasitic **protozoa** found in the intestinal and genitourinary tracts of various invertebrates and vertebrates, including humans.

tricuspid valve, is on the right side of the heart and regulates the blood flow between the right atrium and the right ventricle. the normal tricuspid valve usually has three leaflets and three papillary muscles. Also known as the right atrioventricular valve.

triglyceride (tri-glis´ər-īd) a neutral fat naturally synthesized in the body from carbohydrates for storage in fat cells. Upon enzymatic hydrolysis, it releases free fatty acids into the blood.

trypanosome (tri-pan´o-sōm) a tropical protozoan parasite found in the blood, lymph, and tissues of animals including man.

tuberculosis (too-ber″ku-lo´sis) any of the infectious diseases of humans or other animals caused by species of Mycobacterium and characterized by the formation of a tube-like mass of cells in the infected tissues. Tuberculosis varies widely in its manifestations and has a tendency to become chronic. Any organ may be affected, although in humans the lung is the major seat of the disease and is the usual portal of entry into the body.

tularemia (too″lə-re´me-ə) [Tulare County, California, where it was first described in 1911] an infectious, plague-like disease caused by infection with the bacterium Francisella tularensis, which is found in numerous species of rodents such as rabbits, squirrels, and muskrats. It is transmitted to humans and other animals by the bites of deerflies, fleas, and ticks; by contact with contaminated animals or their products; by inhalation; and by ingestion of contaminated food or water. In addition to a marked reaction at the portal of entry of the pathogen, most cases are characterized by abrupt onset of fever, chills, weakness, headache, backache, and malaise. Also called deer fly, pahvant valley, rabbit fever and francis disease.

typhoid fever, an acute, generalized, systemic illness with fever caused by a strain of salmonella bacteria; it is usually spread by ingestion of contaminated food or water. Characteristics include sustained fever with malaise and later delirium; transient skin rash known as rose spots; abdominal pain, and slow heart rate. Intestinal hemorrhages and perforation may be late complications. Also called typhoid.

typhus (ti´fəs) [Gr. typhos stupor arising from fever] any of a group of acute infections caused by the genus rickettsiac; characterized by severe headache, chills, high fever, stupor, and skin eruption. Can become an epidemic. Also called typhus fever.

ulcer (ul´sər) [L. ulcus, gen. ulceris] a local defect on the surface of an organ or tissue, which is produced by the sloughing of inflammatory necrotic tissue.

ultrasonography (ul″trə-sə-nog´rə-fe) the visualization of deep structures of the body by recording the reflections of (echoes of) pulses of ultrasonic waves directed into the tissues. Diagnostic ultrasonography uses a frequency range of 1 million to 10 million hertz (cycles per second), or 1 to 10 MHz. Such sound waves are transmissible only in liquids and solids. Also called echography and sonography; for the heart, called **echocardiography.**

ultra-sound (ul´trə-sound) 1. sound waves with a frequency above the range of human hearing (greater than 20,000 HZ); see ultrasonics. 2. ultrasonography.

unstable angina is a form of acute coronary syndrome (ACS) where the chest symptoms are similar to stable angina pectoris but occur in an atypical and unpredictable fashion.

valium (val´e-əm) trade name for preparations of diazepam used in the treatment of anxiety disorders and for short-term relief of anxiety symptoms, or as a preoperative or preprocedural medication to relieve anxiety and tension; also used as a skeletal muscle relaxant, anticonvulsant, antitremor agent, antipanic agent, and for treatment of symptoms of acute alcohol withdrawal; administered orally, rectally, intravenously, or intramuscularly.

vasodilator (va″zo-) (vas″o-di´la-tər) a motor nerve or chemical compound that causes dilation of the blood vessels.

vena cava, the large veins that carry deoxygenated blood from the body to the heart's right atrium; there are two of these veins, the **superior vena cava** carries the blood from the upper part of the body and the **inferior vena cava** carries blood from the lower parts. (See "Appendix 3, Diagram of the Heart.")

ventilator (ven″tĭ-la´tər) an apparatus used in artificial respiration, usually with mechanical ventilation.

ventricle (ven´tri-kul) a lower cavity in the heart; **right ventricle**, the lower chamber of the right side of the heart, which pumps venous blood through the pulmonary trunk and arteries to the capillaries of the lungs; **left ventricle**, the lower chamber of the left side of the heart, which pumps oxygenated blood to the body. (See "Appendix 3, Diagram of the Heart.")

ventricular fibrillation, a fatal arrhythmia characterized by uncoordinated contractions of the ventricular muscle due to rapid repetitive excitation of myocardial fibers; with little or no blood pressure created, ventricular fibrillation cannot sustain life.

ventricular pump, see **ventricle**.

ventricular septal defect, a congenital cardiac anomaly in which there is persistent opening in the ventricular wall separating the right and left ventricles, most often due to failure of the wall to close during fetal development.

ventricular tachycardia, an abnormally rapid ventricular rhythm, usually in excess of 150 beats per minute, which is generated within the ventricle.

warfarin (wor'fər-in) [Wisconsin Alumni Research Foundation] a synthetic **coumarin** anticoagulant.

white blood cell, see **leukocyte**.

Wolff-Parkinson-White syndrome, the association of **tachycardia** or **atrial fibrillation** with premature transmission of cardiac impulses to the ventricles.

yellow fever, an acute infectious disease caused by a flavivirus, now limited to tropical parts of Central and South America and Africa. It is considered one of the hemorrhagic fevers and is transmitted to humans by mosquitoes that have acquired the virus from either other humans (urban type) or animals (jungle type). In its severe form it is marked by fever, hemorrhage, renal damage, and jaundice.

xiphoid (zif'oid) (zi'foid) [Gr. xiphoeidēdes sword-shaped, from xiphos sword +eidos form] 1. shaped like a sword; also called ensiform. 2. **xiphoid process**, processus xiphoideus. 3. pertaining to the **xiphoid process.**

xiphoid process, the pointed cartilage formation projecting from the lower end of the sternum, the breast bone.

xylocaine (zi'lo-kān) trade name for preparations of **lidocaine**, a drug having anesthetic, sedative, analgesic, anticonvulsant, and cardiac depressant activities; used as a local anesthetic, applied topically to the skin and mucous membranes.

Zaroxolyn, trade name for metolazone, a long acting diuretic with properties generally similar to the more common **thiazide** diuretics.

APPENDIX 3

Diagram of the Heart

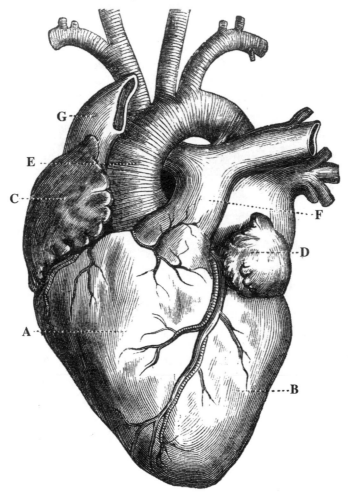

A. Right Ventricle
B. Left Ventricle
C. Right Atrium
D. Left Atrium

E. Aorta
F. Pulmonary Artery
G. Vena Cava, Superior

APPENDIX 4

Norman Makous, M.D., Curriculum Vitae

EDUCATION:

1942-1945	B.S. University of Wisconsin, Madison
1944-1947	M.D. University of Wisconsin, Madison

POSTGRADUATE TRAINING AND FELLOWSHIP APPOINTMENTS:

1947-1948	Research Hospital, Kansas City, MO, Mixed Internship
1948-1950	Resident in Medicine
1950-1951	Fellowship, Cardiovascular Diseases Division Experimental Medicine, University of Vermont, Burlington, VT
1951-1952	Internal Medicine, US Naval Hospital, Camp Lejeune, NC
1953-1955	Fellowship, Cardiovascular Diseases, Pennsylvania Hospital, Philadelphia, PA
1955-1957	Director, Cardiac Catheterization Laboratory, General Hospital, Kansas City, MO

MILITARY SERVICE:

Active Duty

1943-1945	U.S. Naval Reserve, Ensign
1950-1952	U.S. Naval Reserve, Lt., MC
1950-1951	U.S. Army, 10th Field Hospital, Wurzburg Military Post, Germany
1951-1952	U.S. Naval Hospital, Camp Lejeune, NC

Inactive Duty

1945-1950	U.S. Naval Reserve, Lt, MC
1952-1956	U.S. Naval Reserve, Lt, MC
1956-1962	U.S. Naval Reserve, Lt. Cmdr., MC

FACULTY APPOINTMENTS:

University of Pennsylvania School of Medicine, Department of Medicine

1959-1971	Associate in Medicine
1971-1995	Clinical Assistant Professor of Medicine

1994	Thomas Jefferson University Medical School, Clinical Assistant Professor of Medicine

HOSPITAL & ADMINISTRATIVE APPOINTMENTS:

Children's Mercy Hospital, Kansas City, MO

1955-1958	Associate Cardiologist
1959	Cardiologist, Chief of Cardiology

Children's Cardiac Center, Kansas City, MO

1956-1959	Medical Staff
1959	Chairman, Section of Cardiology

Kansas City General Hospital, MO

1955-1956	Director, Cardiac Catheterization Lab
1956-1959	Attending Staff

Kansas City Tuberculosis Sanitarium, MO

1956-1957	Attending Staff

Research Hospital, Kansas City, MO

1956-1958	Associate Staff/Active Staff

Independence Sanitarium and Hospital, Independence, MO

1957-1959	Electrocardiographer and Active Staff

Richards-Gebaur Air Force Base, Grandview, MO

1956-1959	Medical Consultant

Bryn Mawr Hospital, Bryn Mawr, PA

1960-1965	Cardiologist, Outpatient Clinic
1965-1968	Attending Physician, Cardiovascular Section

Pennsylvania Hospital, Philadelphia, PA

1960-1972	Associate Cardiologist
1966-1972	Associate Physician to Hospital
1972-2000	Cardiologist and Physician to the Hospital
2001-2006	Consultant
2006	Retired

SPECIALTY CERTIFICATIONS:

1957	American Board of Internal Medicine
1961	Board of Cardiovascular Disease Subspecialty

LICENSURE:

1948	Wisconsin, No. 10422
1950-1959	Missouri, No. 23746
1959-	Pennsylvania, No. Md005653e

AWARDS AND HONORARY SOCIETIES:

Marquis Who's Who

1962-1967	East

1997-1998	East
2001-2009	America, 55th-63rd Editions
2004-2005	American Education, 6th Edition
2004-2005	Finance and Industry, 34th Edition
1997-2010	Medicine and Health Care 1st-7th Edition
2002-2007	Science and Engineering, 6th-9th Editions
1998-2007	World, 15th-24th Editions

Who's Who in the Delaware Valley
| 1992 | 2nd Edition |

National Directory of Who's Who
| 1994 | Executives and Professionals |

Dictionary of International Biography
| 2006 | 33rd Edition |

The Chapel of The Four Chaplains
| 1980 | Legion of Honor |

American Heart Association, Pennsylvania Affiliate
| 1982 | Distinguished Service Award |
| 1986 | Distinguished Achievement Award |

American Heart Association, Southeastern Pennsylvania Chapter
| 1988 | Volunteer of the Year |
| 1988 | Distinguished Achievement Award |

Southeastern Pennsylvania High Blood Pressure Control Program
| 1988 | Special Achievement Award in Professional Education |

Philadelphia County Medical Society
| 1994 | Cristol Award |

PROFESSIONAL AND SCIENTIFIC SOCIETIES:

American Medical Association
| 1954- | Member |

Missouri State And Jackson County Medical Societies
| 1955-1959 | Member |

Pennsylvania Medical Society
1960-	Member
1982-1983	Co-Chairman, Council on Health Planning
1986-1991	Chairman, Professional Liability Insurance Committee Appeals

Philadelphia County Medical Society
1960-	Member
1980-2000	Member, Board of Directors
1989-1991	Secretary
1980-1986	Chairman, Medical Economics Committee
1980-1981	President, Center City Branch

1981-1982	Chairman, Medical Business Coalition Committee
1987-1992	Vice-Chairman, Hospital Medical Staff Section
1991-1992	Chairman, Bylaws Committee
1991-2000	Chairman, Membership and Organization Committee

Pfahler Foundation

| 1990-2000 | Member, Board of Directors |

American Heart Association

1955-	Member
1965-	Fellow, Council of Clinical Cardiology
1982	Review Committee
1983-1984	Chapter Standards Committee

West Central Missouri Chapter, American Heart Association

| 1955-1959 | Member, Board of Directors |

Southeastern PA Chapter, American Heart Association

1960-	Member
1961-1963	Lois Belber Dickler Research Chairman
1966-1988	Board of Governors
1987-1988	President-Elect And President

Pennsylvania Affiliate, American Heart Association

1970-1991	Member
1966-1969	Cardiac Clinics Committee
1974-1975	Co-Chairman, Risk Reduction Committee
1978-1979	Chairman, Central Program Committee
1978-1988	Member, Board of Governors and Executive Committee
1980-1982	President-Elect, President

Society of Internal Medicine, Greater Kansas City, MO

| 1959 | Member |

American Society of Internal Medicine

| 1974- | American Society of Internal Medicine |

Pennsylvania Society of Internal Medicine

1976-1998	Board Of Governors
1979-1982	Secretary
1982-1984	President-Elect, President

Philadelphia Physiological Society

| 1963-1980 | Member |

American College of Physicians

| 1964- | Fellow |

College of Physicians of Philadelphia

1972-1994	Fellow
1980-1986	Council Member
1980-1986	Chairman, Hall and Grounds Committee

Pennsylvania Hospital
1966   President, Ex-Residents' Association
1972-1975   Secretary, Thomas Bond Society
1975-1978   President, Thomas Bond Society
Philadelphia Academy of Cardiology
1976-1983   Member
American College of Cardiology
1975-   Fellow

OTHER PROFESSIONAL APPOINTMENTS:

Cardiac Work Evaluation Unit of American Heart Association
1961-1965   Director, Pennsylvania Hospital Unit
Edna B. Kynett Memorial Foundation
1963-   Trustee
1994-1996   Vice-President
1997-2004   President
Greater Delaware Valley Regional Medical Program
Advisory Group
1971-1975   Member
Health Systems Agency, Southeastern, PA
1975-1977   Interim Board
1977-1985   West Philadelphia Advisory Council
                Chairman, Education Committee
                Chairman, Advisory Council
Southeastern Pennsylvania Regional High Blood Pressure
Control Program
1978-1980   Founder and Acting Chairman
Keystone Professional Review Organization (KEPRO)
1986-1993   Physician Advisor
Pennsylvania Bureau of Disability Determination
1981-2001   Medical Consultant
Asbestos Litigation Defense Panel
1981-1993   Cardiology Consultant
City of Philadelphia, City Solicitor's Office
1986-2006   Cardiology Consultant
Independence Blue Cross Admission Review
1987-1994   Cardiology Consultant
Journal of Cardiopulmonary Rehabilitation
1990   Peer Review Panel
Visiting Nurse Association of Greater Philadelphia
1996-2000   Member, Pennsylvania Board

MEDICAL BIBLIOGRAPHY:
Published Papers

1. "Pressor effects of epinephrine, norephinephrine and desoxycorticosterone acetate (DCA) weakened by sodium withdrawal." Humphreys RJ, Rabb W, Makous N., Degrandpre R, Gigee W. *Circulation*. 6:373, 1952.
2. "Severe drug sensitivity reaction to phenindione (phenylinadione)." Makous N., Vander Veer JB. *Journal of the American Medical Association*. 155:739, 1954.
3. "A clinical evaluation of the use of a rectal mercurial diuretic in patients with chronic congestive heart failure." Makous N., Jennings P, Funk E Jr., Vander Veer JB. *The American Journal of the Medical Sciences*. 231:86. 1956.
4. "Reversion of atrial fibrillation to sinus rhythm with digitalis therapy." Jennings P, Makous N., Vander Veer JB. *The American Journal of the Medical Sciences*. 235:702, 1968.
5. "Cardiovascular manifestations in progeria. Report of clinical and pathological findings in a patient with severe arteriosclerotic heart disease and aortic stenosis." Makous N., Friedman S, Yakovac W, Maris E. *American Heart Journal*. 64:334, 1996.
6. "Hemodynamics of the master two-step test in hypertension and healed myocardial infarction." Makous N., Cha HD, Taylor E. *Circulation*. 30:77, 1964.
7. "Electrocardiographic leads and techniques in mass screening." Makous N. *JAMA*. 192:801, 1965.
8. "Fever and chills as a reaction to procainamide hydrochloride therapy." Hey EB Jr., Makous N., Vander Veer JB. *Archives of Internal Medicine*. 116:544, 1965.
9. "May cardiacs work?" Makous N. Heart-O-Grams. *Southeastern Pennsylvania Heart Association*. 3:3, 1966.
10. "Ebstein's anomaly and life expectancy. Report of a survival to over age 79." Makous N., Vander Veer JB. *American Journal of Cardiology*. 18:100, 1966.
11. "Rehabilitation and cardiovascular disease." Makous N. Heart-O-Grams, *Southeastern Pennsylvania Heart Association*. 7:1, 1969.
12. "The post two-step electrocardiogram and hemodynamic determinants of myocardial oxygen consumption." Makous N., Gittleman MA, Atencio NEV. *Malattie Cardiovascular*. 10:1-2, 1969.
13. "The diagnosis of coronary heart disease." Makous N. *The Benjamin Franklin Clinic* Letter. 5:1, 1970. Reprinted In The *International Journal Of Industrial Medicine And Surgery*. 39-46, 1970.

14. "Cost of a mobile coronary care unit." Makous N., Binnion PF, Keller W. *American Heart Journal*. 83:723, 1972.
15. "My opinion: mobile coronary care unit: are they effective?" Makous N vs. Moss AJ. *Consultant*. 11:114, 1972.
16. "The Mobile Coronary Care Unit." Binnion PF, Mandal SK, Makous N. *JAMA*. 223:923, 1973.
17. "Exertional xerostomia! Dry mouth during treadmill testing." Makous N. *Journal of Cardiopulmonary Rehabilitation*. 10:45, 1990.
18. "Are gerd sequelae due to reflux or reflex?" Makous, N., *Cortlandt Forum: The Cortlandt Letters*. June 2003.

Published Abstracts.

1. "Hemodynamic changes following the master two-step test in hypertension." Makous N., Chan HD, Taylor ES Jr. *Circulation*. 28:761, 1963.

Reviews, Chapters, Newsletters

1. "Dissecting aneurysm of the aorta. A case report with review of the literature." *Thesis*. 1947.
2. "Biochemical clinics. The Heart." Edited By Kugelmass IN. RH Donnelly Corporation, New York. *Metabolism*. 12: 1054, 1963.
3. "Anticoagulant prophylaxis and treatment. The new emphasis in management." Ingam GIG, Bart JR, Thomas CC in Springfield, Illinois. *Metabolism*. 15:478, 1966.
4. "Angina pectoris." Makous N. *Suspicion In Treatable Diseases*. Edited By Horwitz O, Magee JH. Lea And Febiger. Philadelphia, 1975.
5. "The heart and circulation over fifty-five." Makous N. *A Handbook On Health*. Duncan TG, Editor. Franklin Institute Press, Philadelphia, Pa 1982.
6. *Exercise over fifty-five*. Makous N., Duncan TG, Editor. 1982.
7. *Heart to Heart Health Help Newsletter* from Norman Makous, M.D., Facc, Facp.

   A. "Heart Health Maintenance." Summer, 1984.
   B. "The Diet in Weight Management." Summer, 1985.
   C. "Exercise Stress Testing." Winter, 1986.
   D. "Cholesterol." Fall, 1987.
   E. "Capsules, Pills and Potions." Winter, 1989-1990.
   F. "Cardiac Consultation and Tests." Spring, 1991.

Papers Presented Or Unpublished:
1. "Typhoid fever endocarditis treated with chloromycetin: A case report." Makous N., Asher G. 1949.
2. "Left parasternal systolic murmur of low intensity in acyanotic children and adults. A clinical and right heart catheterization correlation." Makous N. Presented at the *Western Montana Medical and Surgical Society Meeting*. Missoula, Montana. June 28, 1958.
3. "An electrocardiographic response to a valsalva maneuver. A comparison of health, coronary artery disease and the unstable t-wave syndrome." Makous N., 1961.
4. "Experience with ethacrynic acid, a new diuretic." Makous N. Read at The Professional Staff Meeting of Pennsylvania Hospital, Philadelphia, PA. November 18, 1963.
5. "Direct current cardioversion of atrial fibrillation to regular sinus rhythm." Makous N., Vander Veer JB. Read at the *Regional Meeting*, American College of Physicians. Philadelphia, PA. November 22, 1963.
6. "Systemic hemodynamics of the master two-step in hypertension and healed myocardial infarction with some observation concerning the ST-T changes in the recovery electrocardiogram." Makous N. Presented at seminar of "Physiological and Clinical Aspects of Rehabilitation of Cardiac Patient." Sponsored By Council on Rehabilitation of The International Society of Cardiology. Cagliaria, Sardinia, Italy. June 9, 1968.
7. "Systemic hemodynamic changes during and following brief bicycle ergometric exertion in coronary heart disease and hypertension." Makous N. Cagliaria, Sardinia, Italy. June 1968; Ibid.
8. Participant in discussion group for *National Conference on Stress, Strain, and Heart Disease*. American Heart Association. Chicago, Illinois. October 10-12, 1968.
9. "Meeting the cardiac emergency." Makous N. Continuing Education Program. Pennsylvania Hospital, Philadelphia, PA. March 20, 1969.
10. "Information content of limb lead electrocardiography in mass screening." Makous N. 1969.
11. "Unusual presentation of angina pectoris." Presented American College of Physicians Course on "Specifically Treatable Disease." Pennsylvania Hospital, Philadelphia, PA. March 15, 1972.
12. "Risk of passenger motor vehicle operation by driver with coronary disease." Makous N. Prepared for Red Arrow Division of Southeastern Pennsylvania Transportation Authority. 1972.

13. "Mass screening for heart disease." Makous N. American Heart Association, Pennsylvania Affiliate. May 8, 1974.
14. "Rehabilitation following acute myocardial infarction." Makous N. Presented at Seminar on Stress Testing and Rehabilitation in Coronary Heart Disease. New Orleans, LA. February 1977; Atlanta, GA. June 10-12, 1977; Boston, MA. April 14-16, 1978. Sponsored by International Medical Education Corporation.
15. "Indications and contraindications in exercise stress testing." Makous N. Ibid.
16. "Exercise-induced arrhythmia: recognition, significance and management." Makous N. Presented at the symposium on exercise testing and conditioning. Southeastern Pennsylvania Chapter of American Heart Association. Philadelphia, PA. May 16-25, 1978.
17. "The effect of treadmill exercise on the rate of ectopic beating." Makous N. Read at the *Eastern Pennsylvania Regional Meeting*, American College of Physicians. October 6, 1978.
18. "The patient and the profession: partners in the management of hypertension." Makous N., Krehl WA, Co-Chairmen of Workshop at High Blood Pressure Symposium in Philadelphia, PA. November 1, 1979.
19. "Hypertension and the Southeastern Pennsylvania High Blood Pressure Program." Makous N. Lower Bucks County Hospital. March 19, 1980.
20. "The relationship of work and heart disease." Seminar on stress, strain, and coronary risk factors: Workers' Compensation in the 1990's. Valley Forge, PA. May 10, 1990.
21. "When are coronary heart disease and disability work related?" Pennsylvania Bureau of Workers' Compensation Board Advisory Committee Seminar in Philadelphia, PA. November 15, 1990.

Medical Presentations

1   "Congenital heart disease." Makous N. Presented at postgraduate cardiology course. Pennsylvania Hospital, Philadelphia, PA. January 7, 1960.
2. "Closed chest cardiac resuscitation technique." Makous N. Presented to the School of Nursing, University of Pennsylvania, and to Medical Staff Meeting, Pottstown Hospital, Pottstown, PA. March 3 And 17, 1961.
3. "Anticoagulants and fibrinolysis." Makous N. Presented at Postgraduate Program, Wyoming Valley Hospital, Wilkes Barre, PA, October 18, 1961, and Postgraduate Program, WHYY-FM radio, March 14 and 16, 1991.

4. "Office evaluation of cardiac function." Makous N. Postgraduate cardiology program. Pennsylvania Hospital, Philadelphia, PA. January 30, 1963.
5. "Anticoagulants and thromboembolic disease." Makous N. Postgraduate cardiology course for general practitioners. Pennsylvania Hospital, Philadelphia, PA. February 7, 1963.
6. "Pulmonary embolism: A clinical pathology review of sixteen consecutively autopsied cases." Makous N., Fisher GR. Panel and co-moderators. Pennsylvania Hospital, Philadelphia, PA. February 18, 1965.
7. "The cardiac care unit." Makous N. Presented at staff conference at St. Peter's General Hospital, New Brunswick, NJ. September 7, 1965.
8. "Diuretics and the treatment of edema." Makous N. Presented on WHYY-FM radio. Philadelphia, PA, February 15 and 17, 1965, and at the General Staff Meeting, Cherry Hill Hospital. Cherry Hill, NJ. March 15, 1966.
9. "Diuretic applications." Makous N. Presented at *Chester County Academy Of General Practice*. Downingtown, PA. May 18, 1966.
10. "Management of chronic congestive heart failure." Makous N. Presented to Medical Department Meeting. Monmouth Medical Center, Longbranch, NJ. October 13, 1966.
11. "The controversy of periodic health examinations." Makous N. Presented at Seniors' Seminar. Women's Medical College of Pennsylvania. Philadelphia, PA. October 20, 1966.
12. "Effective use of diuretics." Makous N. Long Island Jewish Hospital, NY. May 3, 1967.
13. "Treatment of resistant congestive heart failure." Makous N. Presented at Medical Services Staff of the Coney Island Hospital, Brooklyn, NY. May 18, 1967.
14. "Rehabilitation of the cardiac patient." Makous N. Presented at the *Pennsylvania Medical Society Annual Meeting*. Philadelphia, PA. September 27, 1967.
15. "Physiology of the myocardial infarction patient in the rehabilitative phase." Makous N. Presented at School of Nursing, University of Pennsylvania, Philadelphia, PA. November 17, 1967.
16. "Anticoagulant therapy." Makous N. Presented at Pennsylvania Hospital School of Medical Technology, Philadelphia, PA. November 4, 1968.

17. "Meeting the cardiac emergency." Makous N. WHYY-FM radio seminar. Pennsylvania Hospital, Philadelphia, PA. February 18, 1969.
18. "Meeting the cardiac emergency." Makous N. CME Program, Pennsylvania Hospital, Philadelphia, PA. March 18-20, 1969.
19. "Electrophysiology of the heart and electrocardiology." Makous N. Presented at cardiac arrhythmia seminar for nurses. American Heart Association of Southeastern Pennsylvania, Philadelphia, PA. September 9, 1970.
20. "Newer drugs for treatment of cardiovascular disease." Makous N. Presented to students at Temple University School of Pharmacy, Philadelphia, PA. April 15, 1971.
21. "Acute myocardial infarction and cardiac arrhythmias, cardiovascular disease screening and preventative rehabilitation." Makous N. Program for Philadelphia Association Industrial Nurses by American Heart Association. Southeastern Pennsylvania, Philadelphia, PA. November 16, 23, 30, 1971.
22. "Early recognition of the symptoms of heart attack." Makous N. Presented at *Emergency Intervention Seminar, American Heart Association*. Southeastern Pennsylvania, Philadelphia, PA. March 22, 1972.
23. "Post-tachycardial circulatory insufficiency and sudden death." Makous N. Presented at *WT Longscope Research Seminar of the Pennsylvania Hospital*, Philadelphia, PA. February 12, 1975.
24. "The heart, arrhythmia, and pulmonary hypertension." Makous N. Binnion AT, Kershbaum KB. Presented at the *American College of Cardiology Program on Venous Thrombosis - Pulmonary Embolism Complex*. Sponsored by Council on Thrombosis, American Heart Association, University of Pennsylvania, Jefferson University, and Temple School of Medicine. Philadelphia, PA. September 8, 1976.
25. "The significance of hypertension." Makous N. Presented at the *Delaware County Dental Society Seminar on Hypertension*. October 20, 1976.
26. "Stress testing and coronary disease." Makous N. Presented at Grand Rounds. Abington Memorial Hospital. Philadelphia, PA. September 20, 1978.
27. "The patient and the professions—partners in the management of hypertension." Krehl, W, Makous, N. Workshop symposium on *High Blood Pressure is Everybody's Responsibility,* College of Physicians. Philadelphia, PA. November 1, 1979.

28. "Effect of exertion on cardiac irritability." Makous N. Cardiac Section Conference, Pennsylvania Hospital, Philadelphia, PA. October 1992.
29. "Congenital heart disease in adults." Makous, N. Cardiology Section Conference. Pennsylvania Hospital, Philadelphia, PA. August 1994.
30. "Catabolic heart failure." Makous, N. Cardiology Section Conference. Pennsylvania Hospital, Philadelphia, PA. 1995.
31. "Fifty years of cardiology: an odyssey." Makous N. Cardiology Section Conference. Pennsylvania Hospital. June 1996.
32. "Hemorrhagic/embolic complications from chronic warfarin therapy in patients with multi-etiologic heart disease." Makous N. Cardiology Section Conference. Pennsylvania Hospital, Philadelphia, PA. February 1997.
33. "Is angina pectoris still relevant?" Makous N. Cardiology Section Conference. Pennsylvania Hospital, Philadelphia, PA. April 1998.
34. "Bradycardia? So what?" Cardiology Section Conference. Pennsylvania Hospital, Philadelphia, PA. May 1999.

MEDICAL SOCIOECONOMIC BIBLIOGRAPHY:

Papers And Presentations

1. "Comments on the plan for diagnosis and treatment services and the hypertension plan in the proposed plan of the Health Systems Agency of Southeastern Pennsylvania." Makous N. September 17 And 19, 1978.
2. "Comments on prescription drug products: patient-labeling requirements, in *The Federal Register*." Makous N. July 7, 1979.
3. "Opinion: rationing of medical care." *Bulletin: Health Systems Agency of Southeastern Pennsylvania*. Makous N. July 1979.
4. "CAT Scanners: a response to a KYW editorial." Makous N. KYW Telecast and News Radio. Philadelphia, PA. July 16 and 17, 1979.
5. "The internist, the patient, and third parties." Makous N. *PSIM Report*. Winter, 1980.
6. "Chest radiograph quality study." Makous N. Presented at Pennsylvania Blue Shield Panel Meeting. Camp Hill, PA. March 3, 1980.
7. "Physicians cognitive services." Makous N. Presented at *Annual Meeting of Pennsylvania Society of Internal Medicine*. August 1983.

8. "Crisis in the medical care system." Makous N. Presented at The Pennsylvania Society of Internal Medicine Regional Meeting. Erie, PA. October 26, 1983.

9. "The future of cognitive care." Makous N. Read at The Pennsylvania Society of Internal Medicine Regional Meeting. Philadelphia, PA. November 30, 1983.

10. "A quality of care, cost control, and rationing." Makous N. *PSIM Report*, March 1984.

11. "HealthPASS, The HIO demonstration project for Southwest Philadelphia." Makous N. Presented at *Governors' Conference on Alternative Health Delivery Systems*. Harrisburg, PA. April 30, 1984.

12. "Advocacy for the Internist." Makous N. *PSIM Report*. August 1984.

13. "Proposed revisions of Pennsylvania Blue Shield Bylaws." Makous N. Sent to Division of Healthcare Planning Department of Health and Welfare. Harrisburg, PA. February 20, 1985.

14. "Disability management program for nonoccupational illness." Makous N. Presented at *The Hospital as a Workplace* Seminar. Philadelphia County Medical Society. Philadelphia, PA. March 9, 1985.

15. "Practice standards vs. individualized care." Makous N. *PSIM Report*. August 1989.

16. "Cardiology Presentation." Pennsylvania. Workers Compensation Seminar. May 10, 1990

17. "Healthcare reform: A congressional healthcare briefing." Makous N. *Philadelphia Medicine* 88: (3) 134, March 1992.

18. "Medicare concurrent care." Makous, N. Report for Medical Services Committee, Pennsylvania Society of Internal Medicine. June 1992.

19. "Enhancement of patient care." Makous N. Presented at *Pennsylvania County Medical Society Seminar*. November 4, 1992. *Philadelphia Medicine*, April 1993.

20. Panelist, *Issues Forum*: "Western medicine vs. holistic medicine," Greater Media Cable TV. Philadelphia, PA. June 7, 1993, 7:00-8:00 P.M.

21. "Medical professionalism: fads and fashions." *Philadelphia Medicine*. Makous N. V95:203-205, November 1999.

22. "US health system: think piece, various dissemination," October 2002.

23. "Medical Care" presented at Freedom Village. Brandywine, PA.
    June-July 2003.
        June 2003
            I: "Pre WWII, getting from there to here"
            II. "Post WWII, personal to herd care"
            III. "Contemporary fads, fashion, folklore and
                fantasy"
        July 2003
            IV. "Contemporary/future"
        September 2005
            V. "Should medical care be a right?"
            VI. "Trends and costs of medical care"

Appendix 5

Additional Reading

Henry J. Asron and William B. Schwartz with Melissa Cox, *Can We Say No? The Challenge of Rationing Health Care*, Brookings Institution Press, 2005.

Andrew B. Bindman, "Is There a Personal Doctor in the House?" *Annals of Internal Medicine*, 2009.

Shannon Brownlee, *Overtreated: Why Too Much Medicine Is Making Us Sicker and Poorer*, Bloomsbury USA, 2007.

Arthur L. Caplan, *If I Were a Rich Man Could I Buy a Pancreas?* Indiana University Press, 1992.

Arthur L. Caplan, James J. McCartney, Dominic A. Sisti, *Health, Disease, and Illness: Concepts in Medicine*, Georgetown University Press, 2004.

Tom Daschle, *Critical: What We Can Do About the Health-Care Crisis*, Thomas Dunne Books, 2008.

Alain Einthoven, "Health Care With a Few Bucks Left Over," *The New York Times*, December 28, 2008.

George Ross Fisher, *Health Care and Insurance: Distortions in the Financing of Medical Expenditures*, Beard Books, 2000.

George Ross Fisher, *The Hospital That Ate Chicago: Distortions Imposed on the Medical System by Its Financing*, The Saunders Press, 1980.

Atul Gawande, "The Cost Conundrum," *The New Yorker*, June 1, 2009.

John Geyman, *The Corrosion of Medicine: Can the Profession Reclaim Its Moral Legacy?* Common Courage Press, 2007.

Federico Girosi, Amado Cordova, Christine Eibner, Carole Roan Gresenz, Emmett Keeler, Jeanne Ringel, Jeffrey Sullivan, John Bertko, Melinda Beeuwkes Buntin, Raffaele Vardavas, *Overview of the COMPARE*

(Comprehensive Assessment of Reform Efforts) Microsimulation Model to Evaluate Health Care Proposals—Working Paper, Rand Corporation, 2009.

Richard Gordon, *The Alarming History of Medicine: Amusing Anecdotes from Hippocrates to Heart Transplants,* St. Martin's Griffin, 1997.

Jerome Groopman, *How Doctors Think,* Mariner Books, 2008.

Nortin M. Hadler, MD, *Worried Sick: A Prescription for Health in an Overtreated America,* University of North Carolina Press, 2008.

George E. Halvorson, *Health Care Reform Now: A Prescription for Change,* John Wiley and Sons, Inc., 2007.

David A. Hyman, *Medicare Meets Mephistopheles,* Cato Institute, 2006.

William C. Kashatus, "When Medicine Meant Care," *The Philadelphia Inquirer,* June 6, 2009.

G. Wayne Miller, *The King of Hearts: The True Story of the Maverick Who Pioneered Open Heart Surgery,* Crown Publishers, 2000.

Sharon Moalem with Jonathan Prince, *Survival of the Sickest: The Surprising Connection Between Disease and Longevity,* Harpercollins Publishers, 2007.

Arnold S. Relman, "Medical Professionalism in a Commercialized Health Care Market," *Journal of the American Medical Association,* 2007; 298:2668-2672.

Moises Rivera-Ruiz, Christian Cajavilca, and Joseph Varon, "Einthoven's String Galvanometer: The First Electrocardiograph," *Texas Heart Institute Journal,* 2008; 35:174-178.

Michael F. Roizen and Mehmet C. Oz, *YOU: The Smart Patient: An Insider's Handbook for Getting the Best Treatment,* Free Press, 2006.

Siddharth Singh and Abha Goyal, "The Origin Of Echocardiography: A Tribute to Inge Edler," *Texas Heart Institute Journal,* 2007; 34:431-438.

Henry A. Shenkin, Current *Dilemmas In Medical-Care Rationing: A Pragmatic Approach,* University Press of America, 1996.

Paul Starr, *The Social Transformation of American Medicine: The rise of a sovereign profession and the making of a vast industry,* Basic Books, Inc., 1982.

Joseph B. Vander Veer, *Cardiology at the Pennsylvania Hospital 1920-1980,* Dorrance & Company, Inc., 1986.

Steven H. Woolf, "A Closer Look at the Economic Argument for Disease Prevention," *Journal Of The American Medical Association,* 2009; 536-538.

ACKNOWLEDGEMENTS

I am thankful for the input of the many people who helped in the creation of this book. The comments from the reviewers of the first draft were helpful in providing initial direction. These included my brother, Dr. Walter Makous, a psychologist and physiologist on the faculty of the University of Rochester Medical School; my old friend Harold Braun, M.D., a retired cardiologist in Missoula, Montana; my son Monte Makous, M.D., a family practitioner and regional medical director with the US State Department; and my daughter Catherine Davis.

My son Bruce Makous has been most responsible for helping me establish and maintain the theme and direction of the book. Our copy editor, Susan Courtney, was very helpful in preparation of the manuscript and Victoria Colotta did an outstanding job creating a striking design for the book. I would like to acknowledge the good work of Author Marketing Experts and Monkey C Media in getting the word out about the book.

Finally, I am particularly thankful for the help and encouragement from my loving wife Eleanor throughout the long and sometimes tedious process of creating a book.

About Norman Makous, M.D.

Norman Makous practiced medicine for sixty years. After extensive training and service in the Navy, he started private practice in Kansas City and moved to Philadelphia. He held appointments for many years on the faculties of both the University of Pennsylvania Medical School and Thomas Jefferson Medical University.

Dr. Makous has also served on the boards of several government and health insurance advisory groups. He has received many professional awards, including the Distinguished Achievement Award from the American Heart Association of Pennsylvania.

He is the author of many professional articles. His first book, *The Road Taken: My Life and Times*, was published in 2006 by TowPath Publications.

Dr. Makous was married for fifty-four years to Dorothy Bowlin Makous, until she died in 2003. They have ten children and nineteen grandchildren. He is married to Eleanor Sullivan and lives in Coatesville, Pennsylvania.

About Bruce Makous

Bruce Makous is a published author as well as a leading healthcare fundraiser noted in *The NonProfit Times* in 2009 as one of the most influential and effective fundraisers in the US. He is the author of two novels, including *Riding the Brand*, which received coverage in *The Wall Street Journal* because of its indictment of the venture capital industry for operating like organized crime. Bruce is an enthusiastic supporter of the writing of his father, and lives in Philadelphia with his wife and two daughters.